Health Care and Poor Relief in
Century Northern Europe

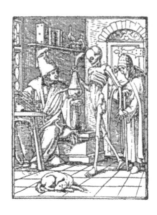

The History of Medicine in Context

Series Editors: Andrew Cunningham and Ole Peter Grell

Department of History and Philosophy of Science
University of Cambridge

Department of History
The Open University

Health Care and Poor Relief in 18th and 19th Century Northern Europe

Edited by

OLE PETER GRELL
ANDREW CUNNINGHAM
and
ROBERT JÜTTE

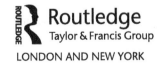

Routledge
Taylor & Francis Group

LONDON AND NEW YORK

First published 2002 by Ashgate Publishing

Published 2017 by Routledge
2 Park Square, Milton Park, Abingdon, Oxfordshire OX14 4RN
711 Third Avenue, New York, NY 10017, USA

First issued in paperback 2017

Routledge is an imprint of the Taylor & Francis Group, an informa business

British Library Cataloguing in Publication Data

Health care and poor relief in 18th and 19th century
  Northern Europe. – (The history of medicine in context)
  1. Poor – Medical care – Europe, Northern – History – 18th
  century 2. Poor – Medical care – Europe, Northern – History
  – 19th century 3. Charities – Europe, Northern – History –
  18th century 4. Charities – Europe, Northern – History –
  19th century
  I. Grell, Ole Peter II. Cunningham, Andrew III. Jütte, Robert
  362.5'094'09033

Library of Congress Cataloging-in-Publication Data

Health care and poor relief in 18th and 19th century northern Europe / edited by Ole Peter Grell, Andrew Cunningham, and Robert Jütte.
    p. cm. — (History of medicine in context)
  Includes bibliographical references.
  ISBN 0-7546-0275-3 (alk. paper)
    1. Medical care – Europe, Northern – History – 18th century. 2. Medical care –
  Europe, Northern – History – 19th century. 3. Public welfare – Europe, Northern –
  History – 18th century. 4. Public welfare – Europe, Northern – History – 19th
  century. 5. Poor – Medical care – Europe, Northern – History. 6. Public health –
  Europe, Northern – History. 7. Social medicine – Europe, Northern – History. I.
  Grell, Ole Peter. II. Cunningham, Andrew, Dr. III. Jütte, Robert. IV. Series.

RA418.5.P6 H3865 2001
362.1'094'09033 – dc21

2001022822

Typeset in Times by Manton Typesetters, Louth, Lincolnshire, UK.

ISBN 13: 978-1-138-26340-6 (pbk)
ISBN 13: 978-0-7546-0275-0 (hbk)

Contents

List of Figures

List of Tables

List of Contributors

Gerda Bonderup, University of Aarhus, Denmark

Anne Crowther, University of Glasgow, Scotland

Andrew Cunningham, University of Cambridge, England

Fritz Dross, Heinrich Heine University, Düsseldorf, Germany

Olivier Faure, University of Lyons, France

Marijke Gijswijt-Hofstra, University of Amsterdam, The Netherlands

David Green, King's College, University of London, England

Ole Peter Grell, The Open University, England

Hubertus Jahn, Clare College, Cambridge, England

Robert Jütte, Robert Bosch Stiftung, Stuttgart, Germany

Øivind Larsen, University of Oslo, Norway

Marco van Leeuwen, University of Rotterdam, The Netherlands

Mary Lindemann, Carnegie Mellon University, Pittsburgh, USA

Rosalind Mitchison, University of Edinburgh, Scotland

Dorothy Porter, Birkbeck College, University of London, England

Matthew Ramsey, Vanderbilt University, USA

Michael Stolberg, Technische Universität, Munich, Germany

Acknowledgements

This volume is built around a conference organised by Ole Peter Grell and Andrew Cunningham, at that time members of the now defunct Cambridge Wellcome Unit for the History of Medicine, in collaboration with Robert Jütte, director of the Robert Bosch Stiftung of Stuttgart, and held at the Stiftung in Stuttgart in June 1998. We are grateful to the Robert Bosch Stiftung for hosting the conference. For financial support of the conference we thank the Wellcome Trust and the Robert Bosch Stiftung.

The editors would especially like to thank Linda Cayford for her sensitive and skilful copy-editing of a challenging set of chapters.

PART ONE

General Themes

CHAPTER ONE

Health Care and Poor Relief in 18th and 19th Century Northern Europe

Ole Peter Grell and Andrew Cunningham

According to Christ, the poor are always with us (Matthew 26: 11). This had been the case in 16th and 17th century Europe and it certainly remained so in the two centuries we are concerned with in this volume. How did the European governments and states cope with the needs of the poorer parts of their populations, during the Enlightenment and industrialisation? What role did such arrangements for the poor play with respect to maintaining social stability and furthering the interests of the ruling classes? How did provision for the maintenance and health of the poor change under rapidly changing economic circumstances? How did the different states of Europe and their people differ in their attitudes to, and provision for, the poor?

This volume offers some answers to these questions by presenting the basis for a comparative view of health care provision and poor relief in northern Europe in the 18th and 19th centuries. Although complete in itself, the volume is also the third of a four-volume survey of health care and poor relief provision in early modern Europe, 1500–1900.[1] In the first two volumes of this series we were particularly concerned with the important role played by the religious impulse in making and shaping provision for the poor in the two centuries after the Reformation. It is clear that, for the most part, the health care provision and poor relief in the north and south of Europe developed along different routes during and after the Reformation and Counter-Reformation. The northern, Protestant, countries came to be characterised by schemes predominantly initiated by local and central governments, while the southern, Catholic, parts of Europe in particular witnessed a reinvigoration of confessional institutions and the creation of new lay and clerical orders dedicated to the poor and the sick.

These two different lines of development continued into the 18th and 19th centuries, although not so directly linked with confessional differences. While in the 15th and early 16th centuries the dynamism of trade and industry had been most evident in the south of Europe, especially in the Italian city states, this state of affairs had begun to change in the course of the 16th century and, as a result, it was the states of northern Europe which by the 17th century, began to lead the way in trade, industry and wealth creation. The Netherlands and Britain were the first to reform their agricultural systems and expand their trade and, in Britain's case, to industrialise. In the course of the 19th century their dominant roles came to be challenged by other northern states, especially Germany and France, as they too underwent agricultural, industrial and trading revolutions. The traditional institutions and arrangements for the care of the sick and poor were themselves put under stress by these developments, especially in the countries where the populations were rapidly expanding. New solutions were needed for both old and new problems.

These two centuries, and especially the 18th century, were a time not only of industrialisation on an unprecedented scale, but also of a revolution in thinking and attitudes, customarily known as the Enlightenment. It was the northern states where these intellectual developments were most advanced, especially in France and some of the German states, but later including Britain, the Netherlands and the Scandinavian countries. Even in the feudally benighted land of Russia attempts were made to introduce enlightened policies and attitudes, but here the movement was led from the top, by the Emperor Peter the Great and the Empress Catherine the Great, and their autocratic versions of Enlightenment did not have a significant effect on the country as a whole. The role that the Enlightenment ideologues played – if any – in modernising poor relief and health care in the northern countries is explored in every chapter of this volume.

The reforms adopted were, for the most part, not very humane by modern standards. There were two primary streams of Enlightenment concern with the health care of the poor and poor relief. From the centralist absolutist German-speaking states, especially Prussia and Austria, came the ideology of *Kameralismus* which preached that the interests of the state had priority over those of the individual, and that it was in the interests of the state to maximise the population and ensure its productivity. From the individualistic, limited monarchy of England came the ideology of liberalism, which advocated the enlightened self-interest of the ruling class. It is these attitudes, rather than any humane concern for the welfare of the whole of society, which we find underlying the reforms of the period. Hence, from a modern perspective, the reforms were, for the most part, surprisingly harsh towards the poor and to the sick poor. It is only at the very end of the period dealt with in this volume – that is, at the end of the 19th and the beginning of the 20th centuries when we find most states opting (or being obliged to opt) for a model where they treated it as one of their positive duties to care for the health and relief of their poor. In effect there was a transformation in what 'liberal' and 'liberalism' meant in the course of the 19th century. For most of the century it meant putting the freedom of the productive individual first, and making this the model for the behaviour of all members of society. Towards the end of the century, however, it came to mean something much more like its modern-day meaning, in which the rights of all individuals within a society are seen as equal and as deserving fair, if not equal, treatment. Thus for the poor, until at least the mid-19th century, the liberals were the reformers who brought them generally harsher conditions in both health care and poor relief than they had previously experienced.

With the secularisation of world outlook in the wake of the Enlightenment, it might be expected that the motives and reasoning behind the supply of health care and poor relief for the growing populations of the European states would become less based on traditions of Christian charity, whether Catholic or Protestant, and more steered by rationality and the needs of a growing industrial capitalism. To some extent this was true, as we shall see. However, in both Catholic and Protestant countries, we still find extensive voluntary care in this period, clearly based on religious impulses. For instance the Society of St Vincent-de-Paul was founded in Paris in 1833 by a group of concerned young Catholic men around Antoine-Fréderic Ozanam in order to help put their vision of a revived Catholicism into practice. Naming their new society after the great French reformer of Catholic welfare provision of the early 17th century, who had founded the Confraternities of Charity, its members resolved to visit the poor in their own homes, the middle-class members of the society giving directly to the poor according to the need they themselves witnessed. Such an action was thought to result in the sanctification of both parties. The movement spread to the Catholic Netherlands, Ireland and elsewhere. Similarly, in Protestant England, the 18th century saw an unprecedented movement, spreading to virtually all significant towns and also at the county level, of founding charitable hospitals (or 'infirmaries') for the poor. The first such 'voluntary hospital', the Westminster Infirmary, founded in 1719, was the creation of High Church Tories excluded from direct political involvement and seeking to exercise Christian charity in their own neighbourhood.[2] But subsequently, religious principles were only marginal to the founding and running of these charitable hospitals in England. The upperclass subscribers typically held an annual church service, and the poor patients on their discharge were expected to thank God and the subscribers for their care, but explicitly religious involvement went no further than that. Rather, the structure of an active body of subscribers providing medical care for the 'deserving poor' of their region, was a focused version of wider class relations in England, with the givers wishing to celebrate their own social position while seeking to promote satisfaction with their lot among the labouring classes.

Throughout this period, health care for the poor was inextricably linked with poor relief, a legacy which has had its effects on modern systems of social welfare. In the first place, the richer classes donated the funds for poor relief, but never drew on it themselves. Similarly, the richer classes never attended hospitals as patients. They made their own arrangements for their own medical care, which was brought to them in their own homes. So the hospitals and infirmaries only contained poor people, supported on the contributions extracted in one way or another from the well-to-do. So 'health care' here refers only to provision for the poor and needy of 18th and 19th century European societies, not to the medical arrangements of the wealthier classes. However, the historic link between poverty and disease that is most evident to the modern eye – that disease, especially epidemic disease, can rapidly reduce the wage labourer and his family to poverty, and thus make them dependent on poor relief – was not readily seen, since poverty was primarily seen as a moral failing, not as a consequence of the vagaries of the economic system as a whole. Some governments, such as those of the German states, had seen the maintenance of general social hygiene as one of their duties. In other states, however, it was really only when harsh new Poor Laws had been enacted in the early 19th century that this link between poverty and disease was noticed and acted upon.

A few technical terms are frequently used by our contributors, and need to be noted. First there is the distinction between 'outdoor' and 'indoor' relief. These particular terms were the ones used in England when workhouses had first been established, but they had parallels in other languages. The distinction began as a practical one and ended as a moral one. Indoor relief was assistance given inside an institution such as a workhouse, or possibly a hospital. By contrast, outdoor relief referred to assistance (in cash, kind or medical attendance) given outside the workhouse – that is, in the homes of the poor. As we shall see, there was continued discussion amongst the giving classes as to which form of relief was most effective, not just for the health and subsistence of the poor, but also for their moral and social improvement. The general trend was to reduce outdoor relief, by enclosing in the workhouse the poor who were unable to work (the 'impotent poor') and the sick poor. When, in time, the workhouse came to be used as a deterrent for the ablebodied poor, then only indoor relief was to be given. Hence the poor were encouraged morally to make every effort to fend for themselves rather than become a burden on society as a whole by entering the workhouse. In fact, indoor relief was always more expensive than outdoor relief because workhouses had to be built and managed, so this growing insistence on giving only indoor relief reveals how highly the giving classes valued the deterrent effect of the workhouse on the moral condition of the poor.

The second distinction of poor relief which recurs in these pages is the distinction between the 'deserving' and the 'undeserving' poor – deserving (or undeserving), that is, of relief, whether the condition that required relief was sickness or poverty and want. Obviously this is a moral distinction, distinguishing between those who, in the eyes of those providing relief, were either truly disabled or temporarily unable to work (the 'deserving' poor), and those who were deemed to be ablebodied but workshy (the 'undeserving' poor).

Finally there is the distinction between the poor, and the so-called 'shamefaced poor'. The first group were those who were forever poor; the second were those who were normally amongst the class of independent labourers or better-off, but had fallen temporarily on hard times and were embarrassed to find themselves seeking poor relief.

As with the previous volumes in this series, we begin with two overviews of the period which deal with some of the issues common to most countries. In these two chapters the general themes of Enlightenment and political ideology are looked at across the whole region, as is the general relationship between the providers and those provided for in the domain of health care and poor relief. Then follow 12 chapters covering the local situation in most of the larger states of northern Europe of the period. We are aware of some gaps in this roll-call, including Ireland, Switzerland, Sweden and Finland, some of which we had hoped to fill but in the event were unable to find contributors for. However, even so, this wide range of states certainly allows comparative consideration of poor relief and health care across northern Europe to an extent not hitherto possible.

The authors of the two overviews both put the traditional historiography of the topic under the spotlight. In Chapter Two Dorothy Porter shows that, until recently, the history of poor relief and health care for the poor had been written in a 'progressivist' way, with historians looking for evidence of early progress towards the modern state-run health care systems with which they themselves were familiar in the mid-20th century. Every provision for the poor, whether ameliorative or punitive, was counted as a step, forwards or backwards, on this historic route towards the establishment of the modern health care systems of Western states. Moreover, the story of the development of state-funded health care for all, which began with provision for the poor, was also taken to be a story of the development of the rights of the individual in a modern democracy. Health care for all and democratic citizenship were two sides of the same historical coin. However, according to recent historians writing from within a different ideological perspective, what had been left out of the story in particular was the continued role of voluntary, public, giving for the poor by the richer classes, and of mutual aid provision for themselves by the working classes – 'voluntarist welfare' as it has been called. According to such historians, of whom in Britain Geoffrey Finlayson has been perhaps the most prominent, these public, participatory, charities were themselves the great nurturers of participatory democracy – 'contributory citizenship', as its historians call it.

Historians are, of course, to some extent inevitably caught up in the dominant ideologies of their own ages, and the history of health care and poor relief is no exception. What we have here is a conflict, played out in the field of the history of health care and poor relief, between two major modern-day positions. On the one hand there has been the collectivist consensus, to which belonged the historians who wrote the 'progressivist' accounts, which celebrated state involvement in provision for the poor as the solution to a historical problem. On the other hand there is the view of social and political relationships – a view which originated with the political right, and which has been dominant in Western societies in the last 20 years – which is opposed to state involvement and favours individualism in all areas of life and society. Historians of this persuasion write accounts of poor relief and health care in the past, which bring to the forefront the voluntarist involvement of individuals. The two groups of historians naturally treat the Enlightenment as something of a battleground: were its principles, when put into practice, statist and democratic, or individualistic and democratic? Of course they were both. Both types of account now exist, and they are not complementary. As Dorothy Porter shows, other modern ideological positions, such as feminism, have also begun to shape yet more new accounts of this area of the past.

A new approach to poor relief and health care across northern Europe is offered to historians in Chapter Three by Marco van Leeuwen. He concentrates on analysing the historic events of health care and poor relief in terms of the modern concern with calculating individual and group actions in terms of *risk*. This approach tends to highlight not only state moves towards providing general health care and poor relief, but also the voluntary alternatives to poor relief which continued to exist – in other words, it stresses the so-called 'mixed economy of welfare'. Moreover, with respect to risk assessment, van Leeuwen presents poor relief as both 'a control strategy of the élites and as a survival strategy for the poor'. Thus, for the élites, providing poor relief was not just a way of coping with social poverty, but also a way of controlling risks to the labour supply and of keeping the peace in early modern society. For the poor, the other main party affected, the option of taking poor relief was one of a range of possible strategies they could deploy for survival. Among these other options were voluntary institutions such as guilds, mutual aid societies and trade unions, all available as strategies for coping with risk from poverty and illness.

Our survey of health care and poor relief in different states begins in the German-speaking states of northern Europe, starting with Prussia. By the end of the 19th century, Prussia was giving the lead in a number of ways to other countries in the replacement of traditional forms of poor relief. Developments in this country during the 18th and 19th centuries are therefore of particular interest. Prussia, an absolutist state, was a centre for the practice of the Enlightenment science of state finances, *Kameralismus*. According to this, the people of a state are its wealth; therefore their productivity needs to be preserved and enhanced and their numbers increased. Promoting these ideals are all primarily state duties. As an enlightened absolutist state Prussia was also an ideal location for pursuing the ideals of 'medical police', expounded by Johann Peter Frank, and first published in his *System einer vollständigen medizinischen Polizei* of 1779.[3] Fritz Dross in Chapter Four shows that poor relief was taken to be a state obligation in Prussia from 1794:

the central government made the decrees, the local administration had to fulfil them. For the most part outdoor relief was used to care for the sick poor, and big hospitals, especially the Charité in Berlin, were used to house the impoverished. From as early as 1699 Berlin had a governmental organisation to ensure care of the poor, the *Armendirektorium*. However, the capacity of the state to continue these policies was greatly reduced by the defeats of Prussia by France in 1795 and 1806 and by the disorder in state finances. Moreover, by the mid-19th century, Prussia was suffering badly from the pauperism which everywhere seemed to stalk industrialisation like a shadow. Among the responses to this in Prussia was the introduction of a system of bourgeois welfare volunteers – 'friends of the poor' – on the 'Eberfeld' system (itself based on the Hamburg system of poor relief). Yet, towards the end of the century, salaried municipal administrators were already taking over these voluntary roles. Under Bismarck, state policy still, like *Kameralismus*, placed the state's needs at the centre of law-making. In particular, policy was aimed as much at providing a flexible and docile industrial workforce as at the beneficent care of the poor. The government introduced insurance against accidents, against ill-health and for retirement and, by the end of the century, these innovations were just beginning to replace traditional poor relief. As Dross writes, 'Consequently, the ideological basis of public welfare changed – from the "charitable citizens' sense of community" to a professionally run public assistance system. The deserving poor were transformed into "needy fellow citizens".'

Bavaria, by contrast, was slow to industrialise. However, as Michael Stolberg shows in Chapter Five, it nevertheless experienced a crisis over the issue of begging in the late 18th century. Although attempts to outlaw begging and almsgiving failed, even when the army was used to enforce the law, a system of public poor relief was brought in and, from 1799 a centralised, state-run system of poor relief was initiated throughout the kingdom. This last measure was part of a short-lived attempt to make Bavaria into an enlightened absolutist state. In a more liberal atmosphere, 19th century Bavarian responses towards the problem of the poor were marked by extensive voluntary involvement in the provision of soup and moral improvement. As in other states, the 19th century was a century of hospital-building to cater to the needs of the sick poor in Bavaria. Most notably, acting as what Stolberg calls 'a vanguard force', from the early 19th century, Bavaria was also establishing medical insurance for the labouring poor which would have served to mitigate the worst effects of the intermittent unemployment of the nascent industrialisation process.

The 'Hamburg system' of poor relief, discussed by Mary Lindemann in Chapter Six, operated in Hamburg between (at most) 1770 and 1810. Hamburg was a trading city which had lost its manufacturing element, and which was prone to trade depressions and hence to unemployment throughout the

18th century. Formally established in 1788, the 'General Poor Relief' involved civic involvement as volunteers on the part of the well-to-do. It took over, as its Medical Deputation, a system of home-based medical relief which in its turn had been an outcome of extensive discussions of the role of disease in causing impoverishment in the previous decades. Thus in Hamburg the poor were visited in their homes by one of two hundred or more individual volunteers, distributing relief on the principle of making up the difference between what the poor person *did* earn by labour and what he actually *needed*. In addition, they were also visited in their homes by volunteer unpaid doctors offering free medical care. All this attention was aimed at getting the poor back to work or keeping them in work. This communal involvement in health care and poor relief did not survive the French occupation, and by the mid-19th century, attitudes towards the poor and destitute had hardened and home-visiting was being replaced by institutionalisation.

Russia promised to be an enlightened state on the Western model with respect to poor relief and health care for the poor under the guidance of Peter the Great. However, as Hubertus Jahn writes in Chapter Seven, this was not to be. The great problems of organisation across the vastness of Russia worked against it, together with the continued dominance of orthodox religion, in which the support of beggars and the poor were part of Christian duty, such that 'beggars were a constituent part of every-day religious practice'. Greater success attended Catherine the Great's attempts to introduce German *Kameralist* practices, through 'social welfare boards'. Later, a combination of state and private initiatives led to the creation of the Imperial Philanthropic Society which promoted philanthropy in general, as well as caring for the poor. Finally the 'beggars' committee' was founded in St Petersburg and Moscow in 1837 under tsarist initiative with the impossible brief of eliminating begging. The absence of private charity and the dominance of the tsar meant that it was the absolutist ruler, whether enlightened or not, who had the role of moderniser in Russia.

Until 1814, Denmark and Norway were one state under Danish domination. During the 18th century, as Gerda Bonderup shows in Chapter Eight, the situation for the poor followed the common pattern, with begging prohibited and the deserving poor supported on outdoor relief paid for by local parishioners and administered by state and religious authorities. Subsequently, workhouses were constructed and the 'Hamburg system' was gradually introduced. However, an 'enlightened' investigation of the whole poor relief system in the 1780s, in the long run led only to a tightening of poor relief conditions, albeit ameliorated by the emergence of many bourgeois societies offering philanthropy to the poor in the 19th century. Norway, separate from Denmark after 1814 but in a semi-voluntary union with Sweden until 1905, had its own particular problems in the 19th century, as Øivind Larsen argues in Chapter Nine. Still predominantly a rural society, with settlements scattered at great distances from each other, Norway nevertheless shared in the population explosion common to most European countries during the 19th century, with the same consequent problems of poor relief.

The Industrial Revolution had its earliest effects in England and Scotland. The great rise in population and the movement of so many people from the countryside to the new industrial towns put the traditional poor law system under great stress. The old system, dating from the 16th century, had made provision for the poor via parish collections. Entitlement therefore depended on residence. The great population movements in the late 18th and 19th centuries therefore made a nonsense of this old system. By the end of the 18th century this system was being widely criticised, and Thomas Malthus, writing in the interests of the country landowners, called for it to be dismantled. However, the Enlightenment ideology that was actually used to reform the old system was that of Jeremy Bentham. Unfortunately, it was enlightened only in the sense that it expressed the interests of the industrial class – in other words, enlightened self-interest. Bentham's approach was thoroughly secular, but nevertheless moralistic, in that he believed that poor relief corrupted the morality of the workers by making them dependent. The workers had to be persuaded to take responsibility for themselves as individuals, both by forming provident societies for themselves, and also by being deterred from dependence on poor relief. So the reform of the old Poor Law, which was carried into effect by Bentham's own secretary and follower, Edwin Chadwick, produced, in 1834, a New Poor Law which aimed to make poor relief literally the last thing the poor would seek; relief had to be received indoors, in workhouses, and it had to be stigmatised. In Chapter Ten Anne Crowther discusses the implementation of the New Poor Law across the country as a whole, while in Chapter Eleven David Green looks at the special case of London: both of them deal with the quite unexpected emergence from this strict new regime of a countrywide system of infirmaries giving free medical service to all the poor, including midwifery and care of infectious diseases.

Scotland, too, underwent the same industrialisation process, being transformed, as Rosalind Mitchison says in Chapter Twelve, from the least urbanised country in western Europe to being second only to England in terms of the proportion of the population who lived in towns. Here, too, reform of the Poor Law, when it came in 1845, was based on Benthamite principles, promoting the ideal of the 'independent' worker. But conditions had been so bad for the poor before that the New Poor Law actually improved the support given to them. Perhaps surprisingly, the ideologues of the Scottish Enlightenment seem to have contributed no theoretical basis to this change.

The Netherlands were commercially very rich at the beginning of this period, but were quite late in industrialising. As in England, the crisis in poor relief in the Dutch provinces came in the 1790s, when the old system broke down. This system had depended on each of the many confessional Churches looking after its own poor, with the charge of those outside the Churches falling on the state. Again, as with England, the relief was offered only locally – that is, to members of the local confessional groups or, in the case of the towns, to those born locally. Consequently, this system could not withstand the strains of economic and social change at the end of the 18th century. In the midst of the frequent political changes affecting the Netherlands during this period, a succession of Poor Laws were passed, from 1800 to 1870. In Chapter Thirteen Marijke Gijswijt-Hofstra shows that it was not until the socially-oriented liberals came to power in the late 19th century that the system began to significantly change for the better. Until then, free-market liberals had joined their voices to confessional parties in proclaiming poor relief to be an encouragement to laziness.

Finally we turn to France, arguably the country which set the political model for Europe in this period. France, and especially Paris, during the central hundred years of this period underwent a series of major political transformations, beginning with the French Revolution in 1789, and including switches back and forth from monarchy to republic, and even the communard rule of the brief Paris Commune of 1871. As Matthew Ramsey shows in Chapter Fourteen, Paris was both a magnet for the poor and sick of France and also by far the best equipped town in Europe in respect of hospitals of all kinds. Here, as elsewhere in the 18th century, begging was criminalised and workhouses introduced for the 'undeserving' poor. But, by contrast, the financial aid available to the 'deserving poor' in Paris was relatively generous. Towards the end of the century voluntary philanthropic societies were the liberal reformers' favourite devices to provide policed care to the poor and sick. In the Revolution there was an attempt to eliminate begging altogether, and to return poor relief to its 'natural' place, the home. Both of these were in line with revolutionary ideology about the causes of illness and poverty; as Ramsey puts it, 'in a regenerated and virtuous society, both poverty and sickness would disappear'. The radical experiments of the Revolution were short-lived; later, care of the poor was returned to the local level, hospitals were re-established, and voluntary philanthropic societies were again encouraged. The Assistance Publique à Paris was created in 1849 to administer hospitals, hospices and the poor relief system, but a combination of public and private financing supported poor relief and the health care of the poor: *la bienfaisance publique* remained a collective and voluntary enterprise throughout the 19th century in Paris.

While Paris was always the political barometer of France and the care of the poor was crucial to avoid revolt, elsewhere in France, as Olivier Faure shows in Chapter Fifteen, poor relief also continued to play a significant role in avoiding popular revolution. Enlightenment attitudes at the time of the Revolution proved 'unhappy' (as Faure puts it) in their outcomes. There was a return to local levels of organisation of hospitals and poor relief, together with religiously-inspired voluntary involvement in charities. The 'return to charity' was interrupted by the cholera epidemics but, despite discussion of the possibility, a compulsory welfare state system did not eventuate. It was only at the end of the 19th century that the public assistance system was organised, although private charity and mutualism were still important elements. Even today, as Faure recounts, the French system is very complicated and is a legacy from the 19th century: 'It is based on private charity, public assistance, compulsory social insurance, mutual and voluntary aid. Each component of the system was created by one of the numerous social and political forces acting during the nineteenth century'.

Taken together, the essays in this volume chart the varying responses of states, social classes and political theorists towards the great social and economic issue of the age – industrialisation. Its demands and effects undermined the capacity of the old poor relief arrangements to look after those people that the fits and starts of the industrialisation cycle itself turned into paupers. In particular, the old principle of relief according to residence, generally based on parish or district of residence, was completely unable to cope with the wandering labourer. The liberal ideological response, whether inspired by Enlightenment thinking or not, tended towards the repressive. The late 18th and 19th centuries were the period of the experiment of the workhouse at its harshest. It was only with the rise of labour as a political force in industrialised states, and the transformation of liberalism into a socially-oriented political approach, that the poor came to be seen as people with rights. Fritz Dross's conclusions for his account of the situation in Prussia (in Chapter Four) can be extended more widely to all the states of northern Europe:

> ... municipal and state poor relief had begun to change in character by the 1870s. A restrictive and exclusive welfare policy gradually evolved into a pacifying and socially integrating labour policy. Financial benefits were replaced by (medical) benefits in kind. These eventually assumed a preventive character. Along with social disciplining and the regulation of behaviour, social security gradually locked poor people into the scientific–technological industrial world: paupers were transformed into the industrial proletariat, then into a predictable industrial labour force. In this development, the medical culture played an increasingly important role: health, as a social good, became a generally accepted ideal in industrial society.

Notes

1. See O.P. Grell and A. Cunningham (eds), *Health Care and Poor Relief in Protestant Europe, 1500–1700*. London, 1997; O.P. Grell, A. Cunningham and J. Arrizabalaga (eds), *Health Care and Poor Relief in Counter-Reformation*

Europe, London, 1999. We are preparing a final volume on health care and poor relief in southern Europe in the 18th and 19th centuries.

2. A. Wilson, 'The Politics of Medical Improvement in Early Hanoverian London', in A. Cunningham and R. French (eds), *The Medical Enlightenment of the Eighteenth Century*, Cambridge, 1990, pp. 4–39; R. Porter, 'The Gift Relation: Philanthropy and Provincial Hospitals in Eighteenth-Century England', in L. Granshaw and R. Porter (eds), *The Hospital in History*, London: Routledge 1990, pp. 149–78.

3. E. Lesky (ed.), *A System of Complete Medical Police: Selections from Johann Peter Frank*. Baltimore, Maryland, 1976.

CHAPTER TWO

Health Care and the Construction of Citizenship in Civil Societies in the Era of the Enlightenment and Industrialisation

Dorothy Porter

At one time, the historiography of welfare states conceptualised them as comprehensive systems of social security, funded and administered by centralised political organisations which first emerged in Northern Europe in the first half of the 19th century following the French Revolution.[1] More recent studies, however, have begun to explore changing forms of welfare provided by myriad agencies, from self-help and mutual aid to various types of collective distribution organised by political, voluntaristic or commercial institutions, in communities with or without a centralisation of power.[2] This chapter will address both of these conceptualisations by examining what determined ideological changes within the mixed economies of welfare in northern Europe in the 18th and 19th centuries – how were ideas about health care and poor relief influenced by the ideologies of the Enlightenment and the force of industrialisation?

The historiography of state and voluntary welfare provision

In order to examine the questions outlined above, it is necessary to explore the historiographical context in which such a discussion can take place. Until recently, far more attention had been paid to the history of state, than voluntary, welfare. One reason for the extensive attention paid to state welfare has been the interest taken by social policy theorists in the history of their own subject. Analysts of contemporary welfare states consistently contextualise their investigations historically[3] and frequently cite the influence of the British model on other European systems. Britain has thus been given prominence within the context of comparative accounts.[4] Consequently, the literature on the history of British welfare has expanded, with numerous historians providing sometimes overlapping, if alternative, interpretations of the same events.[5]

The historian, the late Geoffrey Finlayson, argued, however, that the historiography of the British welfare state had created an intellectual distortion of the subject as a whole.[6] He suggested that most accounts of British welfare history offered Whiggish linear descriptions of progressive state expansion working its way teleologically toward the establishment of what Anne Digby and others have identified as the 'classic welfare state'.[7] This has influenced writing on the history of other European welfare systems, which also give tacit acknowledgement to the existence of a classical model of welfare that experienced a 'golden age' during the first two decades following the Second World War. Finlayson claimed that this historiographical tradition reflected the truth of the belief of the English post-war theorist of social welfare, Richard Titmuss, that 'when we study welfare systems we see that they reflect the dominant cultural and political characteristics of their societies'.[8] The reason for the teleological history of the welfare state in Britain and in other European states, Finlayson suggested, is that it was written by historians who were as much advocates of social democracy as analysts of it.

For example, historians, such as George Kitson-Clarke, Oliver MacDonagh and Henry Paris, writing in the late 1950s on 'the growth in government' in 19th century Britain, shared the values of those who provided the intellectual and political legitimation of the welfare state, such as T. H. Marshall, William Beveridge and Clement Attlee. Throughout the 1970s British historiography perpetuated a linear tradition in works such as those of Maurice Bruce, Derek Fraser, David Roberts and R.C. Birch who gave accounts of *The Rise ...* and *The Coming of the Welfare State*, *The Evolution of the Welfare State*, *The Victorian Origins of the Welfare State* and *The Shaping of the Welfare State*.[9] Finlayson suggests that this tradition of linear, Whiggish, teleological history was based on a belief that modern democratic citizenship was given a new meaning by the establishment of the welfare state. The historians of the growth of government believed that, as the British sociologist T.H. Marshall had pointed out, the welfare state added social rights to the civil and political rights of citizenship in democratic states in the 20th century.[10]

Finlayson claimed that this linear historiography was not challenged until the integrity of the welfare state itself was threatened by the political rhetoric of the New Right in the 1980s, which also questioned the parameters of democratic citizenship.[11] The New Right drew attention to the historical alternatives to statutory welfare provision, and began to highlight the role of contributory citizenship in achieving a citizenship of entitlement – that is, the necessity for rights to be earned through the undertaking of social and economic responsibilities. A New Right political consensus – which in Britain, at least under Margaret Thatcher, dismissed the existence of society – emphasised the value of individualistic resolutions to the provision of welfare through voluntarism, self-help and mutual aid.

Thus, from the 1980s, historians began to pay increasing attention to voluntarist welfare. To begin with, new investigations were undertaken on health care and welfare provision 'before the welfare state'.[12] Peregrine Horden revealed the intricate networks of social provision amongst early medieval European communities.[13] The expansion of this complex web of charity provision has been explored in the late medieval and early modern periods.[14] Jonathan Barry and Colin Jones edited a seminal collection of essays that documented the mixed economies of welfare in Europe up to the beginning of the twentieth century.[15]

One of the themes of the historiography of voluntary welfare has been the public, rather than the private, nature of charity. Sandra Cavallo demonstrated the intricate nature of the relationship of charity hospitals in early modern Italian city-states to local governments, while Anne Borsay illustrated the growth of associative charities, such as the voluntary hospital movement and charity schools in England, that were set up on the model of publicly owned joint stock companies, made possible by financial reforms enacted in the early 18th century.[16] Alan Mitchell and Paul Weindling have shown how mutual aid organisations set up in Germany and France in the 19th century were collectivist 'communities' of skilled workers and artisans founded on the principles of self-help.[17] The public nature of charity highlighted the role of a wide range of social groups in the organisation of health care and charity. Borsay illustrated the way in which associative charity revealed the emergence of a middle class in 18th century English society. Cavallo drew attention to the role of women as both benefactors and recipients in hospital charity in early modern Italy and England.[18] Other feminist historians discussed the participation of women in 'active citizenship' or in a 'citizenship of contribution' through the voluntary organisation of health and social welfare in the 19th and early 20th centuries.[19]

Finlayson believed that examining the history of charity provided a special opportunity for highlighting the democratic advantages of individualistic voluntarism. He contrasted the opportunities for democratic participation in self-governing charities, self-help and mutual aid organisations with the authoritarian implications of expanded bureaucratic welfare provision by centralised governments.[20] He also argued that, in 19th century England, basic provisions such as education, health, housing and social security were largely provided through voluntary organisations, and that the Victorian state simply performed 'an enabling or complementary role, which facilitated the proper discharge of voluntary initiatives, or a residual or supplementary role which filled in the gaps in that provision'.[21]

Restating Titmuss's dictum, Finlayson argued that the new historiography of voluntary welfare reflected new social ideologies of a new era. This historiography investigated the influence of the mixed economy of welfare on transformations in the conceptualisation of citizenship in liberal democratic

societies. Feminist historians used the opportunity to unpack the history of
social citizenship that had previously ignored the role of women. When
Marshall and his contemporaries had identified social citizenship with entitlements to welfare, they mainly had male breadwinners in mind. Feminist
historians in the 1980s and 1990s began to investigate the active citizenship
of contribution which middle- and upper-class women had been able to
express through participation in voluntary and charitable organisations.[22] Investigating contributory citizenship offered historians the opportunity to
reconsider a wide range of ideological motivations for collective action in the
provision of welfare, such as religious consciousness and paternalism. As the
historian of female philanthropy in 19th century England, Frank Prochaska,
pointed out: 'if there was a conviction peculiar to nineteenth-century philanthropic women it was their belief, inspired by Christ, that love could transform
society.'[23] The history of active, contributory citizenship has also offered
historians the opportunity to unpack complex social ideologies of gender in a
new way. The active female citizenry engaged in voluntary welfare provision
did not necessarily link the right to participate in what Lady Violet Greville
liked to call 'slumming' to the right to vote.[24] In fact, significant Victorian
lady philanthropists, such as Louisa Twining, Octavia Hill and Florence
Nightingale, were anti-suffragists.

Finlayson was right to suggest that the dismantling of the older historiography of the welfare state has offered up new opportunities for a new
generation of historians living in a new era. He himself greatly contributed
to the new historiography by linking his investigations of voluntarism in
England to the opportunities it offered for democratic participation and
control in the distribution of welfare. He was wrong, however, to dismiss
the need for further investigation into the history of what he called political
collectivism, or state administered and funded welfare. His critique of what
he identified as the linear, teleological historiography of the welfare state
ignores the fact that, while historians such as Kitson-Clarke may have
implicitly linked the 'rise' of the welfare state to the creation of social
citizenship, they did not write histories of citizenship itself. The investigation of citizenship justifies continued attention to the history of political
collectivism for two reasons.

First, the creators of the classic welfare state based on the principle of
universalism believed that the expansion of central government was the route
to increased egalitarianism in the social and economic relations of industrial
capitalist society.[25] As a result, they assumed that the statutory universal
guarantee of minimum living standards without stigma would act as a
counterforce to structural inequality produced by free-market economies and
would create a citizenship of entitlement for all. But, in so doing, the architects of the modern welfare state did not lose sight of an equally long
tradition within the concept of citizenship in which entitlements were earned

through the fulfilment of social obligations.[26] In order to explore the complexities of the rights and obligations of civil and social citizenship it is impossible to ignore the history of political collectivism and the history of central state expansion. The history of the active citizenship of contribution in the voluntary sector needs to be examined in relation to the 'active' fulfilment of obligations and social responsibilities required before the citizenship of entitlement is granted by the democratic state.

Second, the history of political collectivism and central state expansion has yet further value, especially for historians concerned with the influence of scientific rationalism in the ideological and cultural transformations of modern and post-modern industrial–technological societies. This is really the task of exploring the cultures of politics and the narratives of government as they were constructed and deconstructed through the languages of Enlightenment rationalism and positivistic scientism.

This chapter will examine the influence of ideological forces on the changing configurations of the mixed economies of health care and welfare in the 18th and 19th centuries, concentrating on three issues:

1. the complex history of ideologies of citizenship in civil society;
2. the influence of Enlightenment rationalism on the political cultures of health and welfare provision; and
3. the relationship of positivistic conceptions of science to the systematic organisation of health and welfare by the state and other agencies.

The strength of the state, the rights of man, and self-improvement

I need not restate the commonplace that the Enlightenment was a highly diverse historical movement that was expressed variably in different national contexts – a movement with both a cluster of commonalities and sharp contradictions.[27] Perhaps, as Lester Crocker has pointed out, the greatest common element amongst those who aspired to the status of Enlightened philosophers was not *what* they thought but *how*.[28] As Roy Porter has suggested, 18th century critics liked to think of themselves as 'bringing light into a world too long shrouded in gloom by the forces of ignorance, superstition, political and ecclesiastical despotism and censorship'.[29] And while the Age of Reason is an inappropriate description, because rationalism characterised the spirit of earlier epochs from the medieval world to the 17th century, nevertheless a common project of the Enlightenment was to apply rationalism to the understanding of nature and the organisation of the social world. These latter two projects were linked in the development of Enlightenment social sciences of population health and wealth and in proposals for new forms of collective organisation to promote both.

A further Enlightenment value emphasised the role of philanthropy in encouraging self-help and civic improvement.[30] This was linked throughout Europe to the revival of ancient philosophies of both individual and environmental health improvement.[31] In late 18th century England, the idea of environmental improvement was translated into the expansion of Town Improvement Commissions that sought to bring about the 'civilising process' amongst the wretchedly squalid poor by inducing self-improvement through environmental improvement.[32] The largest commercial economy in Europe also made civic environmentalism a profitable trade, spawning new commercial enterprises in night soil collection, street widening, paving and lighting.[33]

In Enlightenment England the campaign to avoid disease was based on social, as well as environmental, analysis. It was only sporadically translated into public policy through the haphazard proliferation of urban Improvement Commissions. Philanthropic individuals set up Commissions with responsibility for improving paving, lighting and street cleaning in local areas. No central government policy was developed; instead, in this *laissez-faire* society, public health became a commercial enterprise.[34] Elsewhere in Europe, however, Enlightenment rationalism encouraged the growth of political collectivism and activity by central states.

Despite the fact that later Enlightenment thinkers, such as Voltaire, reacted against the rationalism of Leibniz, satirising him in *Candide* as a dogmatist of *a priori* reasoning, the co-founder of the calculus was an early advocate of enlightened actions by the state to increase its strength by analysing and improving population health. Early modern political philosophies of mercantilism and cameralism stressed the need to measure the strength of the state by assessing levels of population health. Various methods of counting the subjects of the state, and measuring the state's size and strength in terms of their number and their health, were introduced by early modern administrations. In the 16th century, Italian cities made elaborate statistical inquiries into population, economic activity and epidemic disease.[35] The Spanish carried out a census of Peru in 1548 and of their territories in North America in 1576. Nova Scotia and Quebec instituted censuses in the 1660s. English intellectuals in the late 17th century developed the idea of a political arithmetic and produced an arithmetical account of Ireland in 1679.[36] The Caribbean Islands reported on trade and populations to their French, Spanish and English rulers. The Constitution of the United States continued colonial practice and required a decennial census. In the 18th century Sweden used its Episcopalian ministry to collect information on births, deaths, cause of death, levels of literacy and levels of ill-health,[37] and France established a bureau of statistical investigation during the Napoleonic era. Imperialism encouraged the development of censuses.[38] Counting and evaluating the strength of the state was based on a form of political book-keeping which not only enabled the state to measure its strength in terms of the size of its healthy population but also guided its administrative goals and objectives.

In the 1680s Leibniz had sought to institutionalise the analysis of population structure in Brandenburg-Prussia by proposing that the state should create a central statistical bureau which could serve various branches of military and civil administration and maintain a register of births, marriages and deaths. He devised 56 categories to evaluate the population, including gender, social status, the number of ablebodied men for bearing arms and marriageable women for bearing children. When Brandenburg-Prussia became a kingdom in 1701, although Frederick I had been impressed by Leibniz's proposals, a statistical office was not created until the reign of Wilhelm I (1713–1740). In 1661 Liebniz had also proposed that a *Collegium Medicum* be set up to regulate the medical profession and the sale of drugs.[39] The *Collegium Medicum* was created by the Elector Frederick William in 1685, and issued edicts which imposed new regulations on medical practice and pharmacy. The *Collegium Medicum* decided who should be admitted to the medical profession and established a state examination system and preparatory courses. It also policed unlicensed practice through a legal system administered by local health bureaucracies. Town and district physicians, set up throughout the German states from the 15th century onwards, were officially appointed as servants of the state to oversee the institutionalisation of qualified practice in their localities, to prosecute unlicensed quacks and to administer new laws on the sale of pharmaceuticals. Town physicians were charged with making sure that a standardisation of fees was established amongst local practitioners.[40] Although the extent to which they fulfilled these functions was, as Mary Lindemann has shown, highly variable,[41] the seeds of systematic regulation of the healing market by the state, with the aim of improving population health, were sown and nurtured throughout the 18th century in the Prussian state. Preventive health measures to avoid epidemic disease, however, were not part of its remit. Instead the cameralist state perceived the route to population growth to be through an efficient state regulation of medical practice and the standardisation of pharmaceutical preparations and sales.[42]

The practice of 'medical police' in 18th century Prussia contrasted with the situation in Sweden, where a different approach to state health intervention was developed before 1800.[43] Health reform in Sweden – which, of course, at that time included Finland – was made possible through the creation of a national census in 1749, the first in Europe. Shockingly low levels of population in Sweden galvanised the state into action on health and pronatalism.[44] Sweden's homogenous society and universal Episcopal bureaucracy enabled the state to institute the first comprehensive system of population registration and census-taking in Europe. The promotion of fertility and personal hygiene education, the policing of sexually and socially transmitted diseases through policies of isolation and treatment, and the development of municipal hospitals, were all instituted in 18th century Sweden in the name of strengthening the state through population growth.[45] These policies were administered through local secular and Episcopal bureaucracies long before Johann Peter Frank included such measures in his theoretical system of medical police.

The concept of medical police also helped found some preliminary forms of health administration under the ancien régime in France, initiated by Louis XIV's minister of finance, Colbert. The Société Royale de Médecine was created in 1772 to police medical nostrums and quackery, distribute medicine chests to rural health authorities and to set up a network for reporting local epidemics.[46] And although the practice of medical police varied, throughout Europe mercantilist concerns over healthy population levels promoted ever stricter enforcement of port quarantines, border sanitary cordons and the policing of public nuisances and civic disorder.

However, mercantilism and medical police were not the only ideological forces stimulating collective action regarding population health and social welfare prior to the 19th century. In the last quarter of the 18th century, collective actions regarding the health and welfare of populations were inherently bound up with the rhetorics of revolutionary democracy on the one hand, and the rational pursuit of individual and collective happiness on the other.[47]

Democratic revolutions in America and France asserted new principles regarding the state and the health of its subjects. Thomas Paine did not include health amongst the property rights to which all free men were innately entitled, but Thomas Jefferson declared that sick populations were the product of sick political systems.[48] According to Jefferson, despotism produced disease, whereas democracy liberated health. Jefferson believed that a life of political 'liberty and the pursuit of happiness' would automatically be a healthy one. He told his co-signer of the Declaration of Independence, the physician and patriot Benjamin Rush, that the iniquity of European absolutism was reflected in its peoples' wretchedly unhealthy and demoralised condition. Democracy was the source of the people's health. Democratic citizens, self-educated in exercising their political judgement, would secure a healthy existence. Furthermore, he claimed, the healthiness of the American people reflected the superiority of democratic citizenship.[49]

It was French revolutionaries who, in 1792, added health and a minimum subsistence to the rights of man, and asserted that a healthy citizenship should be a characteristic of the modern democratic state. The citizens' charter of health, however, was doublesided. The *idéologue*, Constantine Volney (1757–1820), raised the issue of the citizen's responsibility to maintain his own health for the benefit of the state. In the new social order the individual was a political and economic unit of a collective whole. It was a citizen's duty to keep healthy through temperance, both in the consumption of pleasure and the exercise of passions, and through cleanliness.[50]

Democratic rhetoric on health citizenship and new rights to economic welfare failed to translate into a material reality in any late Enlightenment state, even though it was still idealistically burning in the hearts of the German and French revolutionaries of 1848. The mantle of health reform and social reform was inherited, instead, by utilitarian political economists. It was the economic value, to expanding industrial societies of preventing premature mortality which was ultimately responsible for public health reform in early 19th century Europe. And it was the cost of poverty which stimulated 19th century governments to apply systematic rationalisation to the administration of economic relief to the destitute.

Voluntarism in the 19th century

The application of enlightened rationalism encouraged collective actions and collective responsibilities for health care and welfare provision in the 18th century. Even though the force of industrialisation rapidly reconfigured the socioeconomic landscapes of northern European societies, 18th century ideologies continued to influence 19th century political discourses. One Enlightenment legacy was the attempt by some 19th century political reformers to turn government itself into a form of social science rationally trying to pursue a felicific calculus.[51] In the context of health care this stimulated some 19th century reformers to interpret health citizenship as a civil right. In England at least, mid-19th century advocates of state medicine, such as England's first medical statesman, John Simon, equated the right to be protected from an infectious disease with the equal right under the law to be protected against personal violence.[52] While the notion of health rights was not interpreted in the same way throughout Europe, echoes of French revolutionary rhetoric still resounded in the mid-19th century in the definitions of social and political medicine offered in France by Jules Gérain and in Germany by Rudolf Virchow and his fellow health reformers.[53]

European states varied widely in the development of health care in the 19th century and responded to the challenges of industrialisation in different ways. In the first half of the century, France led the field in the development of public hygiene as a science of 'social physics'.[54] While the centralised state retained a firm grip on the legal structure of French society, however, it resisted interfering in the economic and social lives of its citizens to improve population health.[55] The new group of academic sociomedical investigators in France, the *partie d'hygiène*, were wedded to the economic liberalism of the political economist Jean Baptiste Le Say and concluded that responsibility for the relationship between poverty and ill-health lay with the poor. Consequently, they advocated the remoralisation of the poor as the most effective route to disease control and improvement of social conditions.[56]

In England, social reformers also investigated the connection between poverty and disease. The leader of the public health movement in the first half of the 19th century, Edwin Chadwick, believed, however, that disease caused poverty by prematurely killing breadwinners who left widows and orphans to become burdens on the poor rates. Chadwick's utilitarian solution was to reduce the cost of poverty by reducing the spread of epidemic diseases. Inspired by a miasmatic theory of disease he and his contemporary reformer, Thomas Southwood Smith, advocated environmental reform as the most effective means of disease prevention and the reduction of poverty. Utilitarianism was superseded by Christian Socialism as the ideological context for public health reform in Britain in the mid-19th century when John Simon replaced Chadwick as the civil servant in charge of the public health system. As mentioned earlier, Simon equated the right to health to a civil liberty, even though he was prepared to sacrifice individual freedoms for the benefit of the community – for example, in the enforcement of compulsory smallpox vaccination. However, the most powerful determining influence on British public health reform in the second half of the 19th century was the professional ideology of preventive medicine as doctors began to take up local government appointments that laid the foundations of a national public health service.[57]

In Germany, health care policy continued to be a function of the *Polizei* and remained dominated by the civil service rather than influenced by medical expertise.[58] The development of laboratory biomedical science in Germany, however, facilitated the expansion of bacteriological knowledge which became a determining political force in Germany when it assisted the centralisation of health administration in the last decades of the century. Germany's renowned bacteriologist, Robert Koch, legitimated the Prussianisation of the independent city-state of Hamburg in 1892 with a bacteriological explanation of the spread of the last cholera epidemic that took place there.[59] In Sweden, by comparison, the slow growth of industrialisation in the 19th century allowed the state to continue to focus on the individual methods of disease prevention that it had relied on throughout the 18th century. However, with the development of industrialisation towards the end of the century, the Swedish state expanded its role in both public hospital provision and the establishment of a national service of public health officers.[60]

If the costs of industrialisation stimulated European states into addressing the question of health citizenship, the right to receive economic support was not represented in the political languages of industrialising societies until the last quarter of the century. Some central states in Northern Europe had national systems of poverty relief from the 17th century but, in the 19th century, state welfare provision expanded only incrementally within the economic and political reconfigurations of industrialising societies. Although states began to take welfare measures, largely in relation to the destitute, for the first three-quarters of the 19th century protection against the economic insecurities experienced by industrial workers was organised to a greater degree by themselves and to a lesser extent by new forms of philanthropic voluntarism. Mutualism and philanthropy also provided social services in the fields of housing and education.

In France, Germany, Sweden and England, the medieval institutions of guilds evolved into new forms of mutual organisations providing their members with forms of insurance against sickness and unemployment, as well as funeral benefits.[61] In England, mutual aid amongst the labouring classes was organised in a variety of institutions including local and national friendly societies, temporary and more permanent housing clubs and building societies, and through trade unions. In addition to providing funds during times of economic hardship, these institutions were often used as vehicles for organising educational services for both children and adults.[62] When Samuel Smiles published his famous tract on *Self Help* in 1859 he was already talking to a large body of the converted who were seeking to dignify and improve the condition of the labouring classes through thrift, temperance and commitment to the community through the practice of self-interest.[63]

Mutuality in France was a significant force in health and welfare provision from the early 19th century to the first half of the 20th century. Exclusive groups of workers had organised voluntary health funds through mutual aid societies from the time of the late Napoleonic Empire. The early societies were formed for individual occupational groups in different localities, but by the time of the Second Empire, mutuals had become increasingly multiprofessional and regional. Largely, they were voluntary associations of wage-earners with similar social and economic status. Mutual society memberships were often small and restricted usually to about 50 to 60 members. Larger mutuals with 100–150 members were rarer, but later in the 19th century they sometimes became as large as 500 members. Members paid an induction fee to join and a monthly premium and, if they failed to pay it, they would be fined or expelled. The purpose of mutual aid societies was to provide funds for medical diagnosis and income during times of illness. New members were restricted to workers between the ages of 25 to 45. Older workers were refused because the risk of sickness was greater. The societies were designed to protect stable, relatively prosperous breadwinners against the misfortunes of illness; they were not aimed at rescuing paupers from destitution and disease. After the revolutions of 1848, mutuals often required their members not to engage in political agitation or raise religious issues at meetings. In many respects, the mutualist movement represented the values of the artisan and shopkeeper classes in France and, as a result, mutualism became separated from the syndicalism and trade unionism of the industrial proletariat.[64]

In Germany and Sweden a similar outgrowth of the guild system produced mutual aid organisations which could administer voluntary insurance for their members. Indeed in Britain, Germany and Sweden these agencies were initially used for the administration of statutory contributions.[65] The expansion of mutualism in the 19th century was matched by the growth of philanthropic voluntarism. Such charities fulfilled a wide variety of welfare functions from soup kitchens to housing associations and charity schools. Here, the participation of women in welfare organisation was extensive. However, as mentioned earlier, while philanthropy offered women the opportunity to participate in the public sphere, not all who did so acknowledged it to be the case. Similar views were also to be found amongst some of the women attempting to enter professional medicine and nursing. Elizabeth Blackwell, the first woman to qualify as a physician, and Florence Nightingale who professionalised nursing, viewed women's participation in healing as a natural extension of their legitimate authority over the domestic sphere.[66] The separation of spheres was not necessarily challenged therefore by women's 'active citizenship', which is reflected in the fact that numerous pioneering female philanthropists and professional medical practitioners opposed female suffrage.

The voluntary sector also contributed to the development of health care in the nineteenth century through the expansion of the voluntary hospital as a charitable institution. While charitable hospitals had been developing from the Middle Ages, from the early modern period their function as centres for medical therapeutics became increasingly separated from their function as almshouses.[67] In the 19th century the large charity hospitals facilitated the professionalisation of clinical practice and reached ever wider populations as their numbers increased and their reputations improved. By the end of that century, some voluntary hospitals had begun to treat paying middle-class patients as well as working-class patients supported by patrons of the institutions.[68]

Voluntary welfare provision thus expanded throughout the 19th century. In health care, however, the role of the state also expanded, contributing to what George Kitson-Clarke, Oliver MacDonagh and Gillian Sutherland have identified as the growth in government. This was expressed in various developments in different national contexts, but belief in the appropriateness of the protection of population health as a legitimate branch of government gained ground.[69] The organisation of both statutory and voluntary health care and welfare in the 19th century, however, became increasingly determined by a common belief in the value of positivistic rationalisation.

The rationalisation of the mixed economy of welfare

Society in the 19th century responded on many different levels to the paradoxes of industrialisation and extensive urbanisation. The ideological determinants of the mixed economy of welfare in 19th century northern Europe produced new expressions of rationalism. The Enlightenment study of political arithmetic and human longevity evolved into the statistical study of human aggregates and their consequences for both the moral and physical environment. The enumeration of human misery was linked to the social physics of human improvement, inspired by both the Enlightenment pursuit of happiness and an evangelical and philanthropic moral imperative. In the 19th century, health and welfare reform in both the public and the voluntary sector interwove social science with Enlightenment political economy, and was integrated into the politics of social amelioration.

Belief in the value of facts over opinion, and of objectivity over vested interests, increasingly dominated the organisation of health care and welfare by both the state and the voluntary sector. State medicine identified itself as a form of government administration driven by scientific values. Public health developed as an academic discipline in France and Britain, based upon the quantitative science of social physics which turned Condorcet's concept of social mathematics into systematic social statistical inquiry.[70] Quantification facilitated what the philosopher and historian of science, Georges Canguilhem, has identified as the creation of a 'normative citizen', represented in numerical conformity, differentiated from the deviant by 'standard errors' along the Bell curve.[71] This linked health citizenship directly to a positivist agenda. In mid-19th century England and Germany quantitative methods were combined with clinical epistemology in the construction of the idea of social medicine, practised on behalf of communities rather than individuals. Health citizenship therefore, was served by the 19th century state, creating the possibility for a politics of expertise and employing qualified specialists, such as eminent doctors, to guide the policy-making process.[72]

Voluntary philanthropy also harnessed itself to the new positivist spirit as it increasingly sought to systematise methods for identifying worthy subjects for doles, turning charity into social work based on rational social investigation and analysis of need. By the end of the 19th century, the language of systematic, rational and scientific administration increasingly dominated the organisation of statutory and voluntary health care and welfare.[73] Whatever the shape of the mixed economy of welfare, its administration was now legitimated as a science of social amelioration. The implied neutrality and positivist objectivity of scientific social assistance subsequently legitimated a new collectivist hegemony which would underwrite the expansion of social citizenship in the 20th century by establishing an egalitarianising central state providing welfare based on the principles of universalism and the exchange of stigma for entitlements.[74]

Thus, the structure of health and welfare provision in the 19th century was determined by a mixed bag of ideologies. In health care, some central states began to incorporate the idea of state provision into a concept of civil rights, and some political reformers believed that central states should develop expert administrative systems. In economic and social security, central state involvement was limited until the development of German social security in the last quarter of the century. In the meantime, the 19th century witnessed the growth of mutual aid and voluntary and entrepreneurial philanthropy to provide economic security and a variety of social services. A unifying feature between these various modes of health and welfare provision was the growing influence of the positivistic social sciences claiming to replace subjective opinion with objective qualitative and quantitative analyses based on empirical facts.

Conclusion

Recent historiographical accounts of social welfare have rightly drawn attention to the importance of studying mixed economies of health care and social security. However, it is necessary to evaluate the role of both voluntary and statutory provision in the construction of citizenship in civil societies because this offers the opportunity to investigate transmutations in the operation of power. In order to do so we need to look at the changing configuration of knowledge and values which influenced the ideological parameters of citizenship. This allows us to link the politics of epistemology to the politics of material change, giving us a chance to explore the relationship between what Karl Marx identified as the unfolding dialectic between super- and substructural forces of historical transformation.

Notes

1. Douglas Ashford, *The Emergence of Welfare States*, Oxford, 1986; Peter Flora (ed.), *Growth to Limits: The Western European Welfare State since World War II*, Berlin, 1986.
2. Jonathan Barry and Colin Jones (eds), *Medicine and Charity before the Welfare State*, London, 1994.
3. Vic George and Peter Taylor-Gooby (eds), *Squaring the European Welfare Policy Circle*, London, 1996.
4. Gosta Esping-Anderson, *The Three Worlds of Welfare Capitalism*, Cambridge, 1990; idem, 'After the Golden Age? Welfare State Dilemmas in a Global Economy', in Gosta Esping-Anderson (ed.), *Welfare States in Transition. National Adaptations in Global Economies*, London, 1997, pp. 1–31.
5. Rodney Lowe, *The Welfare State in Britain since 1945*, London, 1993; Nicholas Deakin, *The Politics of Welfare: Continuities and Change*, London, 1994; Howard Glennerster, *British Social Policy Since 1945*, Oxford, 1995; Nicolas Timmins, *The Five Giants. A Biography of the Welfare State*, London, 1995.
6. Geoffrey Finlayson, *Citizen, State, and Social Welfare in Britain 1830–1990*, Oxford, 1994.

7. Anne Digby, *British Welfare Policy. Workhouse to Workfare*, London, 1989.
8. Quoted by Finlayson, *Citizen, State and Social Welfare* (n. 6), p. 1.
9. See ibid., pp. 1–3.
10. T.H. Marshall, *Citizenship and Class and Other Essays*, Cambridge, 1950.
11. Ibid., p. 14.
12. Barry and Jones, *Medicine and Charity before the Welfare State*, (n. 2).
13. P. Horden,'The Byzantine Welfare State: Image and Reality', *Society for the Social History of Medicine Bulletin*, **37** (1985), pp. 7–10.
14. R. Palmer, 'The Church, Leprosy and Plague in Medieval and Early Modern Europe', in W.J. Shiels (ed.), *The Church and Healing: Papers Read at the Twentieth Summer Meeting and the Twenty-first Winter Meeting of the Ecclesiastical History Society*, Oxford, 1982, pp. 79–101; Katherine Park, *Doctors and Medicine in Early Renaissance Florence*, Princeton, NJ, 1985; John Henderson, 'The Hospitals of Late-medieval and Renaissance Florence', in Lindsay Granshaw and Roy Porter (eds), *The Hospital in History*, London, 1990.
15. Barry and Jones, *Medicine and Charity before the Welfare State* (n. 2).
16. Sandra Cavallo, 'The Motivations of Benefactors: An Overview of Approaches to the Study of Charity', in Barry and Jones (eds), *Medicine, Charity before the Welfare State* (n. 2), pp. 46–62; Anne Borsay, *Medicine and Charity in Georgian Bath*, London, 1999.
17. Alan Mitchell, *The Divided Path: The German Influence on Social Policy Reform in France After 1870*, Chapel Hill, 1991; Paul Weindling, 'The Modernisation of Charity in Nineteenth-Century France and Germany', in Barry and Jones (eds), *Medicine and Charity before the Welfare State* (n. 2), pp. 190–206.
18. Cavallo, 'The Motivations of Benefactors' (n. 16), pp. 46–62.
19. Jane Lewis, *Women's Welfare, Women's Rights*, London, 1983; idem, *Women and Social Action in Victorian and Edwardian England*, Brighton, 1991; Susan Pederson, *Family Dependence and the Origins of the Welfare State. Britain and France 1914–1945*, Cambridge, 1993; Anne Digby, 'Poverty, Health and the Politics of Gender in Britain, 1870–1948', in Anne Digby and John Stewart (eds), *Gender, Health and Welfare*, London, 1996, pp. 67–90; Lesley Hoggart, 'The Campaign for Birth Control in Britain in the 1920s', in Digby and Stewart (eds), *Gender, Health and Welfare* (*supra*), pp. 141–66.
20. Finlayson, *Citizen, State and Social Welfare* (n. 6).
21. Ibid., p. 403.
22. Ruth Lister, *Citizenship. Feminist Perspectives*, London, 1997.
23. Quoted by Finlayson, *Citizen, State and Social Welfare* (n. 6), p. 48.
24. Ibid., p. 53.
25. Martin Daunton, 'Payment and Participation: Welfare and State Formation in Britain 1900–1951', *Past and Present*, **150** (1996), pp. 169–216; Alan Deacon, 'The Dilemmas of Welfare: Titmuss, Murray and Mead', in S.J.D. Green and R.C. Whiting (eds), *The Boundaries of the State in Modern Britain*, Cambridge, 1996, pp. 191–213; Nicholas Deakin, *The Politics of Welfare: Continuities and Change*, London, 1994.
26. Dorothy Porter, *Health, Civilisation and the State. A History of Public Health from Ancient to Modern Times*, London, 1999.
27. Peter Gay, *The Enlightenment. An Interpretation*, New York, 1969.
28. Lester Crocker, 'Introduction', in John W. Yolton et al., *The Blackwell Companion to the Enlightenment*, Oxford, 1991, pp. 1–10.
29. Roy Porter, 'Enlightenment', in Jeremy Black and Roy Porter (eds), *A Dictionary of Eighteenth-Century World History*, Oxford, 1994, pp. 225–28 at p. 225.

30. Idem, 'Cleaning up the Great Wen: Public Health in Eighteenth Century London', in W.F. Bynum and Roy Porter (eds), *Living and Dying in London: Medical History Supplement No 11*, London, 1991, pp. 61–75.
31. Andrew Wear, 'The History of Personal Hygiene', in W.F. Bynum and Roy Porter (eds), *Companion Encyclopedia of the History of Medicine*, 2 vols, London, 1993, pp. 1283–1308.
32. Peter Borsay, *The English Urban Renaissance: Culture and Society in the Provincial Town 1660–1770*, Oxford, 1989; P.J. Corfield, *The Impact of English Towns 1700–1800*, Oxford, 1982.
33. Roy Porter, 'Cleaning up the Great Wen' (n. 30).
34. Ibid.
35. Gene Brucker, *The Civic World of Renaissance Florence*, Princeton, NJ, 1977.
36. Ian Hacking, *The Taming of Chance*, Cambridge, 1990; George Rosen, *From Medical Police to Social Medicine. Essays on the History of Health Care*, New York, 1974.
37. Karin Johannisson, 'The People's Health: Public Health Policies in Sweden', in Dorothy Porter (ed.), *The History of Public Health and the Modern State*, Amsterdam and Atlanta, 1994, pp. 165–82.
38. Hacking, *The Taming of Chance* (n. 36).
39. Ragnhild Münch, *Gesundheitswesen im 18. und 19. Jahrhundert: das Berliner Beispiel*, Berlin, 1995.
40. Ibid.
41. Mary Lindemann, 'The Enlightenment Encountered: The German Physicus and his World, 1750–1820', in Roy Porter (ed.), *Medicine in the Enlightenment*, Amsterdam and Atlanta, 1995, pp. 181–97.
42. Dorothy Porter, *Health, Civilisation and the State* (n. 26).
43. Johannisson, 'The People's Health' (n. 37).
44. Karin Johannisson, 'Why Cure the Sick? Population Policy and Health Programs within Eighteenth-century Swedish Mercantilism', in Anders Brändström and Lars-Göran Tedebrand (eds), *Society, Health and Population during the Demographic Transition*, Stockholm, 1988.
45. Ibid.; Johannisson, 'The People's Health' (n. 37).
46. Caroline Hannaway, 'The *Société royale de médecine* and Epidemics in the Ancien Regime', *Bulletin of the History of Medicine*, **46** (1972), pp. 257–73; Matthew Ramsey, 'Public Health in France', in Dorothy Porter, *The History of Public Health* (n. 37), pp. 45–118.
47. Dorothy Porter, *Health, Civilisation and the State* (n. 26).
48. George Rosen, 'Political Order and Human Health in Jeffersonian Thought', *Bulletin of the History of Medicine*, **26** (1952), pp. 32–44.
49. Ibid.
50. L.J. Jordanova, 'Guarding the Body Politic: Volney's Catechism of 1793', in Francis Barker et al. (eds), *1789: Reading Writing Revolution. Proceedings of the Essex Conference on the Sociology of Literature, July 1981*, Colchester, 1982, pp. 12–21.
51. Dorothy Porter, 'Public Health and Centralisation: The Victorian State,' in Roger Detels et al. (eds), *Third Oxford Text Book of Public Health*, 2 vols, Oxford, 1997, Vol. 1, pp. 19–34.
52. Ibid.
53. Dorothy Porter and Roy Porter, 'What was Social Medicine? An Historiographical Essay', *Journal of Historical Sociology*, **1** (1988), pp. 90–106.
54. Dorothy Porter, 'Public Health and Centralisation' (n. 51); William Coleman,

Yellow Fever in the North. The Methods of Early Epidemiology, Madison, Wisc., 1978; idem, *Death is a Social Disease*, Madison Wisc., 1982.

55. Ramsay, 'Public Health in France' (n. 46).
56. Ibid.; Coleman, *Death is a Social* Disease, (n. 54).
57. Dorothy Porter, 'Public Health and Centralisation' (n. 51).
58. Paul Weindling, 'Public Health in Germany', in Dorothy Porter, *The History of Public Health* (n. 37), pp. 119–31.
59. Richard J. Evans, *Death in Hamburg. Society and Politics in the Cholera Years 1830–1910*, Oxford, 1987.
60. Johannison, 'The People's Health' (n. 37).
61. Alan Mitchell, 'The Function and Malfunction of Mutual Aid Societies in Nineteenth Century France', in Barry and Jones, *Medicine and Charity before the Welfare State* (n. 2), pp. 149–71; J.R. Hollingsworth *et. al.*, *State Intervention in Medical Care. Consequences for Britain, France, Sweden and the United States, 1890–1970*, Ithaca, NY, 1990.
62. Daunton, 'Payment and Participation' (n. 25).
63. Finlayson, *Citizen, State and Social Welfare* (n. 6).
64. Mitchell, *The Divided Path* (n. 17); idem, 'The Function and Malfunction of Mutual Aid Societies' (n. 61); Ramsay, 'Public Health in France' (n. 46).
65. Hollingsworth et al., *State Intervention in Medical Care* (n. 61).
66. Anne Summers, *Angels and Citizens. Military Nursing in Britain*, London, 1988.
67. Park, *Doctors and Medicine* (n. 14).
68. Lindsay Granshaw and Roy Porter (eds), *The Hospital in History*, London, 1989.
69. Dorothy Porter, *Health, Civilisation and the State* (n. 26).
70. Idem, *Social Medicine and Medical Sociology in the Twentieth Century*, Amsterdam, 1997.
71. Georges Canguilhem, *The Normal and the Pathological*, Reprinted, New York, 1989 (1st edn 1943).
72. Dorothy Porter, *Health, Civilisation and the State* (n. 26).
73. Finlayson, *Citizen, State and Social Welfare* (n. 6).
74. Daunton, 'Payment and Participation' (n. 25).

CHAPTER THREE

Histories of Risk and Welfare in Europe during the 18th and 19th Centuries

Marco van Leeuwen

Introduction

To comprehend all the risks we face is impossible. This is, perhaps, fortunate since such an understanding might easily paralyse us. The realm of human fears – just like that of desires – is almost unlimited. This holds true even if one concentrates solely on material risks of which an almost endless catalogue exists today. In many, but not all, instances such material risks were probably even greater in the 18th and 19th centuries than in the 20th century.[1] Fortunately risks can be countered. Many preventive measures, as well as numerous welfare provisions to soften a blow once it had taken place, have existed. From the Middle Ages to well into the 19th century poor relief administered by churches and civic authorities was probably the single most important welfare provision in Europe. Other such provisions included guild funds, friendly society schemes, trade union funds, factory schemes, help from family and neighbours, sickness funds, commercial life and property insurance and social insurance.

This chapter is about risks and welfare provision in Europe during the 18th and 19th centuries, including the question of how to study these issues. This area of study is large and, in part, new to historians, but important indicators already exist that might assist us in writing histories of risk and welfare.

The chapter begins with a discussion of the functioning of poor relief and the multiple functions that poor relief performed for different groups. It will become clear that poor relief catered both for a variety of risks and for a variety of interests. This is a straightforward but important fact. It implies an emphasis on the multiple interests and interest groups involved in a welfare arrangement, on the problems of collective action and how they were overcome. It also implies an emphasis on the 'mixed economy' of welfare – that is, situating, in this case, poor relief properly among other arrangements covering the same set of risks. To illustrate this point, the chapter discusses an alternative to poor relief – namely, mutual aid by guilds, friendly societies and trade unions. A final focus is on risks as a starting point for analysis. Of course, this does not invalidate studies of institutions, but rather aims to place them in their appropriate context. Welfare institutions are arrangements for risks, and it may often be difficult to understand the functioning of such institutions if we have no eye for the risks they cover. Attention will thus be given to recent approaches in the study of risks in a variety of disciplines – anthropology and sociology among them, but not history. To date, historians, with a few notable exceptions, have not considered risks as a field of study although such studies are not only desirable, but also possible. The final section of the chapter illustrates this by providing a rather limited set of examples of material risks in Europe likely to be of interest with respect to topics discussed in this volume.

The nature of the chapter is slanted towards 'international' history – that is, identifying common traits and problems – as opposed to national or regional history. When weighing the demands posed by truthfulness to historical realities against the exigencies of elegant description and parsimonious ex-planation, local and temporal particularities are sacrificed for the sake of simplicity and clarity.

A general model of poor relief

The term 'poor relief' is used here in a broad sense. It may include outdoor, as well as various types of indoor, relief. It includes both medical and non-medical assistance, the difference between the two often being blurred in practice. The nature, scale and funding of poor relief was not the same across Europe: relief by municipalities and village authorities operated side-by-side with that of ecclesiastical bodies and private institutions. So 'poor relief' is used here as an encompassing term.

A number of theoretical ideas and empirical findings from studies in the fields of history, social sciences and welfare economics have recently been integrated into a simple model of the working of poor relief in pre-industrial societies; see Figure 3.1.[2] In a crude simplification of historical realities, it states that at least two groups of actors operated deliberately in the field of poor relief. Poor relief is viewed as a control strategy of the élites and as a survival strategy of the poor. Both 'sides of the coin' will be discussed here very briefly.[3]

European élites, by and large, could profit in five ways from the existence of poor relief. First, élites could benefit through the ability it gave them to regulate the labour market. A closer examination of the situation in England provides a clearer picture of such a labour-reserve theory. Boyer's analysis of the effects of the Old Poor Law in certain parts of England[4] stresses that landowners wanting to maximise their profits found it cost-effective to pro-vide an allowance for agricultural labourers in the winter. True, there were other means by which landowners could have ensured an adequate labour force at harvest time – for instance, by paying higher wages in summer or

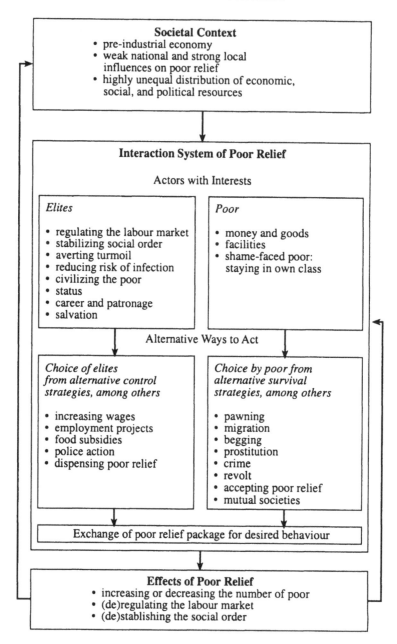

Source: M.H.D. van Leeuwen, 'Logic of Charity: Poor Relief in Preindustrial Europe', *Journal of Interdisciplinary History*, **xxiv** (1994), pp. 589–613.

Figure 3.1   A simple model of the functioning of poor relief in pre-industrial Europe

setting aside small plots of land for the use of agricultural labourers – but these methods were less profitable. Poor relief was so finely tuned that, in combination with other sources of income, it helped to maintain a labour reserve and discouraged the migration of rural labourers to the towns. To prevent such migration, the total annual income of rural labourers, made up of wages and poor relief, had to be higher than the wages they could collect over the year in the town, less the cost of the migration. Boyer's examination of the timing and geographical pattern of outdoor relief for English agricultural workers reveals that this type of relief was only cost-effective in the grain-producing regions of England, where the demand for labour during the sowing and harvesting seasons was much higher than it was in winter. The introduction of the allowance system coincided with the decline of rural industry and with rising land prices; as a result, an alternative source of income for rural labourers became less available and another option – setting aside small plots of land for them – became less attractive to landowners.

Second, relief also helped stabilise the existing social order. Socially, European élites tried to use poor relief as a means of maintaining the existing social order which they presented to the poor as God-given, and hence legitimate and immutable. This conception involved a degree of reciprocity: the well-to-do were under an obligation to assist the poor, and the latter had a duty to resign themselves to their condition. In exchange for handouts of money and goods, the poor were expected to accept the legitimacy of the social order. Their children were obliged to attend pauper schools, where they were taught the justice and immutability of the social order. As Gutton has put it: 'Pauper schools are needed to ensure public order, for they teach children to do their duty to God, their family and their country.... Moreover, free education accustoms the poor to obedience and submission.'[5]

Third, poor relief was politically useful in that it helped to avert turmoil: it could be used as a political instrument for the maintenance of public order and the prevention of unrest. Poverty for the many and prosperity for the few bred discontent. Fear of the poor was widespread among the well-to-do, especially when food prices rose. The title of a book by Louis Chevalier, *Classes laborieuses, classes dangereuses* (1958), reflects the anxieties of the Paris bourgeoisie during the first half of the 19th century. The élites used various strategies to prevent unrest, ranging from repression to the granting of poor relief. Poor relief was preferred if its costs were less than those of other means of maintaining public order and protecting property and lives. Assistance to the needy alleviated their hunger and, to some extent, shielded the rich from the undesirable behaviour of the starving masses: 'Poor relief was the ransom paid by the rich to keep their windows, as well as their consciences, intact.'[6]

The medical use of relief lay in reducing the danger of infection. As the diseases that decimated the poor could also kill the rich, it therefore made sense to ensure that paupers received medical attention, voluntarily or otherwise. Following Edward Jenner's discovery in 1796 that injections of cowpox virus produced immunity from smallpox, compulsory vaccination was made a condition of poor relief.

Finally, poor relief had a moral aspect; élites tried to 'civilise' or 'discipline' the poor – that is, they attempted to curb undesirable behaviour by teaching them 'better' values and standards. This effort may seem odd at first sight – why not leave the poor 'uncivilised'? What seems strange to us, however, was a normal part of the mental universe of many 18th and 19th century authors. Because they considered poverty largely a moral problem – the consequence of living a sordid life – providing poor relief without attaching moral conditions did not strike them as a proper solution to the problem. Assistance without moral conditions was bound to increase squalor. This urge to 'civilise' the poor had a number of corollaries – namely, the work ethos and the promotion of sound family life and education. Because lack of discipline and love of idleness were considered to be major causes of unemployment, poor relief had to be aimed at setting paupers to work. Similarly, the perpetuation of poverty as a result of ill-advised marriages and extramarital sex had to be checked. Thus Malthus counselled the poor to pay heed to 'moral constraints' upon entering into a marriage. In various German states the right to marry was restricted by law during the first half of the 19th century: local authorities were determined that paupers unable to support a family should remain single. Once married, a decent family life shielded people from poverty; an unhappy family life, by contrast, lay at the root of all evil. This was not an unreasonable view, as deserted wives, for instance, regularly succumbed to penury in Europe. Poor relief could be tied to instruction in family ethics, and be withheld from those unwilling to listen. Lack of education was, allegedly, another cause of poverty. As the ranks of the poor included numerous unskilled labourers who had not been to school in their youth, their education became an important issue from the late 18th century onwards. Education seemed to be a good solution to the problem of poverty; the children of the needy could be instructed in vocational skills and in basic reading, writing and arithmetic – but not much more since the attitude of the élite was that one's education ought to be appropriate to one's class. In the area of morals, therefore, poor relief was a tool used to 'civilise' the poor, which, according to many writers at the time, would lead to a diminution of the problem of poverty.

The fact that a group has an interest in a certain welfare arrangement such as poor relief does not mean that it succeeds in operating it, due to problems of collective action. Welfare economics demonstrates that rational members of a social group will not necessarily succeed in purchasing a public good even though the benefits of doing so outweigh the costs. Olson has demonstrated that this so-called *free-rider problem* will lead to the absence or suboptimal production of a public good, unless a third party such as a national government is able to enforce cooperation and punish free-riders, *or* unless selective incentives come into play.[7] In the case of poor relief several *selective incentives* operated.

The first selective incentive was the loss or gain of social standing; those who contributed to poor relief gained social prestige, while reluctance to contribute to this good cause brought opprobrium. The directors of charitable institutions and generous benefactors enhanced their own social status. This is reflected in paintings of charity directors and of generous donors, in eulogies while they were alive and in glowing obituaries thereafter, and also in public privileges such as special pews in the church or the right to walk at the front of processions. In other words, participation in poor relief legitimised the privileged position held by leading members of the élites, or, in the case of the *nouveaux riches*, the privileged positions to which they aspired. In addition, there was the possibility of furthering one's political career and dispensing patronage. Serving on a charity board gave young members of the élite a chance to develop their administrative skills and make contacts likely to further their career. Furthermore, charity directors could help their clients obtain assistance for themselves, for their families and for their friends, but also to get jobs, the more so as charitable institutions provided employment for people in clerical and supervisory positions, for contractors, book-keepers, financial specialists, and for artisans who maintained the buildings.

The final selective incentive was the existence of a religious norm promising eternal salvation to those who helped the poor and threatening those who did not with eternal damnation. Until the 20th century, a significant proportion of poor relief in western Europe was administered by the Churches. Sincere compassion for the poor in one's own village, town, region or country, mostly combined with the biblical command to aid the poor, also induced members of the élite to dispense charity. To some extent this was pure altruism, about which little more can be said here than that it was admirable, but this feature cannot be incorporated into a model of goal-directed actions. There is, however, another, complementary, view of poor relief. Several modern authors consider it a prerequisite of spiritual salvation: 'The poor man is a useful social being…. He enables the rich man to find salvation by giving alms' was how Gutton put it.[8] On poor relief in Aix-en-Provence Fairchild had this to say: 'Charity then was a way for a rich man to buy salvation.' Norberg noted that the Catholic faith acted as a selective incentive for poor relief in Grenoble: 'Catholicism encouraged charitable giving. … It successfully attached personal benefit to the common good by promising benefactors distinct rewards – Eternal Salvation – and misers distinct penalties – Eternal Damnation. In short, Catholicism overcame what political scientists call the "free-rider problem".'[9]

A second party involved in poor relief was the poor themselves. Endemic and large-scale poverty was a fact of life in pre-industrial European societies.

A large number of Europeans lived below the poverty line. They lacked financial resources and were dependent on daily or weekly earnings for their livelihood. The slightest misfortune could mean bitter poverty. Even in relatively prosperous areas and during good times, poverty was either a fact or a concern for most Europeans. Risks to welfare included those of health, the life cycle and the economy (these will be discussed in a final section of this chapter). The poor normally belonged to clearly defined groups: the sick and disabled, the elderly, widows with children, workers – particularly casual workers – in certain occupations, and particularly those who had large families to provide for.

Nevertheless, most of the European poor had developed ways of coping with poverty. A number of studies have shown that, in order to survive, the poor had to draw on a number of survival strategies. It is reasonable to suppose that, depending on their circumstances, the poor chose the assortment of survival strategies that offered them the greatest benefits at the smallest cost. Poor relief might be included in this assortment; it was an alternative to, say, prostitution, theft, begging and other survival strategies. The poor could profit from poor relief in several ways: it helped them try to survive; it also provided them with medical and educational assistance and the means to religious improvement. The poor might try to turn these facilities to their own advantage, regardless of the intentions of those providing them. Thus they could use charity schools to have their children taught reading and writing, without attaching too much importance to the doctrine imparted there that every man must keep to his ordained place. They could also use schools as free crèches. Furthermore, a small number of those from the middle class – the genteel or shamefaced poor – who had fallen on hard times used relief as a means of protecting their class status.

What disadvantages were associated with the acceptance of poor relief? Taking charity meant abstaining from illegal survival strategies and bowing to certain forms of behavioural pressure by the élites. To be deserving of help, one had to behave respectfully and 'decently', could not migrate, nor openly resort to begging, prostitution, crime or looting.

So far, we have been looking at the decision of the poor to accept charity after weighing up the relative advantages of drawing regular assistance and employing other survival strategies. A study by Lees of poor relief in London during the 19th century makes it clear that the type of assistance given partly depended on the strategic behaviour of the poor:

> Low-skilled urban workers in the nineteenth century regularly needed to tap resources beyond those of their immediate household and the state was one of its available sources of help. Since poor law aid came in several forms, potential clients could discriminate and shape demands to what was available. Applying for relief was an active, negotiated process between administrators and the poor.[10]

London paupers regularly applied for assistance when they were ill or unemployed, at the birth of a child, or when faced with the costs of a funeral. They
believed that they had the right to choose the most suitable type of relief:
medical aid when ill, financial aid when out of work, a small pension for their
elderly parents so that they would no longer have to bear the full cost of
keeping them, or even the confinement of burdensome family members in
workhouses, hospitals or lunatic asylums.

The model discussed here is only a model, and a rather simple one. It omits
many details as well as temporal and local peculiarities, as models, like maps,
are supposed to do. More negligent is perhaps the fact that the model is as
crude as it can be in distinguishing social groups. It only discusses two, thus
utterly disregarding the role of the 'middling classes'. This flaw may be
excused on the grounds of simplicity or the state of the literature which
makes European-wide generalisations in this respect even more precarious
than is usually the case with models. More local studies are needed on the
roles of the middle classes before we can model them. It may, however, be
that some of the interests and options that the model attributes to élites, also –
but perhaps in different ways and degrees – hold true for the various kinds of
middle class.[11]

Over the course of time, the consequences of poor relief could change both
the societal context in which it operated and the elements with which it
interacted (these feedback loops are indicated with arrows in Figure 3.1).
First, poor relief influenced the behaviour of élites and the poor; the nature of
relief influenced their choice of strategy. Second, poor relief affected society
as a whole. It could regulate or deregulate the labour market, increase or
decrease the number in poverty, (de)stabilise the social order and affect the
behaviour of the poor. Following the criticisms that mounted from the latter
half of the 18th century, the historiography of poor relief has traditionally
emphasised the negative effects of poor relief, first and foremost the alleged
fact that relief was handed out so freely and was so ample as to encourage
workers who preferred to live idly on the dole than work for wages. Thus, it
has been claimed, poor relief interfered with the labour market in a negative
way. By contrast, recent studies have stressed the positive effects of relief, as
the discussion of the British case has already made clear.[12]

Pre-industrial poor relief functioned as a bargaining mechanism. The élites
gave money, food, goods and services, but only under certain conditions and
as a 'package deal'. They could realise their interests in ways other than by
providing poor relief, just as the poor could draw on survival strategies other
than poor relief. The functioning of poor relief was thus dependent on cooperation between the élites and the poor. If the élites did not use poor relief as
a control strategy, the poor could not use it as a survival strategy, and vice
versa. Poor relief had to be in the interests of both parties. This implies
mutual interdependence (but not equal power or equal benefits). It also im-

plies a certain measure or choice. Although poor relief was the single most important welfare provision in case of misfortune in Europe, other arrangements existed, that, in part, could and did fulfil the same functions. Both the élites and the poor could turn to alternatives (see Figure 3.1).

This conclusion is in line with that of other recent research, all pointing in the direction of a 'mixed economy of welfare' in Europe over the past centuries.[13] In all European countries a patchwork quilt of welfare arrangements existed. To understand the degree to which Europeans were protected against risks, for which reasons and under what conditions, one must study the 'quilt' as a whole, even though in practice this is often difficult to do and may complicate the analyses by casting doubts on simplifications such as the development 'from poor relief to welfare state'.[14]

The mixed economy of welfare: the case of organised mutual aid

Even a simple model of poor relief makes it evident that there existed alternatives for the poor (and for elites as well, for that matter) in the form of savings and strategic bequests, private insurance, family help, assistance from neighbours, mutualism, industrial welfare and state welfare legislation. To understand why and how a certain medical charity or poor relief organisation functioned as it did, it is crucial to place its functioning within that of the alternative welfare arrangements.

This is not the place to discuss in any historical detail the functioning of each of these welfare arrangements in a dozen European countries over two centuries. It would perhaps suffice to merely stress the important effects that these alternatives might have on the operation of the specific charity under study. One might, however, go a little further and discuss a few major developments in mutual institutional welfare in the period we are looking at: the flourishing of welfare provision by guilds in many countries – in some instances axed by the ideologies and troops of the French Revolution, but in all cases definitely on the retreat before the end of the 19th century – the subsequent rise of mutual help by friendly societies, and, later, the rise of trade union welfare.

Guilds have long 'suffered from the libel' of the French Revolution. Strongholds of a privilege-based and ill-fated ancien régime, lowering productivity and harming consumers and workers alike, nearly dead anyway before the revolutionary forces axed their way to a better 'new regime', was the consensus opinion until very recently, and it still is the textbook image of guilds. New research on guilds over recent years has painted a different picture.[15] In most European countries, guilds were certainly not moribund, dwindling organisations during the 18th century. In fact, in many cases they prospered, if measured in terms of the number of members. Quite sizeable parts of the male labour force were organised under the guilds. In some instances the French Revolution cut this short by abolishing guilds, as it did in France in 1791 and between 1798 and 1820 in the Netherlands, although there in some cases guild-like organisations managed to continue until the middle of the century. Until the *Gewerbefreiheit* acts became legally binding for all regions in the German state in 1871, in most German cities – containing more than half of the population – one-third of the total population worked under a guild régime.[16] And even after the legal abolition of guilds their functions were, in some instances, prolonged.

Guilds did not originate to provide welfare, but by the 18th century this had become one of their *raisons d'être*. They dated from before the Reformation and were set up to control production for their members to the detriment of outsiders, to discuss matters concerning labour markets, prices and production with city councils to the benefit of their members, but also for social reasons – to eat, drink and talk shop – and to pay tribute to their patron saint. In Protestant areas before the Reformation, and in Catholic regions afterwards as well, they were also associated with certain religious charities. The Reformation cut these religious tasks short in Protestant countries, and the guilds redirected funds to provide welfare for their members.

It has perhaps not been sufficiently acknowledged until now that many guilds offered welfare arrangements to their members – and, as a consequence, sometimes to a sizable proportion of the male labour force – that were among the best by the standards of the day in terms of amounts supplied and conditions attached.[17] This was first and foremost true for illness. In the Netherlands, for example, guilds 'insured' many of their members and their families for the loss of income as well as the costs of medicaments in case of illness. They generally also 'insured' against burial costs, and sometimes operated widow funds. Only infrequently did they operate pension schemes. The terms 'insurance' and 'insured' have been put in inverted commas for a reason. Some aspects of guild welfare provision clearly rested on insurance principles as we know them today. Often a guild would compel all its members – and thus those working in a certain branch of the economy – to contribute a fixed amount every month or so to a scheme, thus avoiding the problems of adverse selection (see below). In return, a guild member and his family were promised benefits if sick, widowed, or in case of burial. Some insurance principles applied, such as being only eligible for support after having contributed to the funds for some time (period of eligibility), having to fund the first few days of illness out of one's own pocket (*Karenz*-time or waiting period at own risk), and support being dependent on the legitimacy of a claim. All this could count as a form of insurance, and it was often laid down in writing in the form of regulations. What made guild welfare not quite an insurance was that, sometimes, welfare was given over and above what the rules and regulations stipulated, and sometimes support fell short of it, notably when the coffers were empty. When the latter was the case, claims could be put on hold for the moment or even indefinitely, amounts or duration of benefits could be reduced, and contributions for all members be increased. This amounted to a degree of legal insecurity that would lead to a public outcry today in the case of private or social security, but by 18th century standards it was often neither illegal nor unwise. From the legal perspective, as associations with administrators drawn from, and representing, the members, they generally had this decision-making authority. Nor may it have been unwise, since it could very well have been this 'flexibility' that helped guilds sustain their contributory schemes for long periods in the absence of the usage of appropriate actuarial tables.

In the wake of the French Revolution, guilds were abolished in those parts of Europe occupied by the French, often to the chagrin of local authorities, which did not want to lose their grip on the labour market and were fearful of their relief institutions being flooded by those who otherwise would have been supported by the guilds. When the French retreated, guilds were sometimes reinstated, but sooner or later lost their vigour. Even after their demise, the former guilds could still be active as welfare providers if their funds were not nationalised. In the Netherlands, for example, welfare payments were made to former guild members, their families and descendants into the 20th century and, up to the present day, the municipality of Amsterdam controls former guild funds for charitable purposes.[18] In sum, guild welfare remained of importance in Europe throughout the 18th and even in some cases well into the 19th century.

The same was true for assistance by mutual aid societies. The French Revolution proclaimed the poor citizen's right to uniform state assistance but neglected to finance it, while dealing a serious blow to what had been major sources of assistance to that citizen – namely, poor relief and guild welfare. The poor citizen would have to wait more than a century for the promised state help. This interlude between the proclamation and the realisation of high ideals formed the golden age of mutual aid societies (also known as friendly societies, *sociétés de secours mutuel*, *onderlinges* and *Krankenkassen*).[19] These societies were non-profit institutions, organised on a voluntary basis by risk groups themselves. They insured large segments of the European population against the consequences of illness, and in some cases old age, widowhood or even unemployment. Mutual aid societies usually operated locally, although sometimes as a member of a federation. However, they had an incomplete social coverage; the very poor could not afford the contributions. Friendly societies were financed and controlled by the participants themselves. In the event of illness they could compensate the costs of medication, loss of wages, and, finally, burial costs. Sometimes widows might be assisted too. In addition, they took some, if limited, measures to combat *adverse selection* (discussed in more detail below). Thus the potentially poor such as unskilled labourers were barred for fear of enlisting future bad risks. The historical literature on friendly societies has concentrated on descriptions of rules and regulations. Some basic facts are in need of further discussion, such as the costs of contribution as a proportion of working-class income, what proportion of the various risk groups was covered, and the value of benefits in relation to the income of the working class.[20] Relatively little is also known about the demise of friendly societies, or, to phrase it more accurately, both their demise and their evolution into other institutions, such as trade-union mutual funds or agencies administering state welfare schemes.

Trade unions were not just institutions furthering the interests of workers by negotiating wage levels or labour conditions with employers. They also offered their members the opportunity to insure themselves against illness, accidents, strikes and even unemployment.[21] Such provisions functioned as selective incentives to join a union and also combated the free-rider problem of rational workers who might be tempted not to join a union while nonetheless automatically profiting from the higher wages or better working conditions negotiated by this union. Being aware of this potential problem, union officials used their mutual-aid provisions to compete with other unions in enlisting non-organised workers. Unions, in short, functioned as non-profit insurance groups organised by risk groups themselves. They had a high capacity to fight moral hazards, but they were vulnerable to adverse selection and correlated risks. These issues have loomed large in this chapter, and are indeed among the pressing problems of welfare arrangements.

A vocabulary of risks: some terms from welfare economics

The free-rider problem has already been discussed in the case of poor relief. A self-interested group member may attempt, without contributing, to enjoy the benefits of a collective arrangement from which he or she cannot be excluded (because exclusion is impossible or not feasible because of high costs). Even if, for instance, it is assumed that poor relief is, in part, a control strategy for élites, the existence of the free-rider problem still makes it difficult to understand why individual members of the élite would participate, and hence how poor relief can function. Solutions to the free-rider problem include third-party enforcement in general, and state enforcement in particular, and selective incentives – that is, attaching a private good (such as praise in the case of cooperation or shaming in the case of free-riding), to contributing to a collective good.[22]

Moral hazards refer to behaviour that increases the occurrence of the risk for which one is insured. For example, in the absence of unemployment benefits, unemployed workers may be forced to search even more diligently for new work and to be even less particular in accepting another job. This situation is different from search-induced unemployment: it may take time to find another job, however much one would like to find one. Furthermore, moral hazard is not the same as fraud ...

> the boundary between can't work and won't work is necessarily indistinct, and arguably a legitimate reason for insuring is to obtain a degree of discretion ... to quit a job when conditions have become intolerable, and to find the best available new job rather than have to accept the first one that comes along.[23]

Moral hazards increase expenditure, and thus raise contribution levels. For some welfare arrangements, moral hazards are less problematic than for others. Only the truly desperate would cut off an arm in order to receive a disability benefit. In the case of unemployment, however, the problem is more pronounced. Solving moral hazards may take the form of efficient monitoring techniques or coinsurance (where the insurer only indemnifies in part, and the client bears the remaining burden). The waiting period – or *Karenz* time as it is usually termed on the continent – is an example of coinsurance. It is the length of time before which sickness or unemployment benefits can be claimed. It shifts part of the loss of income (for example, due to ill-health or lack of work) to the insured in order to reduce the risk of imaginary ailments or unacceptably high standards when deciding whether or not to accept a new position.

Adverse selection occurs when an insurer finds it impossible or too costly to distinguish 'good' from 'bad' risks, with the result that the latter may profit by paying standard contributions with above-standard returns. As a consequence, good risks find it increasingly worthwhile to leave, or not to join, in order to avoid subsidising bad risks. Without proper measures, adverse selection might thus preclude an insurance scheme being set up, even though there are providers interested in offering it to good risks and good risks able and willing to pay for it.[24] Solutions to adverse selection include compulsory insurance for all risks, good or bad, better screening techniques before a risk is accepted, a differentiation in contribution level according to risk category, and stipulations that the insurer will not indemnify if wilfully misled.

Correlated risks refer to risks that are clustered or interlinked. For example, the chances of workers becoming unemployed (or ill) are not independent but correlated, because economic cycles (and epidemics) can put a large proportion of workers in a certain segment of the economy out of work (or incapacitated from work) at the same time. When, for example, the demand for steel falls, an engineering union might find that many of its members are eligible for an unemployment allowance. This may cause grave financial problems for the union, and, in extreme cases, bankrupt union welfare arrangements.

Approaches to the study of risk

The fact that a variety of welfare arrangements covered risks leads one to assume not only that a study of the full spectrum of such arrangements might be fruitful, but also that it might be advantageous to start by studying risks as opposed to institutional reactions to risk. This chapter has already gone in this direction by identifying some phenomena likely to be central to most histories of risk and welfare, in the form of the above vocabulary of risk. This is only one modest step in the right direction. To develop a framework for the study of risks in past societies, historians may further borrow from disciplines that already have a tradition in researching risks. A few general approaches to the study of risk may be discerned, elaborating upon a recent classification by Tierny.[25]

Most familiar to historians, at least those working in the field of economics, demography and morbidity, is an approach that technicians, statisticians and policy-makers favour for present-day risks. It involves the estimation of the probability distribution associated with a certain risk, and the magnitude of the adverse affects of those risks. Questions asked include: what is the probability of getting a certain disease? How long does one stay ill? What are the chances of recovery? How does illness affect the income position of the person involved and his family? Or, what is the chance of a young man or woman reaching old age? How long will they remain in old age? What is the life cycle course of earnings and expenditure? To what extent does old age imply poverty? Some decades ago, even these seemingly simple questions would probably have been thought by many historians to be unanswerable, given the historical record. Today this is no longer so. Interesting examples exist of studies developing a methodology appropriate to historical data and applying it to case studies. The final section of this chapter will give a few examples. Of course, there may be many problems associated with these studies, if only because of peculiarities of the historical records and the relative novelty of some of the methods used and the debates on interpreting the results and improving the methods. Even in comparison with seemingly less problematic research on current societies – for example, in estimating hazards of modern traffic, there exist large controversies.[26] Scientists often disagree and historians are no exception.

Geographers have been interested in the spatial distribution of risks and in linking these to variations in social, economic and other resources. Historians can only follow this approach if sufficiently large, roughly comparable historical data exist for regions or countries which can be treated with a common method. This has limited historical research somewhat.[27] It is not impossible, however, that the ongoing creation of large-scale electronic databases, in combination with methodological advances, will stimulate historians to work in the geographical tradition. There certainly has been an interest in spatial variation – for example, in historical studies trying to explain why Western civilisations, once dwarfed by those in the near and far East, have risen to their present-day ranks. Such studies often discuss East–West differences in the occurrence of 'natural' risks, such as diseases, earthquakes and flooding, before turning to social and cultural explanations.[28]

Social scientists – notably psychologists and social psychologists – analyse how humans estimate risks and losses – and thus their willingness to take one risk rather than another – in the face of very incomplete information. In very many instances one has to choose a course of action when it is simply impossible, or not feasible due to pressures of time and resources, to even roughly estimate hazard probabilities or the magnitude of losses. Somehow humans manage – but how? Which mental procedures– 'short-cuts' or 'frames' – do they use? How efficient are those procedures? Are there systematic errors? Are there systematic differences between certain groups of people?[29] Whereas, today, experiments in laboratories – where behaviour can be controlled – are a main source of data-gathering, this approach has been difficult to adopt for historians.[30] Alongside mental procedures to cope with incomplete information, exist social procedures. These may take the form of a norm prescribing and thus facilitating choices for an individual:

> In risk perception, humans act less as individuals and more as social beings who have internalised social pressures and delegated their decision-making processes to institutions. They manage as well as they do, without knowing the risks they face, by following simple social rules on what to ignore: institutions are their problem simplifying devices.[31]

Institutions may also make life simpler by creating predictable courses of action, reducing conflicts between individuals. This topic has been researched by rational choice sociologists like Schelling.[32] It has also attracted the attention of economic historians working in a neo-institutional tradition, notably North.[33]

Another tradition of risk research focuses on how risk assessment, risk attribution and risk behaviour is tied to predetermined *Weltanschauungen* – that is, social, cultural and political ideologies on how the world is, or ought to be, structured. This may be labelled an anthropological tradition. The following extracts from the work of Douglas and Wildavsky may give an impression of some of the central concerns of scholars working in this tradition:

> Pollution ideas are the product of an ongoing political debate about the ideal society ... Children die, there must have been adultery; cows die, food taboos must have been broken; the hunters come back empty handed, there must have been quarrelling in the camp. Pollution beliefs trace causal chains from actions to disasters.
>
> For studying beliefs in mysterious pollution, the anthropologist asks: what is being judged impure; then, who is accused of causing the impu-

rity; and who are the victims? What are the processes for removing the stain, washing out or cancelling the impurity?

> No doubt the water in fourteenth century Europe was a persistent health hazard, but a cultural theory of perception would point out that it became a public preoccupation only when it seemed plausible to accuse Jews of poisoning the wells.[34]

A pivotal theme in this approach to the history of risks is that even if, by some stroke of magic, we could estimate exactly all the losses and gains of all courses of action in the face of risk, there would never be one single 'best' solution we could single out – as, for example, in the economic technique of 'cost-benefit' analysis. The best solution, in this view, depends on the premises from which we start – the *Weltanschauungen* in which we are rooted. While this approach may resonate with many cultural historians, it is not one which has yet engendered a great many studies on risks in past societies. Perhaps historical studies on the decline of magic or on the interpretation of nature and natural disasters could be interpreted in this fashion.[35]

A final approach listed by Tierny and which she labels 'critical sociology of risk' is related to the anthropological approach but is sufficiently different to be listed separately.[36] This approach also casts great doubt on estimates of risks as measuring reality, although, of course no sound scholar would wish to deny that, for instance, epidemics, hurricanes or floods make victims. Those working in the tradition of critical sociology instead wish to link these estimates, and the courses of action consequently taken, to political economy and social inequality. Statements in a recent article by Tierney make this clear. Two main themes are: first, what are the 'social and cultural factors that influence the selection of ... "risk objects", a term encompassing event probabilities, event characteristics, resulting impacts and losses, and the putative sources of those events and losses'; and, second, how does 'the social construction of formal risk analyses' take place – that is, 'the social processes and institutional constraints that influence the manner in which analyses are carried out'?[37] Scholars working in this tradition point out that, and try to explain why, estimates of risk fail to take into consideration options that, with hindsight, appear important if not crucial. They also believe that sometimes the most appropriate estimates are not made, or not made public due to ignorance or even malice:

> ... that the risks associated with asbestos exposure are real and can be theoretically measured is less important sociologically than what asbestos manufacturers did for decades to keep the public ignorant about those risks.

> political power, organizational agendas, and economic interests drive the science of risk assessment ... . Decisions about large-scale technologies and projects are not driven by scientific considerations regarding

risks. Rather, the opposite is the case: judgements about risk and safety should more appropriately be viewed as the by-products of decisions made on economic and political grounds. Once a decision is made to understand a project, and to do that project in a particular way, then studies are conducted that show how necessary it is – and how safe it is.[38]

It is not easy to present examples from historical works which would fit in this tradition, except perhaps those from a somewhat related field – that of the social history of science.[39]

In principle all the above approaches to risk are open to historians, although they have not yet been eager to see risk as a topic worth attention in its own right. Historians might gain by consulting works in other disciplines. But what may historians, in return, have to offer? Or to put it differently, why does history matter? This is not an easy question to answer, given the relative lack of historical risk studies. The relevance of historical studies would be easier to gauge were we to have them in abundance. Perhaps it is thus best to discuss the *potential* value history might have.

On the statistical side, enlarging the time span may greatly increase the availability of data. This may be advantageous if data are scarce or if, say, one is dealing with slowly changing processes – for example, those where a single cycle takes decades or even centuries. The global rise in temperature is an obvious example in which use is frequently made of historical data from a wide range of sources, such as the freezing of canals, the starting date of grape harvests, the month of flowering of special trees, or the thickness of annual growth rings of trees. These sources enable the researchers to estimate temperatures over a long time span – longer than that covered by thermometers. Demographic processes are another example. Present-day processes in developing countries are sometimes studied by looking at their historical counterparts in pre-industrial Europe, for which we have better data. In this respect, it may be noted that some demographic processes appear so slow that it takes data on two centuries to study only one full cycle.[40] Of course, it should be added that uncritical use of historical data would not be of much value. Both an awareness of the reliability of the sources and a careful consideration of the validity of the historical context for present-day purposes are, naturally, essential.

By the same reasoning, long-term data may facilitate *explanations*. Societies change, and long-term data may thus cover many different situations with regard to variations in explanatory phenomena. In this respect it makes no difference whether one considers some form of statistical multivariate analyses or qualitative case comparisons. A statistician might benefit from historical data, just as might an anthropologist or a sociologist trying to link risks to *Weltanschauungen* or to root it in the political economy or in inequalities in resources.

Given the relative absence of historical studies, it may not be very useful to continue this *oratio pro domo* much further: the proof is in the pudding. One final remark may perhaps still be permissible. In neo-institutional economics the notions of 'path-dependency' and 'historical lock-ins' are in use.[41] These refer to situations where a certain longstanding institutional arrangement is clearly inefficient, in the sense that if one were to start from scratch, one would choose an alternative arrangement. Yet it cannot easily be changed because the costs of alteration – financial and otherwise – are too high. It is believed that such a lock-in may occur because, at the time the arrangement came into being, it was (or was believed to be) among the most efficient, but over time this became no longer the case (or was found out to be not so efficient after all). In cases of path dependency, historical studies are absolutely essential. For then it would be clear that it is past development that to a large extent shapes present institutions, which could not be understood and would, in some cases, look utterly incomprehensible, if one did not have knowledge of their origin. Does this apply to the 'patchwork quilt' of welfare arrangements?

Risks to welfare in Europe in the 18th and 19th centuries

Having broadened the focus of this chapter to encompass the various approaches to risks, it will now shrink to a brief discussion of certain, important, material risks to welfare in Europe during the 18th and 19th centuries. The state of historical writings, as well as the limited focus of this chapter as an overall introduction to material risks, warrant such a reduction. Now that the much broader potential research agenda has been sketched, the reader can easily discern the large chunks of risk history missing from the following, although they are no doubt to some measure provided for in the various studies in this volume.

What do we know about the nature and developments of sources of risks to material security in Europe in the 18th and 19th centuries? It is important to take stock of our knowledge in this field, as the answers to these questions are very relevant to the demands which had to be made to health care provision and poor relief. In a recent article Johnson has divided the risks to welfare in the following rubrics: health, life cycle, economic risks and environmental risks. Let us discuss all but the latter risk category briefly here, while acknowledging both the lack of comparative data as well as a certain degree of overlap between the categories. In principle we would like to have at our disposal comparative data on the – possibly changing – nature of each hazard, on its frequency, perceptions of risks, effects on the welfare of Europeans in the past, and pressures on welfare regimes, both perceived and real. Yet, on the other hand, we often do not know what we would like to know, in part precisely because interest in a shift to a risk-centred history of welfare arrangements is of recent date.

Risks of the economy

Work protected many from destitution, but also posed its own risks, including those of insufficient earnings, un- and underemployment, loss or partial loss of means of production, and lack of demand for goods and services. Work-related illnesses or accidents – the *risque professionel* – may also be included in this list. Although all these are labelled economic risks here, it should also be pointed out that they, as well as measures of prevention and welfare arrangements, are embedded in political and moral issues. The organisation of production partly reflects differences in political power between various groups. This is testified to, for example, by the long political battles for safety measures on the workfloor, minimum wages, laws setting a limit on the maximum hours of work per day or regulations covering child labour, unemployment benefits and benefits in case of work-related accidents.

Comparative macro-economic data do exist on the world of work in Europe, but they generally offer only indirect clues on those changes that had most impact on welfare provision and arrangements. It is well-known, for example, that the proportion of the labour force engaged in agriculture declined in the 19th century and that numbers working in industry generally rose.[42] Industrialisation caused problems of its own but it did not necessarily lead to poverty or, for that matter to an increase of the *risque professionel*.[43]

Some brief comments follow on the problems of un- and underemployment, on the transition from the *crise de type ancien* to the modern industrial cycle, on wage levels and on accidents at work. In the latter case both new methods of estimating these risks in the past are discussed, as well as the importance of the public perception of risks – right or wrong – in shaping the political debate and preparing the ground for state action.

Today, wage levels are important determinants of relative poverty and affluence, and the past was no different in this respect. It may be important to stress that, in the 18th century, a very large proportion of Europeans worked for wages, and that this proportion increased over time. One estimate states that around 1500 some 30 per cent of all Europeans worked for wages (as opposed to being farmers or self-employed); this increased to around 67 per cent by 1800 and around 1900 to 70 per cent.[44] Regional variations in wage levels are a problem if one wants to sketch a general pattern for Europe. Another difficulty is that while we do have series of nominal daily wages, we often do not know how many days were worked by each member of the family.[45]

Comparative estimates of levels of un- or underemployment in Europe have yet to be made, but some more general remarks can nonetheless be made. Structural underemployment existed in many European towns from the later 18th century until the mid-19th century. Descriptions abound of large numbers of casual labourers – for example, those working in the docks or transporting goods through the city – roaming the streets and quays for work and having irregular incomes.[46] However, while irregularity of income did not automatically lead to poverty – a few weeks of high earnings could compensate for a bad spell – in most instances it probably did imply poverty during this period. In addition, even if the overall yearly income was the same, regular earnings were to be preferred to an irregular income, due to problems in spending it evenly and, if that failed, sometimes having to buy more expensive products from shopkeepers who demanded an extra margin on their products to cover bad debts.

Seasonal unemployment had traditionally been high in Europe. Pre-industrial markets experienced sharp seasonal and cyclical fluctuations, resulting in marked increases in the demand for labour in summer and during economic upturns, and in sizeable decreases in winter and during economic downturns. In his study of 19th century London, Stedman Jones mentions three causes of seasonal fluctuations in the demand for labour.[47] To begin with, the demand for certain articles, such as luxury garments, was seasonal. Next, the flow of base materials was often interrupted during the winter. Finally, cold or frost could prevent outdoor work, particularly work on the land. However, given the shift from agriculture to other sectors of the economy, seasonal unemployment – though, as stated, by no means restricted to agriculture – may have declined for the labour force as a whole.

A gradual overall change in the nature of (un)employment related to the decline of what Labrousse has termed the *crises de type ancien* and the rise of crises of the modern, cyclical, industrial type. Labrousse demonstrated that, in France under the ancien régime, grain prices could fluctuate markedly from year to year with corresponding cycles in purchasing power.[48] Furthermore, in times of famine and dearth, the demand for 'luxury' goods such as clothes and other artisanal products fell much more sharply than the demand for basic essentials such as bread. Thus periods of high grain prices not only led directly to poverty for those unable to buy what they needed to feed their families properly, but also indirectly as others, namely artisans, were faced with a serious decline in the demand for their products. This pattern of *crises de type ancien* gradually gave way to a newer pattern, familiar to us today, of industrial cycles.

Much more information is needed to discern how changes in the economy affected demands on welfare, including knowledge of the hazards of accidents when working on the land, in the workplace, in the factory or on the street. A good example of the type of information needed, as well as an example using a rather novel combination of method and sources, is given by Table 3.1 which relates to the risk of an individual being killed in a range of

Table 3.1   Risk of a lethal accident in a range of occupational sectors in London, 1654–90

Economic sector	Probability per year per person
Transport	1:200
Transport, excluding drowning	1:530
Construction	1:780
Brewing	1:960
Street activities	1:5500
All	1:3400

Source: G. Spence, 'Accidentally Killed by a Cart: Workplace Hazard, and Risk in Late Seventeenth Century London', *European Review of History*, 3 (1990), pp. 9–25.

occupational sectors in London at the end of the 17th century. The table is based on data on causes and localities of death skilfully extracted from the London bills of mortality and related to other data on the population at risk. It makes clear that, in London, transport and construction workers were under a relatively high risk of accident (which, incidentally, may hold true for other places and epochs given the nature of the work, and see also, in this respect, Table 3.2). This fact alone may partly explain why these groups could figure prominently as recipients of poor relief, although other factors may also have been of importance, such as labour market concerns and public perception of the rightfulness of the claims. An example of labour market concerns has already been given when discussing the economic reasons for local élites to support poor relief to ablebodied workers. An example of public perception is provided by the public debate on the hazards of steam. Steam engines in workplaces caused considerable public anxiety – as did trains, for that matter.[49] The overall public image of steam was decidedly bad, but not inevitably correct. Table 3.2 gives the probabilities of having an accident in branches of industry in the Netherlands which had few steam engines as opposed to those with many. The probabilities are contrary to contemporary expectations, but the concerns about safety in a steam engine environment nevertheless did shape the public debate and led to laws governing working conditions in factories and, in 1901, to the first social security law in the Netherlands, covering accidents at work. Although this example illustrates that estimating the hazards of work in past societies may tell us which groups knocked on the doors of welfare agencies, and why, it does not automatically tell us that they were given relief: welfare agencies had their own agendas too.

Table 3.2 Risk of an accident at work in the Netherlands, 1899

Economic sector	Probability in %	
	All accidents	**Fatal accidents**
Low steam engine density		
Building trades	38.6	1.3
Shipbuilding	19.2	0.2
High steam engine density		
Paper industry	3.5	0.0
All sectors	5.3	0.1

Source: R.J.S. Schwitters, *De Risico's van de Arbeid. Het Ontstaan van de Ongevallenwet 1901 in Sociologisch Perspectief*, Groningen, 1991, p. 235.

Risks of the life cycle

Rowntree mapped the risks of the life cycle shown in Figure 3.2, and described them as follows:

> The life of a labourer is marked by five alternating periods of want and comparative plenty. During his early childhood ... he will probably be in poverty; this will last until he, or some of his brothers or sisters, begin to earn money and thus augment their father's wage sufficiently to raise the family above the poverty line. Then follows the period during which he is earning money and living under his parent's roof; for some portion of this period he will be earning more money than is required for lodging, food and clothes. This is his chance to save money. ... This period of comparative prosperity may continue after marriage until he has two or three children, when poverty will again overtake him. This period of poverty will perhaps last for ten years ... . While the children are earning, and before they leave the home to marry, the man enjoys another period of prosperity – possibly, however, only to sink back again in poverty when his children have married and left him, and he himself is too old to work, for his income has never permitted his saving enough for him and his wife to live upon for more than a very short time.[50]

It is worth noting that Rowntree's concept of life cycle poverty is restricted to a unit consisting of a married couple with children staying intact until the parents reach old age. Strictly speaking, this strongly limits the applicability of the concept as it excludes significant sectors of the population such as single men and women, those without children and incomplete families.

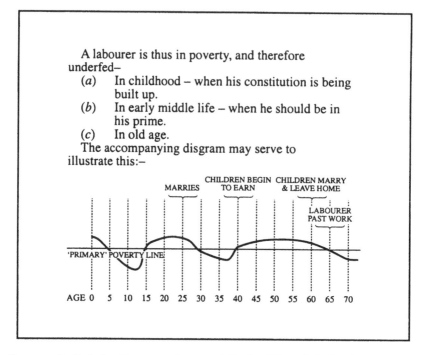

A labourer is thus in poverty, and therefore underfed–

(a)   In childhood – when his constitution is being built up.

(b)   In early middle life – when he should be in his prime.

(c)   In old age.

The accompanying disgram may serve to illustrate this:–

Source: B. Seebohm Rowntree, *Poverty: A Study of Town Life*; London 1922 (1st edn 1901).

Figure 3.2   Life cycles of poverty according to Rowntree

Practically speaking, it is often not easy to find data for 18th and 19th century populations to make a Rowntree graph. Tax data in combination with census material may be of use, but has rarely been used in this way. Calculations according to models on lifetime consumption and production family patterns are another way of approaching this matter, but model outcomes may crucially depend on initial assumptions and, to 'fine tune' these, we often need the empirical data we lack.

The first problematic phase of Rowntree's life cycle concerns a family with many young children. In conditions of 'natural' fertility – that is, in the absence of contraceptive techniques – having a large number of children to support may be considered a risk. It is the rise of a mass market in contraceptives that brought family limitation under individuals' control. From the later decades of the 19th century onwards, it has become more debatable whether having children was a risk to the European masses. If procreation is limited to marriage – which is not entirely the case for our period as testified by the rise of illegitimacy at the end of the 18th century – and in conditions of natural fertility, the only options to limit the number of children born is to marry late or never. The number of children to be supported in a family depend, in addition, on conditions of infant and child mortality, ages at leaving home, and the costs of child-rearing versus income generated by the children themselves. This is a long list, and not surprisingly, it has been difficult to estimate the problems young families faced by looking at aggregate levels of fertility and mortality alone.[51]

The final phase of poverty in Rowntree's life cycle is that of old age. It is known that life expectancy was generally higher at the end of the 19th century than it had been at the beginning of the 18th, although, of course, marked differences could exist between countries, across the social spectrum and between town and country. In addition, it is often noted that the rise began as an effect of a drop in infant and child mortality, and can only later be attributed to the lowering of the mortality of adults and the elderly. Nonetheless, the probability of reaching age 70 from age 25 in, for example, England stood at .31 in 1691–95, at .34 in 1791–95, at .37 in 1881–95.[52] This is no small probability. And life expectancy was generally on the rise from the second half of the 19th century (see Figure 3.3). This may have led to greater demands on welfare, since old age was often associated with ill-health (as Table 3.3 demonstrates) and low wages. Some of the extra lifespan gained by European populations were, in no small measure, years of ill health and poverty. As yet we know little about the development of lifetime savings and earning capacities at old age in the 18th and 19th centuries. Earning capacities depended on physiological processes, and on the availability of such arrangements as 'retirement on the job', where, for example, a farm hand or a shopkeeper's assistant was given less demanding tasks as his earning capacities declined with age, with no corresponding (or only a small) reduction in wages.[53] Other arrangements could also protect the elderly from poverty, such as a rural retirement contract as was the case in parts of 18th century northern and middle Europe where it was customary for a farmer to give the usufruct of their farm to someone else, usually a son, in return for the regular provision of food, shelter and perhaps also an allowance for as long as the farmer/parent lived. A written retirement contract could set out the amounts to be provided and other conditions in considerable detail. During the 19th century retirement contracts became increasingly problematic and, by the end of the century, many had fallen into disuse.[54]

Risks to health

Risks to health are defined here as the consequences of illness and infirmity for the earning capacity of the worker in question and his or her family. If earnings collapsed and savings were insufficient, poverty and an appeal to charitable provisions were often the result. Small wonder that we find the

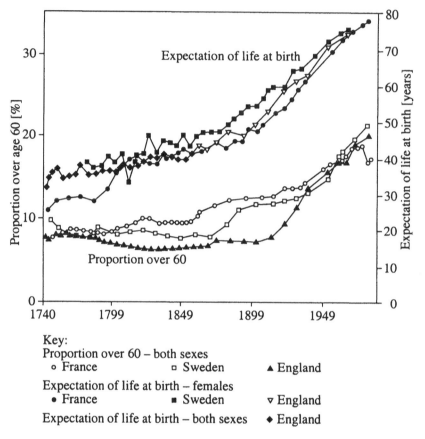

Key:
Proportion over 60 – both sexes
   o France   □ Sweden   ▲ England

Expectation of life at birth – females
   • France   ■ Sweden   ▽ England

Expectation of life at birth – both sexes   ◆ England

Source: P. Laslett, 'Necessary Knowledge: Age and Ageing in the Societies of the
Past', in D.I. Kertzer and P. Laslett (eds), *Ageing in the Past: Demography,
Society, and Old Age*, Berkeley, 1995, pp. 3–77.

Figure 3.3   Life expectancy at birth and the proportion of population aged over 60
in England, France and Sweden, 1740–1990

sick and infirm figuring prominently on the lists of charitable institutions in
our epoch. Is it possible to single out a few core phenomena on the nature of
diseases on the one hand and the level and volatility of morbidity on the
other?

General information on the nature of diseases and medicine is provided by
Table 3.4, showing ten common – but not necessarily the most common –
diseases in Europe between 1600 and 1870. The ten are the roundworm
disease ascariasis, atherosclerosis, dysentery, cholera, influenza, plague, smallpox, the fungal disease sporotrichosis, tuberculosis and typhoid fever. Only

Table 3.3 Periods of sickness and health among foresters according to age

Age	Sick (%)	Health (%)
20–24	1.6	98.4
25–29	1.6	98.4
30–34	1.9	98.1
35–39	2.2	97.8
40–44	2.6	97.4
45–49	3.3	96.7
50–54	4.3	95.7
55–59	6.2	93.8
60–64	8.8	91.2
65–69	15.3	84.7
70–74	23.0	77.0
75–79	33.8	66.2
80–84	40.1	59.9

Source: J.C. Riley, *Sickness, Recovery and Death: A History and Forecast of Ill Health*, London, 1989, Table 3.4.

one of these, atherosclerosis, is not an infectious disease. The other nine are. Of these one, namely the plague, need not concern us here as, by the period with which we are concerned, it already belonged to the past in Europe. All the others were still active, and cholera in Europe was particularly associated with 19th century European cities. It may be of interest to note that, with the exception of smallpox, little progress was made in combating these diseases by means of an effective curative treatment during the 18th and 19th centuries, although there were, of course, important medical developments: public health, for example, became a political issue in the 19th century.

In a seminal article, Omran has sketched a general model of change in the nature and frequency of diseases.[55] This model is usually referred to as the epidemiological transition, analogous to the demographic tradition. The epidemiological transition went from a regime of predominantly infectious diseases with volatile mortality rates to a less volatile regime of predominantly chronic, non-infectious diseases, including cancer and diseases of the heart and arteries. The general validity of such a transition is not in doubt, but as yet we have little information about its Europe-wide chronology, extent and precise nature. Which types of infectious diseases declined when, and which did not? Until recently there was little way of estimating morbidity risks over time, and certainly not from a comparative perspective. Of course, mortality rates, causes of death statistics and general information on the

Table 3.4   Ten prominent diseases in Europe 1600–1870

Disease	Primary age of risk	Course	Clinical fatality rate	Cause
Ascariasis	1–13	Chronic	Low	Ringworm
Atherosclerosis	35+, esp. 65+	Prolonged with sudden resolution	Variable	–
Bacillary dysentery	1–4, adults	1 week	1–25%	Bacterial
Cholera	None	1 week	up to 50%	Bacterial
Influenza (Type A)	None	1–3 weeks	0–7%	Viral
Plague	10–29	4+ weeks	up to 60%	Bacterial
Smallpox	1–4	3–4 weeks	10–50%	Viral
Sporotrichosis	Adults	Prolonged	Very low	Fungal
Tuberculosis (pulmonary)	Infants and young adults	Prolonged	–	Bacterial
Typhoid fever	Under 30, esp. 15–25	1–8 weeks	Circa 10%	Bacterial

Source: J.C. Riley, *Sickness, Recovery and Death: A History and Forecast of Ill Health*, London, 1989, p. 111.

development of diseases and medicine were available, but offered only very partially comparative data on morbidity. Mortality is not morbidity, and most episodes of disease during a human life do not end in death but in recovery.

Riley has recently opened up a new source for the comparative study of morbidity levels – namely, the registers of mutual aid societies. Guilds, friendly societies and trade unions often offered protection to their members in case of illness, as has already been discussed. Such schemes involved the payment of dues by members and made them eligible to claim support in case of illness. Whether they received such support depended on insurance conditions and on the financial situation of the mutual aid society concerned (sometimes a claim was deemed honourable but not honoured as the society's coffers were empty). These factors may have differed from one mutual aid society to another and from one year to the next, with or without a historical researcher being able to know about such differences. This may make comparisons difficult and, indeed, a current ongoing debate concerns the advantages and the pitfalls of using mutual aid sickness registers to measure morbidity levels over time, between places and across occupational groups.[56] Furthermore, as Riley himself has pointed out, the registers usually, but not invariably, relate to male members of the labour force only, to the neglect of women, children and the elderly. However, in the absence of conclusive proof to the contrary, it seems wasteful not to use the data we have on morbidity levels. Riley constructed, for example, sickness rates for an Antwerp printing shop between 1654 and 1765, demonstrating a high degree of volatility in morbidity levels. He further claims, with empirical examples from the Belgium printing shop and more from British friendly societies in the 19th century, that morbidity and mortality did not move hand-in-hand.[57] While mortality fell in the last quarter of the 19th century, morbidity, when measured in sickness time, rose. Fewer people died of a disease, fewer contracted a disease, but those that did were ill for longer periods. The fact that such data exist reminds us again that poor relief agencies were not the sole providers of benefits in case of illness.

Conclusion

Some changes of emphasis in the historiography of welfare may prove refreshing. One such change of emphasis is to locate any particular welfare arrangement firmly in the 'mixed economy of welfare'. Another is to model carefully the multiple purposes that a particular welfare arrangement could have for social groups, and also to model how these interest groups could overcome classic problems plaguing welfare arrangements. If the welfare of certain groups of Europeans was threatened, it does not follow that these groups obtained benefits in practice. At the very least, the identity and interests of those who funded and administered welfare has to be taken into account. Why were risks to welfare a concern to them? Often accepted in principle, but only infrequently encountered, this change in perspective amounts to studying the interest groups involved in a certain welfare arrangement, their aims and the constraints they were under, as well as potential alternative ways available to them to achieve these aims other than through the welfare arrangement in question. The simple model of poor relief in this chapter is an example of this approach.

A final change of emphasis is that on risks. Both the demand for welfare and what a certain welfare arrangement offers may often be difficult to understand if first we fail to ask: for which risks are the welfare arrangements provided? Although historians may not be very familiar with histories of risk, scholars of other disciplines are, and a number of approaches to the history of risk has to be singled out: notably those of technicians, statisticians and policy-makers providing estimates of hazards; geographers interested in documenting and explaining spatial variation; psychologists interested in mental short-cuts in estimating risks in the face of incomplete information; anthropologists researching how risky behaviour and risk attribution is tied to predetermined *Weltanschauungen*; critical sociologists interested in how risk assessments are rooted in institutional constraints, social inequalities and political economies; welfare economists debating problems of welfare arrangements such as those of free-riders, moral hazards and adverse selection. The research agenda is thus much broader than the rather elementary and brief sketch of risks of the economy, life cycle and health given here. That sketch only provides a bare and short general outline of issues likely to be fundamental for other chapters in this volume, providing much richer case studies.

Notes

1. For what is sometimes seen as a counter claim, see U. Beck, *The Risk Society: On the Way to an Alternative Modernity*, Newberry Park, 1992; translation of *Risikogesellschaft. Auf dem Weg in eine ander Moderne*, Frankfurt-am-Main, 1986. For my own recent work on the history of risks in the Netherlands 1500–1890, see M.H.D. van Leeuwen, *De rijke Republiek. Gilden, assuradeurs en armenzorg 1500–1800*, Amsterdam, 2000; and M.H.D. Van Leeuwen, *De eenheidsstaat: onderlinges, armenzorg en commerciële verzekeraars 1800–1890*. Both works are part of a four-volume history of risk and risk management in the Netherlands 1500–2000 which bears the series title, J. van Gerwen and M.H.D. van Leeuwen eds, *Zoeken naar Zekerheid. Risico's, preventie, verzekeringen en andere zekerheidsregelingen in Nederland*, Nederland, 2000.
2. See M.H.D. Van Leeuwen, *The Logic of Charity*, Houndmills, 2000, and idem, 'Logic of Charity: Poor Relief in Preindustrial Europe', *Journal of Interdisciplinary History*, 24 (1994), pp. 589–613, esp. p. 611. This model has been based on a number of studies. The general idea of analysing societies in terms of the purposive actions of persons, developing strategies to realise perceived interests in a given social context, is taken from Boudon: see R. Boudon, *La logique du social. Introduction à l'analyse sociologique*, Paris, 1979; and idem, 'Subjective Rationality and the Explanation of Social Behaviour', *Rationality and Society*, 1 (1989), pp. 173–96. Olson formulated an innovative theory relating to conditions favouring or barring individuals' creating collective goods: see M. Olson, *The Logic of Collective Action. Public Goods and the Theory of Groups*, Cambridge, MA, 1982. De Swaan has provided an original analysis of the development of social welfare in Europe

and the United States, in part based on Olson's work: see A. de Swaan, *In Care of the State. Health Care, Education and Welfare in Europe and the USA in the Modern Era*, New York, 1988. See also J.P. Gutton, *La société et les pauvres en Europe (XVIe–XVIII siècles*, Paris, 1974; C. Lis and H. Soly, *Poverty and Capitalism in Preindustrial Europe*, Hassocks, 1979. These studies have demonstrated the manifold similarities in the functioning of poor relief in pre-industrial Europe. Boyer has shed much light on why, and how, English rural élites made use of charity: see G.R. Boyer, *An Economic History of the English Poor Law 1750–1850*, Cambridge, 1990. See also S. Cavallo, *Charity and power in early modern Italy: benefactors and their motives in Turin, 1541–1789*, Cambridge, 1995. The strategic behaviour of the poor has been particularly stressed in studies by Popkin on Vietnamese peasant communities and Portes on the inhabitants of Latin American slums. A multitude of survival strategies for the pre-industrial poor in Europe has been documented by Hufton and Lis, and Lees has described the pragmatic use of the poor law by the English poor: see O. Hufton, *The Poor of Eighteenth-Century France, 1750–1789*, Oxford, 1974; C. Lis, *Social Change and the Labouring Poor, Antwerp 1770–1860*, New Haven, Conn., 1986; L.H. Lees, *The Solidarities of Strangers. The English Poor Laws and the People, 1700–1948*, Cambridge, 1998; idem, 'The Survival of the "Unfit": Welfare Policies and Family Maintenance in Nineteenth-Century London', in P. Mandler (ed.), *The Uses of Charity. The Poor on Relief in the Nineteenth-Century Metropolis*, Philadelphia, 1990, pp. 68–91. See also the recent collection of essays in L. Fontaine and J. Schlumbohm eds, 'Household strategies for survival 1600–2000: fission, faction and cooperation', supplement of the *International Review of Social History*, 8, 2000.

3. For more details, see van Leeuwen, *The Logic of Charity* (n. 2), and the studies listed there.
4. Boyer, *An Economic History of the English Poor Law* (n. 2).
5. Gutton, *La société et les pauvres* (n. 2), p. 156.
6. P. Matthias, 'Adam's Burden: Diagnoses of Poverty in Post-Medieval Europe and the Third World Now', *Tijdschrift voor Geschiedenis*, **89** (1976), pp. 149–61 at p. 154.
7. Olson, *The Logic of Collective Action* (n. 2).
8. Gutton, *La société et les pauvres*, (n. 2), p. 143.
9. C. Fairchild, *Poverty and Charity in Aix-en-Provence, 1640–1789*, Baltimore, 1976, p. 27.
10. Lees, 'The Survival', (n. 2), p. 69; see also idem, *The Solidarities of Strangers* (n. 2).
11. See, for example, A. McCants, *Civic Charity in a Golden Age: Orphan Care in Early Modern Amsterdam*, Urbana, 1997.
12. Including those of Boyer, *An Economic History* (n. 2); P.M. Solar, 'Poor Relief and English Economic Development before the Industrial Revolution', *Economic History Review*, **48** (1995), pp. 1–22, and van Leeuwen, *The Logic of Charity* (n. 2).
13. See, for example, the essays in M. Katz and C. Sachse (eds), *The Mixed Economy of Social Welfare. Public/Private Relations in England, Germany and the United States, the 1870s to the 1930s*, Baden-Baden, 1996, and those in M. J. Daunton (ed.), *Charity, Self-interest and Welfare in the English Past*, London, 1996. Earlier examples of this notion exist, for example, J. Halpérin, 'La notion de sécurité dans l'histoire économique et sociale', *Revue d'Histoire Economique*

et Sociale, **30** (1952), pp. 7–25, but these have tended to be programmatic rather than providing substantive examples.

14. Compare P. Johnson, 'Risk, Redistribution and Social Welfare in Britain from the Poor Law to Beveridge', in Daunton, *Charity, Self-interest and Welfare* (n. 13), pp. 245–46, for the English situation:

> Once the multi-dimensional character of welfare instruments is recognized, the picture of a progressive evolution of welfare provision across the twentieth century becomes blurred. The Victorian poor law, for all its faults, was based on the idea of a comprehensive risk pool, of a solidaristic rather than a contractual system of entitlement, and on a substantial interpersonal redistribution. The combination of social insurance and social assistance since the Second World War has, in the main, continued to be comprehensive, solidaristic in practice and broadly supportive of interpersonal redistribution. But the Edwardian development of national insurance was a move towards an exclusive risk pool, towards contractual entitlement, and towards a self-financing system of intra-personal redistribution. Viewed from this perspective, the neat lineages of welfare development from the poor law to [the social security following] Beveridge are seen to be an erroneous historical construct.

15. See S. Bos, *'Uyt Liefde tot Malcander.' Onderlinge Hulpverlening binnen Noord-Nederlandse Gilden in Internationaal Perspectief (1570–1820)*, Amsterdam, 1998; and idem, 'The Mutual Benefit System of the Guilds in the Dutch Republic in an International Perspective', paper for the ESTER seminar on guilds at the International Institute for Social History, November 1996, for both Dutch case studies and an international comparison. See also Van Leeuwen, *De rijke Republiek. Gilden, assuradeurs en armenzorg 1500–1800*, pp. 104–14, 166–79 and 419–22 on the nature and extent of guild insurance in the Netherlands 1500–1800.

16. J. Lucassen, 'In Search of Work', in A. Carreras and H.G. Haupt (eds), *The Economic and Social History of Europe in the Nineteenth and Twentieth Centuries*, forthcoming.

17. See Bos, *'Uyt Liefde tot Malcander'* (n. 15).

18. C. Wiskerke, *De Afschaffing der Gilden in Nederland* (Amsterdam, 1938), and Bos, *'Uyt Liefde tot Malcander'*, (n. 15), p. 139.

19. The monumental collection of essays, M. van der Linden, *Social Security Mutualism. The Comparative History of Mutual Benefit Societies*, Bern, 1996, forms a useful starting point for research into these matters. A recent overview for the Netherlands is provided by J. van Genabeek, *Met Vereende Kracht Risico's Verzacht. De Plaats van Onderlinge Hulp binnen de Negentiende Eeuwse Particuliere Regelingen van Sociale Zekerheid*, Amsterdam, 1999. For a theoretical discussion of nineteenth-century mutual aid societies see de Swaan, *In Care of the State* (n. 2).

20. For the Netherlands, these issues are discussed in Van Genabeek, *Met Vereende Kracht* (n. 19). See also Van Leeuwen, *De eenheidsstaat: onderlinges, armenzorg en commerciële verzekeraars 1800–1890*, pp. 82–97, 169–81 and 380–381.

21. See, for example, the articles: G. R. Boyer, 'What did Unions do in Nineteenth-Century Britain?', *Journal of Economic History*, **48** (1988), pp. 319–32; M.H.D. van Leeuwen, 'Trade Unions and the Provision of Welfare in the Netherlands

1910–1960', *Economic History Review*, **50** (1997), pp. 764–91, and the studies cited in these articles.

22. The problem of free-riding with respect to collective goods was introduced to welfare economics by Olson, *The Logic of Collective Action* (n. 2). Olson's analysis is valid for a single prisoner's dilemma faced by two parties with no prior knowledge. Many real-life situations depart from this situation and Olson's analysis may in real life often be a worst-case scenario. See M. Taylor, *The Possibility of Cooperation*, Cambridge, 1987 for an example. For instance, actors may have prior knowledge on which to base their expectations. They may face a dilemma more than once and thus have to take into account the effect of present 'defection' on future relations. They may play several connected games at once and expect to be punished for defection in one game through retaliation in another.

23. H.R. Southall, 'Neither State nor Market: Early Welfare Benefits in Britain', in B. Pallier (ed.), *Comparing Social Welfare Systems in Europe, Vol. 1, Oxford Conference*, Paris, 1995, pp. 59–92 at p. 77.

24. See G.A. Akerlof, 'The Market for "Lemons": Qualitative Uncertainty and the Market Mechanisms', *Quarterly Journal of Economics*, **84** (1970), pp. 488–500.

25. K.J. Tierny, 'Toward a Critical Sociology of Risk', *Sociological Forum* **14** (1999), pp. 215–42 at pp. 217–19, while continuing to neglect single idiosyncratic studies, even influential ones, for example, by Beck, *The Risk Society* (n. 1), and N. Luhmann, *Risk. A Sociological Theory*, New York, 1993, that as yet seem to defy classification. Tierny does not discuss studies on welfare economics and rational choice sociology on problems individuals face when trying to create and maintain institutions providing welfare. Problems of free-riders, adverse selection, moral hazards and solutions for these problems of collective action in the field of welfare are among the themes discussed here. As they have been discussed previously in this chapter, these themes do not need further attention here. The distinction between the various research traditions is, as one would expect, sometimes blurred in practice. For another review of research on risks, see, for example, D. Golding, 'A Social and Programmatic History of Risk Research', in S. Krimsky and D. Golding (eds), *Social Theories of Risk*, London, 1992, pp. 23–52.

26. See, for example, J. Adams, *Risk*, London, 1995.

27. But see, for example, R. Woods and N. Shelton, *An Atlas of Victorian Mortality*, Liverpool, 1997; for a different example covering an earlier period, see E.A. Wrigley and R.S. Schofield, *The Population History of England and Wales 1541–1871. A Reconstruction*, London, 1981, Appendix 10.

28. See E.L. Jones, *The European Miracle. Environments, Economies, and Geopolitics in the History of Europe and Asia*, Cambridge, 1981; and J. Diamond, *Guns, Germs and Steel. A Short History of Everybody for the last 13, 000 Years*, London, 1998.

29. H. Simon, 'A Behavioural Model of Rational Choice', *Quarterly Journal of Economics*, **59** (1955), pp. 99–118; Boudon, 'Subjective Rationality' and *La logique du social* (n. 2); A. Tversky and D. Kahneman, 'The Framing of Decisions and the Psychology of Choice', *Science*, **211** (1981), pp. 453–58; and the essays in D. Kahneman, P. Slovic and A. Tversky (eds), *Judgement under Uncertainty: Heuristics and Biases*, Cambridge, 1982.

30. For interesting examples of historical work asking the same questions, although answering them in different ways, see T. Doerflinger, *A Vigorous Spirit of*

Enterprise: Merchants and Economic Development in Revolutionary Philadel-phia, Chapel Hill, 1986; and D.S. Smith and J.D. Hacker, 'Cultural Demography: New England Deaths and the Puritan Perception of Risk', *Journal of Interdisciplinary History*, **27** (1996), pp. 367–92.

31. M. Douglas and A. Wildavsky, *Risk and Culture. An Essay on the Selection of Technological and Environmental Dangers*, London, 1983, p. 80.

32. There need not be an institution in the formal sense of the word; a norm or a tacit agreement is also possible, such as Schelling's 'focal points':

> Most situations ... provide some clue for coordinating behavior, some focal point for each person's expectation of what the other expects him to expect to be expected to do. Finding the key, or rather finding *a* key – any key that is mutually recognized as the key becomes *the* key – may depend on imagination more than on logic; it may depend on analogy, precedent, accidental arrangements, symmetry, aesthetic or geometric configuration, casuistic reasoning, and who the parties are and what they know about each other ... it is the intrinsic magnetism of particular outcomes, especially those that enjoy prominence, uniqueness, simplicity, precedent, or some rationale that makes them different from the continuum of possible alternatives. ... One has to have a reason for standing firmly on a position. ... The rationale may not be strong at the arbitrary 'focal point', but at least it can defend itself with the argument 'if not here, where?'' (T.C. Schelling, *The Strategy of Conflict*, Cambridge, MA, 1960), pp. 57 and 70).

33. 'Institutions reduce uncertainty by providing a structure to everyday life'; D.C. North, *Institutions, Institutional Change and Economic Performance*, Cambridge, 1990, p. 3 and *passim*.

34. Douglas and Wildavksy, *Risk and Culture* (n. 31), pp. 36–37 and 7.

35. For example, K. Thomas, *Religion and the Decline of Magic*, London, 1971; and idem, *Man and the Natural World*, Harmondsworth, 1983. Praying, for that matter, can be considered as a way of risk management. See, for early studies with this suggestion, L. Febvre, 'Pour l'histoire d'un sentiment: le besoin de sécurité', *Annales ESC*, **11** (1956), pp. 244–47; and J. Delumeau, *Rassurer et protéger: le sentiment de sécurité dans l'Occident d'autrefois*, Paris, 1989.

36. Tierney, 'Toward a Critical Sociology of risk', (n. 25).

37. Ibid., p. 220.

38. Ibid., p. 224.

39. For example, L. Daston, 'The Domestification of Risk: Mathematical Probability and Insurance, 1650–1830', in L. Kruger (ed.), *The Probabilistic Revolution*, Cambridge, 1987, pp. 237–60; G. Gigerenzer et al., *The Empire of Chance. How Probability Changed Science and Everyday Life*, Cambridge, 1989; I. Hacking, *The Taming of Chance*, Cambridge, 1990.

40. Wrigley and Schofield, *The Population History* (n. 27), p. 483.

41. On the notion of path dependency, see W. B. Arthur, 'Positive Feedbacks in the Economy', *Scientific American*, February 1990, pp. 80–85; and P.A. David, 'Understanding the Economics of QWERTY: The Necessity of History', in W.N. Parker (ed.), *Economic History and the Modern Economist*, Oxford, 1986, pp. 30–49. For a criticism on the example of QWERTY, see S.J. Liebowitz and S.E. Margolis, 'The Fable of the Keys', *Journal of Law and Economics*, **33** (1990), pp. 1–25.

42. See, for example, H. Kaelble, 'Was Prometheus most Unbound in Europe? The Labour Force in Europe during the late XIXth and XXth Centuries', *Journal of European Economic History*, **14** (1985), pp. 65–102.

43. W. Abel, *Massenarmut und Hungerkrisen im Vorindustriellen Europa*, Hamburg, 1974, for instance, sees industrialisation as ending the pre-industrial cycles of poverty, culminating in the era of mass pauperisation in the early 19th century.

44. C. Tilly, 'Demographic Origins of the European Proletariat', in D. Levine (ed.), *Proletarianization and Family History*, Orlando, 1984, p. 36.

45. P. Scholliers et al., *Real Wages in 19th and 20th Century Europe. Historical and Comparative Perspectives*, New York, 1989, offers various series of wages, but no comparison could be offered of real wage levels, let alone of family earning, in Europe in the 19th century. See, however, J.L. van Zanden, 'Wages and standard of living in Europe, 1500–1800', in J. Bongaarts et al., *Family demography. Methods and their application*, Oxford, 1987, pp. 65–80.

46. See, for example, Abel, *Massenarmut und Hungerkrisen* (n. 43); Van Leeuwen, *The Logic of Charity* (n. 2); C. Sachse and F. Tennstedt, *Geschichte der Armenfürsorge in Deutschland. Vom Spätmittelalter bis zum 1. Weltkrieg*, Stuttgart, 1980, pp. 185–95; Hufton, *The Poor* (n. 2), p. 97.

47. G. Stedman Jones, *Outcast London. A Study in the Relationship between Classes in Victorian Society*, New York, 1976, pp. 33–51.

48. C.E. Labrousse, *Esquisse du mouvement des prix et des revenus en France au XVIIIe siècle*, Paris, 1933; and idem, *La crise de l'économie française à la fin de l'ancien régime et au début de la Révolution*, Paris, 1944.

49. On the negative public image of steam, see R.J.S. Schwitters, *De Risico's van de Arbeid. Het Ontstaan van de Ongevallenwet 1901 in Sociologisch Perspectief*, Groningen, 1991, pp. 230–39.

50. S. Rowntree, *Poverty. A Study of Town Life*, London, 1922 (1st edn 1901), pp. 169–70.

51. It is known that fertility in Europe generally started to decline from the second half of the 19th century: see, for example, M. Livi-Bacci, *A Concise History of World Population*, Oxford, 1992, p. 122. It was probably earlier in some countries: see M.W. Flinn, *The European Demographic System 1500–1820*, London, 1981; the latest word on England can be found in E.A. Wrigley, R.S. Davies, J.E. Oeppen and R.S. Schofield, *English Population History from Family Reconstitution 1580–1837*, Cambridge, 1997). It is also known that mortality generally declined in Europe over the course of the 19th century: see, for example, Livi-Bacci, *A Concise History of World Population* (n. 51), p. 109.

52. P. Laslett, *A Fresh Map of Life. The Emergence of the Third Age*, London, 1989, p. 86.

53. E. Bulder, *The Social Economics of Old Age. Strategies to Maintain Income in Later Life in the Netherlands 1880–1940*, Amsterdam, 1993.

54. D. Gaunt, 'The Property and Kin Relations of Retired Farmers in Northern and Central Sweden', in R. Wall et al. (eds), *Family Forms in Historic Europe*, Cambridge, 1983, pp. 249–79; O. Löfgren, 'Family and Household among Scandinavian Peasants: an Exploratory Essay', *Ethnologica Scandinavia*, **17** (1974), pp. 17–52.

55. A. Omran, 'The Epidemiologic Transition. A Theory of the Epidemiology of Population Change', *Milbank Memorial Fund Quarterly*, **49** (1971), pp. 509–38.

56. See the recent debate by J.C. Riley, 'Why Sickness and Death Rates do not

Move Parallel to One Another over Time', *Social History of Medicine*, **12** (1999), pp. 101–24 and 133–37, versus B. Harris, 'Morbidity and Mortality during the Health Transition: A Comment', *Social History of Medicine*, **12** (1999), pp. 125–31, and the articles cited in these studies.

57. J.C. Riley, *Sickness, Recovery and Death: A History and Forecast of Ill Health*, London, 1989; and idem, 'Why Sickness and Death Rates do not Move Parallel to One Another over Time' (n. 56).

PART TWO

The German States

CHAPTER FOUR

Health Care Provision and Poor Relief in Enlightenment and 19th Century Prussia

Fritz Dross

The labouring poor and poverty in Prussia

The history of Prussia in the 18th and 19th centuries has, in many ways, been considered the pattern for German history of this period. The history of health care provision and poor relief is no exception, as revealed by a glance at the pertinent and synoptic literature, which primarily contrasts the situation in Prussia with non-Prussian 'exceptions'. This is somewhat surprising, since it is hardly possible to speak of a uniform and continuous territorial existence of Prussia from the mid-18th century to the founding of the Second Reich in 1871 – except for the core lands of Brandenburg and East Prussia.[1]

The territories added to the Prussian state as a result of military and diplomatic activities retained regional identities which were not solely based on traditions pre-dating Prussian influence. They also followed their own particular economic and social paths. Hence, the history of the Prussian Rhineland during the 19th century has little in common with that of East Prussia; similarly disparities exist between the history of Silesia and that of the former diocese of Hildesheim, to name but a couple of examples.

Consequently, a review of Prussian health care provision and poor relief will have little choice but to begin by focusing on government measures and central legislation. Even here, however, the continued existence of French legislation in the Rhenish territories awarded to Prussia at the Congress of Vienna, presents obstacles. With regard to the actual implementation of new legislation, the present study relies on existing local studies. Such studies, however, are only available for the cities of the Rhineland and Westphalia, as well as for Berlin – which makes it difficult to generalise for Prussia as a whole.

Hence the problem of how to interpret Prussian poverty statistics – a problem which had already been identified in 1853[2] – remains. Thus it still seems inadvisable to attempt to present a unified view of the entire Prussian monarchy in the light of the enormous discrepancies in socioeconomic development, including the widely differing welfare provisions, as well as the wide variations in the basic demographic and sociohistorical data (population development, cost of living, wages). Personally, I am of the opinion that the production of sociohistorical averages and aggregated statistics for the entire Prussian state impedes historical insight rather than facilitates it.

Accordingly, this study will describe the legal foundations of local health care provision and poor relief, as well as discussing the rationale and context of the legislation. To this end, in addition to specific welfare legislation, commercial and industrial legislation will be considered, as well as insurance legislation. Likewise, the important measures taken by police authorities to tackle epidemics will be considered. Special attention is devoted to the inter-relationship between work, poverty and illness. Hence, the health care obligations of artisans and other employers, as defined in the *Allgemeines Landrecht*, towards workers' insurance schemes in the 1880s, will be discussed. Problems arising from the implementation of these laws will be illustrated by an analysis of specific developments at the local level.

Poverty had, of course, been a major concern to the magistracies of most European cities well before the Enlightenment. Above all, in Germany the Imperial cities and the cities of the Hanseatic League had endeavoured to establish a system of public poor relief since the Reformation.[3] Often, however, practical, direct assistance remained the responsibility of communal, fraternal organisations (such as guilds, or neighbourhoods) or religious corporations (parishes or confraternities).[4] Although the early modern city-state was increasingly concerned with regulating and improving poor relief, the actual care for the poor remained, in the first instance, a task for the family, the community, the Church and – only in the event of their failure – a municipal obligation.

In the Prussian–German case, the new administrative and·political teachings of *Kameralismus* were influential in promoting the new perception of people as a source of each state's wealth and political power. Starting from the assumption that the sum of goods produced in a country depended on the size of the productive labour force, the new 'population policy' came to be the primary mercantile precept. Thus, the Prussian kings pursued a systematic policy of resettlement and colonisation of those regions which had long remained depopulated as a consequence of the devastation caused by the Thirty Years' War. Evidently the enlightened absolutist state, in addition to territory, had discovered people as a major factor in power politics and economics.[5] Leibniz, who referred to the health of the subjects as one of a state's primary welfare responsibilities along with justice, prosperity and religion, in the 17th century, had called for demographic descriptions of states.[6]

In order to maximise the desired economic advantages, a large population did not merely have to be well-educated, or enjoy its industriousness free from 'inappropriate' tasks or regulations by guilds or estates, but first of all it should consist of people who were dedicated to commercial activity: thus the population should be 'healthy'. Accordingly, governments should not only be concerned with the overall size of their populations – quantity – but also with their general state of health – the quality of the population.[7] The state's responsibility to ensure 'common happiness' extended to the physical well-being of its subjects.[8]

Progressive physicians concerned with health care provisions provided by the state personally witnessed the social inequality of illness and death in their dealings with health care measures administered by the state. The pioneer of Prussian population statistics, Johann Peter Süßmilch, early on in his study of the high mortality rate in 1757, recognised that rising prices, and in particular the relationship between wages and prices, were major causes of inadequate nutrition and resulting high death rates. It first affected the labouring poor, especially those who worked on daily contracts or were paid per piece.[9] The leading theorist and spirit behind the medical police, Johann Peter Frank, called misery 'the mother of illness' in his speech given in Pavia in 1790.[10] Picking up on Rousseau's concept of differentiating between 'natural' and 'deserved' illness (the latter being attributable to civilisation), Frank branded villeinage as a cause of illness and consequently as an unacceptable source of 'deserved' illnesses.

Even though the resulting sociorevolutionary consequences easily went beyond what could medically be justified in the context of the late absolutist state, the medical and political literature of the medical police nevertheless demonstrates the existence of a comprehensive disciplinary project which sought to encourage and direct the population's behaviour in a 'healthy' direction, encompassing all aspects of life from birth to death.[11] Hence, the medical police is rightly considered the originator of the public health care system in the German-speaking areas of Europe.

Besides the lengthy debate among doctors, administrative experts and the educated public about the proper safeguarding of the population – increasingly seen as a biological resource – and the state's focused employment of doctors to this end, the wealth of pertinent regulations passed at the height of the regulatory frenzy of late absolutism, is impressive. The implementation of these regulations was to be monitored by a local bureaucratic apparatus of physicians via the *Provinzial Collegia Medica* until the establishment of the central *Ober-Collegium Medici* in 1725, whose political and administrative influence remained slight, however.[12] The attempts of the medical police to impose a healthy lifestyle on the population reflects the universal responsibility of absolutism as much as it opens a specific medical perspective on the social world. Neither enlightened doctors nor the absolutist state were, however, capable of effectively changing nutrition habits or for that matter the way people dressed, their housing or sexual habits, within a reasonable timeframe.

Begging was often a profession in the second half of the 18th century.[13] However, it would make little sense to construct a uniform image of a 'beggar' because areas of activity, and the survival strategies of wandering beggars or labourers, differed fundamentally from those of the resident poor and beggars who were bound to specific locations.[14] People who were dependent on public and private support, on alms from the Church and state, and whose living expenses were covered essentially by these means, nevertheless had a defined and widely accepted position in the ancien régime society of the Enlightenment era. This can be seen from the dealings of the poor among themselves and with those from whom they expected alms, which correspond to the rules of the contemporary code of honour.[15] The matter-of-course manner in which wandering journeymen (and those who claimed to be so) were given travelling money, in which sheriffs refused to do their duty and perform arrests, in which priests and ministers consecrated illegal weddings among the poor, and in which citizens of good repute issued poverty certificates to their clients and stuck to traditional tithes, all speak for the enormous difficulties of reforming attitudes to poor relief. Partial reform was only achieved on a communal, local level well on into the 19th century.

Poor relief reforms of the late 18th century

A major and wide-ranging discussion of poverty and its causes arose in the last third of the 18th century, which – in contrast to the poverty debate of the Reformation era – had more concrete political and administrative measures as its explicit goal.[16] Semi-public poor relief facilities of a new sort organised in so-called associations were established in several cities.[17] They were characterised by centralisation and volunteerism as well as by a relatively bureaucratic and uniform procedure for a) defining poverty, b) measuring the extent of poverty in their area, and c) distributing benefits in predetermined amounts.[18]

Princes and enlightened urban–patriotic circles provided the initiative leading to new poor relief facilities, which were then formally put into effect by municipal or state authorities.[19] In Prussia poor relief became a general responsibility of the state in the framework of the *Allgemeines Landrecht* of 1794.[20] It committed itself 'to provide for the nutrition and feeding of those citizens who are unable to provide for themselves, and who are unable to receive provisions from others who are bound to provide care in accordance with other special laws'.[21] The responsibilities of local communities, especially the municipalities, were laid down. Central government did not in any way commit itself to the extension of benefits, but only provided the parameters for the lawful regulation and administrative control of poor relief carried out by local communities under the control of central government.

They provided the legal base until Bismarck's social legislation defined the state's sovereignty in this regard. The communities, for their part, were explicitly not obliged to make welfare provision vis-à-vis the poor, but rather vis-à-vis the state.[22]

While the *Allgemeines Landrecht* fundamentally followed the *Heimatprinzip* of poor relief (the principle by which the community of origin, usually the place of birth, determined the relief agency), it did, however, contain several regulations which were intended to limit the foreseeable financial consequences. For instance, the municipalities were forbidden to expel the non-resident poor, a procedure which nevertheless continued to be favoured by the local (police) authorities well into the 19th century.[23] On 8 September, 1804 a 'decree on the more precise definition of the principles of responsibilities for relief for the local poor in Kurmark, Neumark and Pommerania' was passed, which obliged local government to make poor relief payments available to new residents from the day on which claimants had taken up their new domicile.[24] In 1828 the Prussian ministry of the interior stated that a journeyman with scabies had to be cured in the location where the illness was discovered. Only journeymen who had immigrated from abroad could be deported.[25]

However, the costs connected with the transport or imprisonment of arrested beggars, while their communities of origin were being determined, exceeded the financial capabilities of numerous municipalities.[26] Furthermore, villages were not permitted to have non-native poor and sick people cared for in the nearest large city. It was not the existence of medical facilities in the city – in contrast to the countryside – which determined the standard of caring for the poor and sick, 'but solely the availability of doctors and other medical provisions'.[27] In 1800 it was already apparent at the ministerial and governmental level that poor relief provided in accordance with the *Heimatprinzip* could not adequately solve the problem.

The basic unit of social security remained the family. When no relatives could be called upon to support an impoverished person, the responsibility for welfare fell to the village or city, 'where this person last contributed to the common burden'.[28] A fundamental problem remained of caring for migrating journeymen or servants who fell ill. As members of their masters' or employers' households, they did not personally contribute to the 'common burden' while their masters and employers, who should have been responsible for their care, tended to remove staff who were dangerously ill or unable to work from their homes. Hence, local authorities were to 'see to it with their own representatives that an apprentice without means who falls ill shall not be abandoned or expelled before he has successfully or adequately recovered'.[29]

While, on the one hand, Prussian municipalities were denigrated as *Staatsanstalten* (facilities of the state)[30] during the 18th century, and characterised as 'privileged corporations' with a virtually civic status in the

Allgemeines Landrecht, on the other hand they remained burdened with the state's responsibility of poor relief in accordance with the *Heimatrecht* (home law). Communalisation of the welfare system meant the localisation of the widely lamented 'poverty problem' in the cities and communities, which were required by the state to 'solve' it. This changed with the Municipal Code (*Städteordnung*) of 19 November, 1808, by which the municipalities were compelled to establish communal authorities on a uniform, corporate legal basis, while the state withdrew completely from certain areas of responsibility. Among these were the welfare system: 'The entire welfare system will be entrusted to the hands of the citizenry, the civic sense and charity of the urban residents.'[31]

Relief efforts for the poor and sick intensified dramatically in the Prussian capital and royal residence of Berlin, which was growing into a European metropolis by 1800. In 1750, out of a total of 113 289 residents in Berlin, 1384 poor received relief (1:82) while, in 1801, 173 000 residents provided relief for 12 254 poor (1:14).[32] The expenditures of Berlin's poverty funds rose from 3391 thalers in 1778 to 21 144 thalers 11 years later – a sixfold increase.[33] The first organisational steps were taken around 1700: the large Friedrich Hospital was founded in 1697, followed two years later by the *Armendirektorium* which coordinated local welfare efforts, and poverty directives were passed in 1703 and 1708. By 1727 the poor sick could be transferred by the *Armendirektorium* to the newly established hospital, the Charité. When the *Polizeidirektorium* was established in 1742, a new authority was created, which centralised poor relief and appointed city physicians.[34] The year 1787 witnessed the passing of a regulation proposed by Councillor von der Hagen, head of the *Armendirektorium*, which introduced a regime for children in care who were to be set to work spinning wool by the age of six, while girls of 12 were to be sent out as servants; alien, non-resident, unemployed servant girls were to be removed from the city.[35]

However, the special conditions of Berlin should be borne in mind. Here the *Polizeidirektorium* did not constitute an arm of the magistracy, but rather functioned as an intermediate authority of the state. Moreover, the presence of the royal government in Berlin – especially the ministry of the interior – resulted in an unusual awareness of local conditions within central government. Consequently, Berlin's welfare issues were negotiated in a triangle consisting of the magistracy, the *Polizeidirektorium* and the ministry of the interior.[36]

This constellation, in addition to the relative weakness of the magistracy, resulted in a lack of an organised and philanthropically motivated citizenry, which, for instance, was the decisive factor in implementing new forms of poor relief in Hamburg.[37] Hence the introduction of voluntary poor relief deputies within the framework of communal poor relief remained a much discussed topic after 1786, even if it was not put into practice until the 1820s

– and then on the order of central government. Likewise, the example of Hamburg was invoked by Frederick William III, when in 1803 he invited the Hamburg merchant Caspar Voght to Berlin. Voght was internationally respected as the father of the reformed welfare system in Hamburg and was invited to study the conditions in Berlin and submit proposals for their improvement.[38] He suggested the founding of a 'Society of the Friends of the Poor in Berlin' (*Gesellschaft der Berliner Armenfreunde*) as well as the division of the city into 306 poor districts, in which voluntary poor relief deputies (*Armenfreunde*) were to take over activities under the central leadership of the society. The establishment of communal poor relief, as called for in Stein's Municipal Code (*Städteordnung*) of 1808, was not, however, successfully introduced until 1819. In 1796, Ludwig Formey had praised the variety of facilities and foundations available, but at the same time lamented their inadequate organisation and lack of central administration and supervision of the poor.[39]

Poverty had been stripped of all its previous religious significance – that is, poverty as an ideal, poverty as a fate determined by God, or poverty as punishment. Instead, it was seen as a moral problem – often as a moral defect of the poor themselves.[40] Manual labour,[41] recognised by the students of *Kameralismus* – and by Adam Smith and the French physiocrats – as a basic element in the national economy, came to be seen as the universal cure for poverty and explicitly as the main therapy (even in medical practices) for poverty.[42] Since poverty evidently resulted from the lack of work, then it followed that every poor person's duty to work could be considered to be the logical solution to the problem. To the extent that income-related work was the main source of an individual's existence according to bourgeois thought, poor relief had to differentiate between the deserving and undeserving poor. Illness as an explanation for failing to work, and therefore for earning a living, was increasingly questioned from a moral, as well as a legal, perspective by those in authority.[43]

Consequently, it is no surprise that caring for the sick poor was one of the central concerns of the new poor relief facilities established towards the end of the 18th and at the beginning of the 19th centuries. The care of the sick became a central task of the agencies dedicated to combating poverty, since quick recoveries guaranteed the earliest return to work. Two avenues were pursued in this respect: the medical treatment of the poor sick in their homes in the framework of the *Krankenbesuchsanstalten* (domiciliary care) as favoured by Hufeland,[44] and medical care in the newly established early modern hospitals for the poor.[45] As early as 1800 – more than a generation before the connection between poverty and industrial wage labour became evident – the primary and essential aim of medical care offered to the poor was to restore their ability to work. Doctors in Bielefeld explained that over 80 per cent of their poor patients were regularly released as 'cured' between 1807 and 1810 because most of their patients were eager to break off the treatment in order to return to work.[46]

As a rule, medical care for the poor in Berlin[47] took place in their homes or in the Charité hospital. Built as a plague house in 1710, it eventually served as a garrison hospital, as well as a poorhouse, since the plague never reached Berlin. The institution carried the name 'Charité' from 1727 and, in addition to its two older functions, it provided education for doctors and surgeons, medical care of poor people, treatment for prostitutes with venereal diseases and a maternity ward which offered training for midwives.[48] To the extent that the admission of patients by the *Armendirektorium* also meant the super-vision of the (financial) administration of the hospital, notable conflicts regularly arose between the *Armendirektorium* and the doctors working and teaching at the Charité. In 1778 the President of the *Armendirektorium*, Theodor Wilhelm von der Hagen, curtly declared: 'The sick poor shall be given free medication and care, the impoverished however, shall be taken to the Charité.'[49]

In 1798 Frederick William III issued a cabinet order emphasising that the 'Charité [shall be] governed in medical and surgical regards by the head of the medical facility and the *Armendirektorium* together'. The *Ober-Colle-gium Medicum* was expressly excluded from the administration of the Charité.[50] The hospital was notoriously overcrowded because of its broad responsibili-ties. Its expansion during the period 1785 to 1800 did nothing to alleviate the problem. As a response, greater emphasis was placed on providing the sick poor with domestic medical care. In 1800 one poor-doctor and seven sur-geons cared for the sick among the approximately 10 000 poor in Berlin.[51] The patient list for the years 1794 to 1799 of Ernst Ludwig Heim, who was not active as a poor-doctor, contained one-tenth 'wage labourers', of whom half were servants whose treatments obviously were paid for by their em-ployers. With Heim earning an average of 11 thaler and 20 groschen per patient, it is hardly surprising that craftsmen and minor merchants were far from prominent among his clientele.[52]

A plan submitted in May 1806 emphasised the importance of avoiding further admissions to the Charité and called for the division of the city into 20 medical districts, each of which was to have a doctor in charge.[53] The organ-ised care provided by poor-doctors not only gave them fairly precise insights into the living conditions of the poor in the populace, but also led to a transfer of many decisions to those with medical competence – such as decisions on the amount and kind of food distributions. The debate about the advantages and disadvantages of treating the sick poor in hospitals was still running at the beginning of the 19th century.[54] The founders of poor relief in Hamburg decided in favour of a *Krankenbesuchsanstalt*. Likewise, Christoph Wilhelm Hufeland, since 1801 the leading doctor of the Charité and a member of the *Armendirektorium* in Berlin, also actively supported such domiciliary care.[55]

Poverty and disease during early industrialisation: pauperism

With the laws of the Prussian reform era[56] – the regulations of the *Bundesakte* of 1815, as well as the German Customs Union of 1834 – domestic migration by those seeking work became easier. The freeing of peasants and the dissolution of the traditional guilds (*Zünfte*) liberated workers from the restrictions of previous generations. In the transition from a traditional commercial society (manufacturing) to an early industrial society (factories, especially textiles), towns and cities witnessed increased immigration from an expanding landless rural population, particularly from the eastern, agricultural provinces.[57] From the 1840s at the latest, especially in the wake of the Silesian weavers' riot of 1844,[58] 'pauperism' became a spectre of civic life, treated in literature, art and political debates,[59] and accordingly was the lamented dark side of early industrialisation.[60] Marx and Engels attributed pauperism to the conditions of production and claimed that it was only removable by revolutionary means. The manifestation of pauperism led increasingly – in liberal as well as in conservative circles[61] – to the realisation of the structural character of poverty, which was simply presenting itself in new forms.[62]

Privy Councillor Meding, who was in charge of the reform of Prussian poverty legislation in Berlin, concluded with regard to the disconcerting growth of 'proletarians', as he called those dependent on public poor relief that 'This is an evil which appears to be inseparable from the progress of civilisation itself'.[63] The principles of traditional late-absolutist administrative poor relief did, in fact, fundamentally contradict the new proto-industrial or early industrial social order, just as the liberal economic policies contradicted the conservative domestic policies of Prussia.[64] Freedom of movement, and contractual freedom as a foundation of commercial freedom, were irreconcilable with the *Heimatprinzip*. Moreover, the social conflicts, as well as the political interests of the local leading classes of the estate owners east of the Elbe and the Rhenish Prussian cities, were fundamentally different. Thus the dreaded consequences of a policy of freedom of movement were debated from irreconcilably opposed interests and principles.[65]

On 31 December 1842, the law on the incorporation of newly arrived individuals superseded the *Heimatprinzip* in Prussia, although it had been an object of discussion since 1824.[66] It introduced more or less unlimited freedom of movement and commercial freedom of settlement, thereby eliminating those obstacles standing in the way of an open labour market. The only person excluded from the freedom of movement was any individual, 'who possesses neither sufficient means or strength to provide a meagre living for himself and his dependants'. Moreover, the law also explicitly laid down that 'The *concern* of a newcomer's potential impoverishment in the future, does not suffice for turning him away'.[67] Poor relief was adapted to these new conditions with the law on the obligation of poor relief, also of 31 December

1842: if no other obligated parties, such as relatives, could be drawn upon, then the registered domicile was obliged to assist the poor person. If the poor held neither municipal citizenship nor had established a residence in accordance with the law on the incorporation of newly arrived individuals, the duty to provide poor relief took effect if the supplicant had 'reached the age of majority within three years of the point in time when his helplessness arose where he had his usual domicile'.[68]

If a paradigmatic shift was intended in Prussian poor law, then it excluded those sections of the population who were most in need of it – servants, journeymen and factory workers.[69] In questionable cases the legislature gave the municipalities the option to treat the impoverished person as a beggar or vagrant according to the poor law. A law on the punishment of vagrants, beggars and the slothful was passed on 6 January 1843, one week after the two laws mentioned above.[70] In this respect, the municipalities became 'judge and witness in their own case'.[71]

For the municipalities these changes meant the nearly unhindered settlement of potentially needy individuals. The magistracy in Berlin had been complaining of the 'ease of settling here' since the 1820s.[72] The municipalities (especially in the Rhenish cities) objected to this, demanding from the state's poor law and municipal legislation 'protection for the propertied classes from the onrush of the proletariat'.[73] They developed strategies for tackling the influx and its potential obligations, which included the avoidance of regulations.[74] In response, the Municipal Code of 1853,[75] as well as the amendment of the poor laws in May 1855,[76] laid down that poor relief should begin only after a year in residence at a new location and that any benefits before then had to be extended at the cost of the so-called community of origin. The workers' freedom of movement in accordance with the principle of the supporting domicile was not, however, surrendered in any way.

In case of incapacitating illness, the municipalities were definitively obligated to carry the costs (of lost wages) for at least three months. The support was always to remain below the level of the (lost) earned income. Nevertheless, the municipalities' problems when faced with mass poverty were hardly manageable: in those towns and cities where no wealthy, old foundations could be called on, the share of the entire municipal budget expended on poor relief exceeded half of the cities' total expenditures and, at times, even comprised two-thirds.[77]

The North German Confederation adopted the Prussian regulations in the law on the supporting residence (*Unterstützungswohnsitz*) of 6 June 1870.[78] In addition to the equal treatment of all 'northern Germans', it was laid down that public support was to be carried out by local *Ortsarmenverbände* and regional *Landarmenverbände* (welfare associations). Not every municipality (or manorial estate) was forced to form an independent welfare association; the formal fusion of several municipalities into a single association was left up to the local authorities. In similar fashion to the older Prussian regulations, the regional welfare associations assumed the care of people whom no local welfare association was obliged by law to support, especially those needy individuals who had not obtained a supporting domicile after a two-year residency, by marriage or by descent. Pursuant to a supplementary law of application,[79] the Prussian regional welfare associations were obliged to care for – in their poorhouses, but for compensation – those cases of impoverishment that were beyond other local welfare associations, as well as to support the financially weak local welfare associations in their own district.[80]

Similarly, early forms of health insurance were less concerned with the risk of illness as such, but rather with the risk of impoverishment arising from inability to work. The members of so-called *Krankenladen* or *Unterstützungsladen* took out insurance for themselves (not so much for their families) to avoid having to face abject poverty and hunger in case illness prevented them from work. Doctors' bills or expenses for drugs were not usually part of the coverage.[81] The insurance funds established by the new guilds (*Innungen*) in Berlin concluded agreements with the Charité on the treatment of sick, unmarried journeymen as early as the first half of the 19th century. In 1846, 44 of these journeymen's insurance funds, with a total of 14 000 members, jointly shared ten doctors.[82]

In contrast to the state health insurance which came later, the independent health insurance and burial funds, which became common in the 1840s and 1850s, were private insurance associations based on reciprocity, with their payments being directly and exclusively borne by the insured members. This did not mean that membership was always voluntary. Workers and craftsmen were, in fact, often obliged to join by labour contracts, factory rules and guild regulations. This sort of insurance corresponded to the continuing view of poor relief as a moral obligation. The idea that it could be a social obligation in a legally binding form and that the poor should not be deferentially grateful, but rather stubbornly stake their claim to their rights, still unsettled the urban bourgeois and upper classes in the mid-19th century.[83]

It was of particular importance to the municipalities to have journeymen, day labourers, servants and factory workers – who were now far more mobile than before – cared for outside the overstretched municipal budgets, since they were often young and single and had no family or relatives to care for them when illness struck in their new place of residence. In addition to these newcomers, there were also craftsmen who had become directly dependent on public support when they had surrendered their guild membership[84] by having accepted an often better paid job in a factory. Furthermore, 'health care' provision by guilds was being viewed less positively. In 1842 artisan masters in Bielefeld complained that healthy apprentices were being infected by sick ones in the apprentices' lodgings. They combined these complaints with proposals on the financing of a hospital.[85] The oversupply of artisans, particularly in the 1830s and 1840s, also led to a situation where many independent artisan masters barely earned a subsistence-level income.[86] In Elberfeld, where the legal framework for mandatory membership of all journeymen and factory workers did not exist, different means were used: a formal pledge to support their artisans in case of illness was required from the employer. Since such a pledge was generally not provided, the journeymen were essentially compelled to join the *Gesellenauflage* (journeymen's insurance association).[87]

In 1843 the Rhenish provincial estate assembly appealed to the legislature to grant them the possibility of placing newcomers seeking employment under the obligation of joining a support fund or health insurance organisation.[88] With the Prussian *Gewerbeordnung* (Industrial Code) of 1845,[89] the legislature in Berlin for the first time allowed for commercial support organisations at a local level in contrast to voluntary health insurance associations. In a supplementary directive of February 1849,[90] this was expanded to include factory workers in addition to journeymen and assistants. The municipalities could force the people in question to join an insurance organisation, as well as demand contributions to the organisations from the companies, although this was seldom done in practice. In contrast to the widespread view that the *Unterstützungskassen* were to relieve the strained municipal poor, a completely new view was formulated by the commission concerned with the law passed on the commercial *Unterstützungskassen* in March 1854:[91] 'The returns of work must nourish and support the worker not only in times of health, but also in times of illness.'[92] Through this law, the regional governments (Bezirksregierungen) were empowered to introduce mandatory membership when needed. It did not call for compulsory insurance in general, but rather for mandatory membership for certain professional groups. The *Gewerbeordnung* of 1869 of the North German Confederation[93] left the legal regulations in place but freed those workers who could prove that they belonged to a voluntary insurance association from compulsory membership of an insurance association.[94] Besides the mandatory insurance associations that were established by the municipalities by local statute, the independent insurance organisations continued to exist as associations without any set of benefits fixed by the state. Because these independent associations were not prohibited from forging alliances, some of them became important platforms for the workers' movement (particularly for the social–liberal movement).

In light of the state's inability to address the situation adequately by means of poor laws[95] – or the problems of the municipalities, which had been burdened by the legislation – the Prussian legislature attempted to alleviate the situation through a new industrial policy. Going beyond the regulation of the *Hilfskassen*, Prussian industrial policy generated a central regulatory authority for social problems. As early as the 1830s, the Prussian state began intervening in the chaotic development of early capitalism with legislation and administrative initiatives. Besides the *Allgemeine Gewerbeordnung* (Industrial Code) of 1845, protection of children played an important role. The 'Prussian Regulation on the Employment of Youth Workers in Factories' of 1839 proclaimed the 'morality' of young people working as its highest goal.[96] Schooling was defined as a prerequisite for work (and the ability to work). Concealed behind this goal was – at least according to legend – the concern about the bodily 'fitness' of recruits for the Prussian army.[97] This law remained utterly ineffective until means of control were introduced by factory inspectors by the law of 1853; and, even then, its effects were minimal.[98]

The laws on the protection of children as well as the Prussian Industrial Code (*Allgemeine Gewerbeordnung*) influenced the concept of the ability to work and compensation for loss of wages in case of illness. As a consequence of these measures, 'health' remained an issue subordinated to interventions which were intended and legitimised in other ways. Their overriding concern was with the impoverishment of sick workers unable to work. The concern for the education of children was aimed at providing future qualified employees, as were the corresponding regulations of the insurance associations.

The measures taken against epidemics, however, differed in that they were primarily concerned with the prevention of cholera.[99] In this case, 'health' served to legitimise a bundle of measures, from military to welfare and health educational activities. Cholera came to be seen as the 'scandalised illness' (*skandalisierte Krankheit*),[100] which contained a number of interpretations of disease within it. First, it was considered an illness of the poor, which could be explained not only by inadequate housing and nutrition, but also by immorality, alcoholism and impurity. Second, it was seen as a contagious disease. What the early 1830s showed, with dramatic clarity, was that neither military cordons nor medicine could do much to counter the march of cholera.[101] Hence, avoiding cholera meant protecting oneself from its potential carriers, the poor, who consequently were placed under tighter control and supervision.

On 1 September 1831 the *Gesundheits-Comité* (health committee) of Berlin stated that the city was infected, and within a matter of days multiple isolation measures were introduced. While only 13 beds were available for cholera patients in the smallpox hospital at the time of the statement, by the end of the month the city had acquired four civil field hospitals and an equal number of military medical facilities which treated cholera patients.[102] The committee had been established by royal decree on 5 June, and on 2 August the administrative authority was set up, which prepared military, police, civic and hygienic measures under the chairmanship of the chief of police. Special *Schutzkommissionen* (protection commissions), each of which was in charge of one of the 61 poor districts, were assigned the task of local administration; the heads of the poverty commissions, which were elected by the municipal council, often assumed the additional duties of protection commissioner.[103]

Following the cholera epidemics the government introduced a number of new laws dealing with public health. The Prussian *Sanitätsregulativ* (hygiene regulation) of 1835[104] provided the framework for public preventive measures during future epidemics. In accordance with the regulation, it was now possible to isolate chronically infectious individuals – especially syphilis and scabies sufferers, and particularly prostitutes – for a lengthy period of time. In the case of acute epidemics, such as cholera, typhus, dysentery or smallpox, the aim was to be able to quickly isolate a maximum number of affected individuals – or those suspected of being infected – if need be. The municipalities were obliged to make a sufficient number of isolation wards available by drawing on a previous period's public health regulations in times of epidemics. This usually meant the classification of hospital beds for the purpose of isolation. This new regulation gave rise to numerous activities, including the expansion of hospitals.[105] As soon as cholera or one of the other diseases mentioned above was reported anywhere in Europe, the regional governments arranged for a review of the local precautionary measures. The hospitals in particular were often subjected to harsh criticism on the occasion of such reviews. In this way, investigations executed by the state triggered changes in the hospital system at the municipal level.[106]

The cholera directive of June 1831 merely suggested the establishment of hospitals in order to isolate and care for members of the 'poorer class' in case of illness.[107] The cholera regulation of 1835 did not go beyond that.[108] Even though the municipalities were not directly obliged to establish hospitals, the lack of real alternatives was glaring, particularly in the densely populated cities, as long as it was held that 'Experience has shown isolation of the ill to be the safest means of preventing the further spread of infectious diseases'.[109]

The number of hospitals in Prussia actually more than doubled in the 1830s and 1840s, from 209 in 1831 to 480 in 1849. At the same time the ratio of inhabitants per doctor improved from 3005 to 2874, as did the ratio of inhabitants to medical facilities from 62 388 per facility in 1831 to 34 023 per facility in 1849.[110] However, the figures tell us little about the actual care of hospital patients, as the size and quality of the individual facilities varied greatly. While it can be noted that hospitals were almost exclusively to be found in the cities of the monarchy,[111] this indicates that the larger municipalities reacted in a specific manner to the requirements of the state: they established hospitals. How these hospitals looked, what they were capable of doing, and whether they existed for more than a short time, depended on circumstances that varied greatly from one location to the next. Some influential factors included: the existence of older facilities which could be rebuilt or expanded; finance being available independently of the municipal coffers – for instance, from private foundations or religious orders; the committed involvement of prominent doctors; and pressure from middle-level government authorities.[112]

Poverty and disease in municipal politics in the age of industrialisation: towards a welfare city (*Sozialstadt*)

By the 1850s many Prussian cities had introduced a decentralised and non-uniform system of municipal poor relief by relying on and combining voluntary (bourgeois) activities, in which welfare volunteers were assigned no more than four supported households in their district. This so-called 'Elberfeld system'[113] was based on the subdivision of the cities into as many welfare areas as possible, which then became easier to supervise. The volunteer relief officers, who were local people, were expected to prevent indiscriminate long-term distribution of poor relief by virtue of their relatively intimate knowledge of local circumstances. It is, however, problematic to speak of an innovative 'system'. The distribution of support by (volunteer) relief officers ('aid from person to person') corresponded with the system of charity which had been in place in Hamburg since the reform of 1788. It reflected the tradition of neighbourly support already known from many early modern civic communities.[114] The establishment of the 'Elberfeld system' in Berlin had much to do with the size of the city and with the advanced social segregation of its population.[115]

Poor relief based on the Hamburg model was established in Elberfeld in 1800. Here the principle of volunteerism was eventually given up in 1811[116] with the introduction of the Imperial decrees on welfare facilities of 3 November, 1809,[117] at a time when the welfare system in the Grand Duchy of Berg was still organised according to a French model.[118]

Some serious conflicts over the future organisation of the welfare system in the formerly French and Grand Ducal territories arose when they were awarded to Prussia, and these conflicts played themselves out on different levels. At a local level, as part of the contempt for 'French conditions' in 1814–17, the pastors and parishes felt particularly obliged to demand the return of their old responsibilities for poor relief, especially because they wanted once more to control and dispose of such considerable means independently. In contrast, the *Bezirksregierung* (regional government) in Düsseldorf preferred poor relief to be part of the municipal administration under the supervision and leadership of the mayor. In Berlin, not only did competition arise between the ministry of the interior and the ministry for spiritual, educational and medical matters,[119] but both sides were quite unfamiliar with the legal and organisational conditions in the formerly French or Grand Ducal territories.[120]

The municipalities exploited the confusion in unconventional ways. In Düsseldorf, when it became known that a cabinet order had revoked the Imperial decree of 1809 on charity facilities, where no institution existed in accordance with the decree, such a facility was re-established in 1823 – despite having been dissolved only eight years earlier.[121] In Cologne there was no fundamental revision of the poor relief administration in the years following 1814.[122] The poverty legislation of the city of Cologne, which was based on French law, did not lose its validity until the Prussian application law of 8 March, 1871.[123] Due to the intensified efforts in connection with the famine of 1816–17, a reorganisation of the welfare system was achieved, which essentially combined the *'bureau de bienfaisance,'* responsible for outdoor relief, with the *'commission des hospices'* into one welfare authority. Under this 'main association', ten (later 14) 'district associations' were set up at the parish level. Between ten and 24 poor relief officers were serving each of these district associations, each of whom had to care for between 15 and 30 poor families.[124] In contrast to Düsseldorf, Cologne had a considerable number of wealthy, old foundations; the welfare administration of the former free city of the Holy Roman Empire endeavoured to obtain its independence by having its own financial administration separate from the city council and the municipal budget.[125] It was not until the introduction of a salaried representative as chairman of the welfare administration in August 1865 – after years of conflict and great resistance on the part of the welfare administration – as well as the introduction of the law on the supporting domicile of January 1872, that the municipal administration in Cologne assumed control over the welfare system there.

In Elberfeld in 1850, the welfare commission saw itself compelled to propose to the city council the complete return of public poor relief into the hands of the church parishes. Classic arguments were cited, which had previously led, in the years after 1814, to the dissolution of several 'central poor relief facilities' which had been based on the French model: regular poor rates improved not only already declining bourgeois charity but also led to an expectant attitude on the part of the poor.[126] The 'Elberfeld system', which was introduced on 1 January 1853, represented the end of the long conflict between clerical and lay poor relief in that it drew on the principle of small areas and volunteerism of the former, while depending on the overall organisational structure of the latter. 'Hence, even in Wupperthal, a strongly religious city imbued with a very pronounced parish consciousness, protests were reduced to mumbling and grumbling.'[127]

In Düsseldorf poor relief was reorganised in 1851. The central welfare authority was abolished and, in accordance with a municipal directive of 11 March, 1850, a deputation selected by the city council took over its activities under the chairmanship of the mayor. The city with its population of 40 412 was divided into 20 districts. A poor relief provider, three 'friends of the poor', and a minister from each confession – Catholic and Protestant – were responsible for the distribution of benefits, preferably in kind, in each district.[128] In 1877 the 'Elberfeld system' was introduced in Düsseldorf, when the city was divided into 15 poor districts subdivided into 139 quarters. This, however, did not make it possible to reduce the funds distributed.[129]

A reorganisation of poor relief also took place in Münster when major changes were made in the Municipal Code. The introduction of the Revised Municipal Code in 1831 eventually led to the welfare authority (*Armenkommission*) being put on an equal footing with other committees serving the magistracy. This did not happen until ten years after preliminary by-laws of the local *Armenkommission* were agreed upon after extensive negotiations in August 1838. While the administration of the numerous and wealthy private foundations was separated from the general poor relief administration, it came to be dependent on local government. The Westphalian city was divided into 29 poor areas as early as 1842. The volunteer poor relief officers, who were local residents, could lighten their workload by hiring so-called benefit-recipients as messengers – a job which, for the first time, could also be done by women.[130]

The introduction of the 'Elberfeld system' in Münster is, however, associated with the general reform of poor relief there of 1 September 1894, when the *Armenkommission* achieved a cooperative agreement with the Catholic Vinzenz-Joseph Society. This was the only way to recruit the 205 supervisors and poor relief providers after the initial 15 welfare districts had been increased to 66 in 1883, even if only one poor relief provider was initially active in each district.[131] The supervision and coordination of the welfare workers, however, required the employment of 'relief attendants'. Hence, paradoxically, Münster, with the introduction of the 'Elberfeld system', became one of the first cities in the Reich to employ full-time welfare workers.[132]

On 1 January 1820 the administration of poor relief in Berlin was transferred to the municipality, in accordance with a cabinet order of 18 May 1819, which finally implemented the Municipal Code of 1808.[133] The municipal poor law of 1826 stipulated the creation of 59 welfare commissions across the city, whose supervisors exercised decentralised control.[134] With the introduction of the Municipal Code of 30 May 1853,[135] poor relief became the responsibility of a municipal committee which consisted of elected members, subordinate to the magistracy. The members of the now 109 welfare commissions – consisting of six to 22 members – fulfilled their duties without a salary and were elected for six-year terms by the city assembly. Consequently, they functioned as volunteer municipal civil servants.[136] However, as early as the 1860s, the Berlin magistracy felt compelled to hire salaried 'assessors' in order to control the work of the welfare commissions which, as a rule, performed their duties without any remuneration.[137]

Since the mid-19th century, a process of communalisation had become apparent on the organisational level of poor relief. While the ideological principles had hardly changed since their formulation in the late 18th century, and the local elite who took on the voluntary work remained indispensable, the municipal governments were simultaneously forced to try to bring poor relief under administrative control, if only because of the rapidly accelerating costs. In many respects, the new Prussian territories in the west should be recognised for their pioneering role. Concrete experience with early communalised poor relief from the 'French period' was available, and the confessional diversity of the population made care according to denomination difficult. Furthermore, the early industrialisation (Elberfeld/Barmen) as well as the rapid industrialisation and urbanisation in the second half of the century – particularly in the Düsseldorf *Regierungsbezirk* (government district) – led to the formation of distinct working-class areas, where the authority of the Churches was declining and where family members of dignitaries, who could be trusted with the voluntary welfare posts, no longer lived.

As early as the middle of the century, the participation of the urban middle classes in civic poor relief was clearly structured according to social status and proximity to poverty.[138] In Cologne in 1849, for instance, about half of the members of the *Hauptverein* (main association) were bankers and major merchants, while in the *Bezirksvereine* (district associations) the figure was 40 per cent and among the *Armenväter* (welfare ministers) they constituted 36 per cent. Craftsmen and minor merchants, the largest section in this latter group, comprised 40 per cent. More than half of the 226 *Armenväter* belonged to the third tax class (divided by income): a third of them did not reach the minimum tax level of 400 thaler required to have the vote. The 17 members of the *Hauptverein*, all of whom earned enough to have the vote, were fairly equally divided among the three tax classes.

Towards the end of the century a fundamental change was becoming evident. As the enormous number of volunteer welfare workers needed could no longer be recruited, volunteer activity had shifted to the bourgeois' associations and clubs which were becoming increasingly differentiated.[139] The growing municipal administrations adopted welfare systems administered by full-time employees, who occasionally developed detailed concepts of a genuinely communal social policy (the 'Strasbourg system'), which was becoming ever more specialised, as part of a general system of public services.[140] Gradually the administration of Prussian cities by notables was superseded by a professional civic, administrative elite with growing confidence and self-awareness. Consequently, the ideological basis of public welfare changed from the 'charitable citizens' sense of community' to a professionally run public assistance system. The deserving poor were transformed into 'needy fellow citizens'.[141]

'The municipality possesses the entire sphere of activity or the complete responsibility.'[142] This autonomy characterised the rise of the communal administrations from around 1870. Many communal benefits expanded rapidly during this time. The communal activities were expressed using the concepts of 'communal socialism' or 'municipal socialism'. They represented the transition to communal administration of public services with their range of responsibilities 'from the well-being of the whole to the material interests and spiritual development of the individual'.[143] The municipal hospital system deserves mention in this context. Municipal hospitals, like public health care, advanced to become an integral and expected part of communal social policy. As before, the Prussian cities continued to spend substantial amounts of money on health care for the poor. For poor relief and health care provision – inseparable in the fund-raising process – the sum of 150 million marks was allocated in 1907; this corresponded to 7.6 per cent of the cities' total expenditures.[144]

Hospital care in particular was costly,[145] even though the municipalities were often not directly in charge of the facilities.[146] Above all, it was parishes and religious communities and orders that established and supported hospitals. Their continued economic basis was secured by contracts with the municipal poor relief administration. Municipal hospital policy can be interpreted as a fine example of a 'mixed economy of welfare'. It was possible for religious communities and charitable foundations to obtain significant sums through donations, bequests and collections, in contrast to civic administrations. Such funds essentially covered the high costs of establishing and expanding hospitals. By means of contracts on the care of the ill and impoverished at fixed daily rates, a safe financial basis could be established, which was further secured by the inclusion of sponsors and so-called 'paying' patients. In the end, medical care depended on the confessional orders – the Protestant *Diakonie* and the Catholic *Barmherzige Schwestern* – which established new standards of medical care in the medium term.[147]

Since the middle of the century, the 'healthy city'[148] had increasingly developed as a topic discussed outside the domain of health care for the poor, and which specifically had the living conditions of the 'lower classes' in mind, which for reasons of health were in urgent need of improvement. The protagonists of the medical reform debate[149] (including Salomon Neumann and Rudolf Virchow) had already complained that the administration of the health care system for the poor was neither willing nor able to take action against the social causes of illness. Far removed from direct sociopolitical demands, and therefore much less susceptible to attack, Max von Pettenkofer's experimental hygiene was a scientifically, socially and politically acceptable instrument for investigating the living conditions that jeopardised health, as well as for proposing measures for improving these conditions. Pettenkofer's comprehensive hygienic approach was developed along the lines of his *Gesundheitswirtschaftslehre*,[150] which was also intended to guarantee the biological resources of an industrial society.

Municipal civil servants, engineers and doctors consequently developed a programme of urban sanitary reform which incorporated[151] the scientific investigation and public—technological improvement of the immediate and environmental living conditions in industrial cities. This had indirect effects on the situation of the lower classes in general, and especially that of the poor. The practice of hygiene in urban public buildings and houses, in factories and commercial zones, the removal of garbage, burials, food inspection, water supply and wastewater management – all of these created the hygienic technological infrastructure of the (industrial) cities.

By the end of the century the larger cities had begun to develop a health care system that was organisationally and financially further and further removed from poor relief administration. Besides municipal health care, the role of charitable associations grew in importance, which increasingly filled the areas of social responsibility. Specific support was offered to target groups, including care for mothers and children, care for infants, toddlers and schoolchildren, for pregnant women and women in childbed as well as for tuberculosis patients. Through police efforts, the cities offered assistance to alcoholics and those with venereal diseases. Welfare for the homeless and jobless[152] was not, however, systematically built up in many cities before the First World War. This differentiation within municipal care was, among other things, due to the creation of state social insurance. The risks and those at risk who were not covered by state social security were picked up by the care offered by the communal and private associations. Police functions were increasingly separated from welfare functions within the municipal administrations.[153] In addition to lawyers, engineers and doctors in particular were also being entrusted with the corresponding responsibilities. At the same time, the charitable associations began to rely on professionals including civil servants, teachers and doctors. Outside of the administrations, the middle-class women's movement laid claim to the professional exercise of care services: 'mothering as a job'.[154] In the end, the goal was to find structures on the municipal level which combined public with private charity exercised through private associations, as the Zentralen für private Fürsorge (Centres for Private Welfare) succeeded in doing in Berlin and Frankfurt-am-Main in the 1890s.[155]

Labour policy as social policy: on the path to a social welfare state

The state of Prussia was not unique in finding itself increasingly unable to bring the problems associated with poverty under control by means of uniform legislation. In fact, the 'social question', which had been vehemently articulated since the mid-19th century, presented a challenge that could no longer be adequately addressed through traditional methods of poor relief. Hence, the Sozialpolitik[156] that arose in the Bismarck era of the German Reich should not only be seen as a continuation of state regulation of poor relief through other means. During the consultations on the reform of the law concerned with residential support (Unterstützungswohnsitz) in March 1877, the Imperial Chancellor realised that pushing through the Heimatprinzip as a simple reform of the welfare legislation was not achievable: 'This is not a matter of combating individual, obvious social ills, but rather a revision of the leading principles of the law.'[157]

Spectacular accidents involving poor labourers caused a public outrage and consequently the protection of workers became part of the agenda of state politics, just as the discussion on child labour had become the focus of factory inspections since the 1830s.[158] However, the introduction of legislation on the protection of workers was opposed by Bismarck who thought that the personal freedom of workers to earn money should not be curbed by unnecessary legislation.[159] A civil law compensation ruling based on the Imperial Liability Law of 12 May 1871,[160] failed because the basic idea of the employers' general risk liability and that of presumptive guilt of the employer contradicted the legal perceptions of the day. In questionable cases, the worker injured in an accident – or his survivors – were required to produce legally admissible evidence of the employer's fault in order to receive any compensation payments. If a satisfactory ruling was not possible in the framework of the liability legislation,[161] then a political solution had to be found, in order to cut the 'Gordian knot of legal principles'.[162] This resulted in the formulation of a labour policy in the form of plans for accident insurance and the compensation of workers.

On another level, considerations were connected with the so-called internal establishment of the Reich (innere Reichsgründung). The successful external establishment of the Reich guaranteed the existence of the new state in international power and foreign policy terms. In the eyes of the government, an attitude among the people[163] that demonstrated adequate loyalty to the emperor did not automatically follow. Bismarck intended to remedy this situation with concrete benefits for the Reich. Largely free of scruples in his battle against the 'internal enemies of the Reich' (innere Reichsfeinde) – especially the workers' movement organised in unions, social democracy, as well as political Catholicism – Bismarck placed great importance on winning over their supporters. As early as January 1872 Hermann Wagener expressed the conviction that 'The social emperor is stronger than the social Pope in the face of the material tendencies of today'.[164] Correspondingly, the often-quoted Imperial Address of 17 November 1881, which promised the three laws on accident, health, retirement and invalidity insurance, contained the formulation: 'The healing of social damage will not be found exclusively in the repression of social democratic rioting, but rather steadily in the positive advancement of the workers' well-being.'[165]

The Prussian–German reform of social insurance was implemented by means of three laws in the 1880s. The law on accident insurance enacted in 1884[166] represents the central piece of the legislation and consequently was the most controversial.[167] In contrast, health insurance law, which was introduced a year earlier,[168] owes its creation to the fact that Theodor

Lohmann, in the second bill on accident insurance of February 1882, extended the waiting period for the start of benefits 'intentionally and against instructions' from 14 days to 13 weeks.[169] The health insurance law was intended to bridge this time gap. Without generating any complicated negotiations, the bill on health insurance passed the preliminary legislative trials in the 'slipstream' of the discussion on the controversial accident insurance.[170] With the passage of the invalidity insurance and the retirement insurance laws in 1889,[171] the legislative part of the reform of social insurance/security was finally completed.[172]

The political objectives[173] of the legislation were varied, and health care did not feature prominently among them. On the other hand, the protection of workers was among them because accident insurance incorporated compensatory aspects of a state-wide workers' protection policy which, however, was not effectively implemented in the Bismarck era. The political intentions vis-à-vis workers are most apparent in the subsidies given to the invalidity and retirement insurance, paid directly by the Reich. The Reich was thus active and visible to the insured as a principal supporter. The political objectives were rooted in the desire to keep the insured clientele of factory workers from abject impoverishment in case of accident, illness or old age, and not only in order to relieve the municipal poor relief burdens. The establishment of workers' social insurance stipulated by state legislation is characterised by the anti-liberal impetus of a socially conservative policy of pacification. This policy hoped for the reconciliation of the class antagonists, as well as for 'a possible model for a new constitutional body outside of parliament',[174] to comprise representatives of workers and employers.[175]

The health insurance companies were financed by premiums paid two-thirds by the employees and one-third by the employers. The independent administrations of the compulsory insurance companies were filled according to the same ratio.[176] Initially, the focus was on compensation for the loss of earnings in case of illness after the fourth day of incapacity to the amount of half the average local wage for a day, in addition to medical treatment, medications and drugs and, under certain circumstances, admission to a hospital. While at first the independent insurance funds enjoyed a growing membership[177] who were exempted from joining the compulsory insurance companies, the *Ortskrankenkassen* (local insurance companies) eventually became the most commonly selected type of health insurance around the turn of the century.[178] The amendment of 1892 put an end to the registered supplementary insurance funds (*Hilfskassen/freie Unterstützungskassen*) which had paid out three-quarters of the average local daily wage instead of covering only medical care and medications.[179] The shift away from the concentration on compensation in favour of medical treatment led to a structural disadvantage for the independent insurance funds, which were often occupation-related and whose local chapters often had relatively few members.[180]

The state health insurance developed into an institution which primarily financed medical services for insured individuals, thus becoming detached from poor relief in terms of both organisation and content. The insurance benefits corresponded closely to the legal right of the insured and were totally different from traditional, discriminatory public poor relief (see Figure 4.1, and Tables 4.1 and 4.2).[181]

With the health insurance companies, a completely new sort of account-able organisation appeared in the field of health care, which was also becoming more specialised. Internally, they served to balance the interests of employees and employers; externally, in the field of health care policy, they were powerful representatives of their members vis-à-vis the state, the municipalities, and the suppliers of medical services, particularly doctors.[182] With the extension of compulsory health insurance to salaried employ-ees,[183] and finally to the majority of those employed and dependent on wages,[184] as well as the introduction of insurance for family members with the Reich Insurance Code of 1911[185] – anticipated as an option as early as 1883 and 1892[186] – from 1885 to 1911 the revenues and expenditures not only climbed parallel to the growth in membership, but also the average

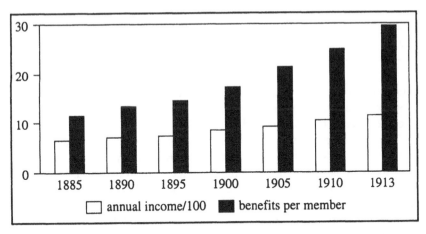

Source: Gerd Hohorst, Jürgen Kocka and Gerhard A. Ritter, *Sozialgeschichtliches Arbeitsbuch. Volume 2: Materialien zur Statistik des Kaiserreichs 1870–1914* (Statistische Arbeitsbücher zur neueren Geschichte) 2nd edn, München, 1978. p. 22: Population of the German Reich; p. 107: average annual income (nominal); p. 154: Members and benefits of the health insurance; p. 155: Members and benefits of the accident insurance. (All data relate to the German Reich, not to Prussia.)

Figure 4.1 Health insurance benefits and average annual income (in marks), 1885–1913

Table 4.1   Health insurance benefits and average annual income (in marks)

Year	Nominal average annual income	Average benefits per member
1885	58,100	10.94
1890	65,000	12.76
1895	66,500	13.95
1900	78,400	16.59
1905	84,900	20.74
1910	97,900	24.48
1913	108,300	28.82

Table 4.2   Insurance members as a percentage of population

Year	Health insurance	Accident insurance
1885	9.16	
1890	13.31	27.67
1895	14.39	35.17
1900	16.89	33.51
1905	18.44	33.38
1910	20.12	42.43

benefits per member paid by the state insurance associations rose from approximately ten to nearly 30 marks,[187] and those for doctors' treatments from 2.1 marks to 6.2 marks.[188]

The benefits extended within the framework of the accident and retirement insurance also satisfied the legally established rights of the insured and was not considered to be poor relief. The reimbursements from the social insurance to the communal welfare coffers represented a new and not insubstantial item in the municipal poor relief budgets.[189] The accident insurance in particular resulted in the expansion and improvement of surgical hospitals, as well as stimulating the development of rehabilitative and functional treatments. Moreover, *Berufsgenossenschaften* (professional associations), established within the framework of the accident insurance, had a fundamental interest in the prevention of occupational accidents, and – parallel to the state's factory inspections – in the long term contributed to the reshaping of the workplace while taking health aspects into account.[190]

After their reformulation of 13 July 1899,[191] the retirement and invalidity insurances generated a new form of medical care: the preventive rehabilitative hospital and the treatments resulting from it, not to mention the corresponding demand for medical facilities – at the time especially for patients with bronchial ailments, particularly tuberculosis. Organisationally, these hospitals or sanatoriums were set up at the country or provincial level.[192] This type of insurance is also seen as influential for the functional specialisation of the health care system, especially with regard to the differentiation of special rehabilitative and preventive sanatoriums.

In fact, the benefits initially paid by the social insurance were quite meagre and, in questionable cases when no relative could be called upon for support, did not protect the insured from falling back on public poor relief. The retirement insurance in particular, which distinguished according to wage groups, had little more than a symbolic effect, since it provided a pension that did not cover the cost of living. This was the case even when workers had contributed for 30 years and qualified for support only when they had turned 60 – an age which hardly any workers attained at that time.[193] Although membership of the state health insurance scheme rocketed, we should not forget that only one-fifth of the German population was insured by 1910.[194]

The systemic shift achieved with the introduction of social insurance as workers' insurance was decisive. The real innovation lay not in the introduction of an insurance based on social security as such. It was of greater significance that the state introduced a comprehensive, obligatory and uniform scheme bringing together employees, employers and the state in a publicly sponsored system. Thus the insured workers obtained rights to benefits which were uniformly laid down by law for the whole nation, vis-à-vis the state-administered insurance. As premium-paying members, workers participated in its administration.

Poor relief, which continued to be administered primarily on a communal level, did not become obsolete. Since the duration of health insurance benefits was limited, sickness remained the most common factor in poverty and accordingly for claiming poor relief.[195] A specific division of responsibilities developed between social insurance on the one hand and welfare care on the other.[196] While the receipt of insurance benefits and one's identity as an insured party was (and is!) connected with having a regular job (that is, a position linked to compulsory insurance), welfare, which was conducted by charitable organisations and in particular by the municipalities, focused increasingly on specific problems.

Summary

A discourse extends from the Reformation into the second half of the 19th century, which, within the framework of the debate on poverty, relied on man's ambition and obligation to work. The suppression of begging rested on this basis, while adequately providing for the labouring poor became a religious, moral and political problem. With the implementation of social insurance as workers' insurance, both health care provision and poor relief took on modern features, while their relationship changed fundamentally. Social insurance can be considered an achievement of the German Reich. Its conception and discussion, introduction and modification took place at the national level. Accordingly, from a systematic perspective, it makes little sense to follow its further development from a purely Prussian angle.

The developments described in this chapter show that municipal and state poor relief had begun to change in character by the 1870s. A restrictive and exclusive welfare policy gradually evolved into a pacifying and socially integrating labour policy. Financial benefits were replaced by (medical) benefits in kind. These eventually assumed a preventive character. Along with social disciplining and the regulation of behaviour, social security gradually locked poor people into the scientific–technological industrial world: paupers were transformed into the industrial proletariat, then into a predictable industrial labour force. In this development, the medical culture played an increasingly important role: health, as a social good, became a generally accepted ideal in industrial society.[197]

Along with the differentiation of the general risk of poverty into specific risks to the social state, the system developed a tendency to encompass more and more contingencies and to reach into more and more areas of people's lives. After the basic conditions of the system had been laid down, many other political facts, social and economic developments, as well as political interests, played a role. It became an issue when politics encountered its ideologically loaded borders of intervention: state–city–family. Historical and cultural contrasts – between the cities and the state, as well as between regions that industrialised earlier and faster and those that industrialised later, slower and to a lesser degree – were nourished by different economic interests. Consequently the social policies directed at the industrial workers were circumscribed by the political structures of Prussia and the Reich. Laws and regulations, the classic means of state intervention, were suspended in the conflict of interests between industry and agriculture.

In contrast, the relatively clear conditions at the local level, traditional procedures for settling conflicts between municipal administrations and urban society, as well as the powerful position of mayors, which was laid down in the municipal constitutions, made it possible for large Prussian–German cities to become confident protagonists of welfare and health policy at the communal and intercommunal level.

A system of clubs, associations and societies developed, which achieved considerable significance, as a response to what society at large perceived to be scandalous risks to industrial workers. Various local, regional and national interest groups came together in such associations: bourgeois activists, the women's movement, professional groups such as doctors, local politicians and so on. Leading civil servants and politicians in municipalities, independent states and in the Reich recognised that these interest groups, with only limited financial means and non-material support, could help solve relevant social problems and discover and occasionally repair shortcomings in the gradually developing social state. The associations and clubs became an important experimental field for new state social and medical benefits, as well as an important mechanism for the integration of divergent social groups.

Any attempt at an overview of health care provision and poor relief in Enlightenment and 19th century Prussia, however, will remain incomplete and unsatisfying. Regional differences within the Prussian monarchy were not only consequences of local peculiarities, but rather indicate divergent structures of the political, social, economic and cultural conditions. Only in the urban situation do certain similarities arise in the second half of the 19th century, which make it possible to provide an overview. The metropolis and royal residence of Berlin has to be regarded as atypical for Prussian cities in general, even if exemplary in other respects.

The rural and agricultural regions of Prussia, where three-quarters of the Prussian population lived as late as 1900,[198] have scarcely been researched with regard to health care and poor relief. In light of the structural differences between such rural regions as the Cologne–Aachen region and those in West and East Prussia, it is doubtful whether one would be able to speak of a single rural development, which could be compared with the urban development. The consequences of attempts like this would seem to suggest that the phenomenon of poverty was a specifically urban one or, even worse, that poverty did not exist 'in the countryside'. Both would be false conclusions. The lack of medical care for the sick and impoverished, especially the lack of hospital beds, was extremely grave in rural areas as late as 1900. Those incapable of obtaining appropriate care in the nearest, large town usually had to go without treatment.[199]

The implementation of comprehensive ideological and legislative prescriptions on welfare, as well as the changing balance between state responsibility and municipal enforcement, can, at least, be illustrated. The questions regarding survival strategies of the poor and sick, and those experiencing poverty and illness, however, remain unanswered. It is also unclear what the role of doctors was, especially that of the locally active poor-doctors. Although normative sources are available and known in the form of the pauperism literature of the day, doctors' reports, poverty directives, rules for welfare doctors and so on, too little is known still about the practices of poor-doctors to enable a contrast to be made between the literary figure of the heroic welfare doctor[200] and a more inconsistent – and consequently more realistic – image.

Notes

1. Gerhard Köbler, *Historisches Lexikon der Deutschen Länder. Die Deutschen Territorien und Reichsmittelbaren Geschlechter vom Mittelalter bis zur Gegenwart*, 5th edn, Munich 1995, pp. 477–80.
2. *Tabellen und amtliche Nachrichten über den Preußischen Staat für das Jahr 1849*. Vol. 4, Berlin 1853. Quoted by Christian Sachße and Florian Tennstedt in *Geschichte der Armenfürsorge in Deutschland*, Vol. 1: *Vom Spätmittelalter bis zum 1. Weltkrieg*, 2nd edn, Stuttgart, 1998, p. 269. See also Ernst Bruch, 'Königreich Preußen' in Alfred Emminghaus (ed.), *Das Armenwesen und die Armengesetzgebung in europäischen Staaten*, Berlin, 1870, pp. 25–67.
3. Robert Jütte, *Poverty and Deviance in Early Modern Europe. New Approaches to European History*, Cambridge, 1994; idem, *Obrigkeitliche Armenfürsorge in den deutschen Reichsstädten der frühen Neuzeit. Städtisches Armenwesen in Frankfurt am Main und Köln*, Köln, 1984; Thomas Fischer, *Städtische Armut und Armenfürsorge im 15. und 16. Jahrhundert. Sozialgeschichtliche Untersuchungen am Beispiel der Städte Basel, Freiburg im Breisgau und Straßburg*, Göttingen, 1979.
4. Ole Peter Grell and Andrew Cunningham (eds), *Health Care and Poor Relief in Protestant Europe 1500–1700*, London, 1997; Annemarie Kinzelbach, *Gesundbleiben, Krankwerden, Armsein in der frühzeitlichen Gesellschaft. Gesunde und Kranke in den Reichsstädten Überlingen und Ulm, 1500–1700*, Stuttgart, 1995.
5. See the entry 'Bevölkerung' in the *Deutsche Encyclopädie oder Allgemeines Real-Wörterbuch aller Künste und Wissenschaften von einer Gesellschaft Gelehrten*, Vol. 3, Frankfurt-am-Main 1780, pp. 511–16. See also 'Berechnung des Volkes im Lande' in Johann Georg Krünitz, *Oekonomische Encyclopädie oder allgemeines System der Staats- Stadt- Haus- und Landwirtschaft, in alphabetischer Ordnung*, Vol. 4, Berlin, 1783, pp. 210–28.
6. Alfons Labisch, *Homo Hygienicus, Gesundheit und Hygiene in der Neuzeit*, Frankfurt-am-Main and New York, 1992, pp. 77–79.
7. See Ragnhild Münch, *Gesundheitswesen im 18. Jahrhundert. Das Berliner Beispiel*, Berlin, 1995.
8. August Winkelmann, *Kenntniß der öffentlichen Gesundheitspflege. Zum Leitfaden seiner Vorlesungen über die medizinische Polizei*, Frankfurt-am-Main, 1804, p. 2.
9. Johann Peter Süßmilch, *Gedancken von den epidemischen Kranckheiten und dem größeren Sterben des 1757ten Jahres*, Berlin, 1758, p. 53. Cited from the facsimile in Herwig Birg (ed.), *Ursprünge der Demographie in Deutschland. Leben und Werk Johann Peter Süßmilchs (1707–1767)*, Forschungsberichte des Instituts für Bevölkerungsforschung und Sozialpolitik (IBS) Universität Bielefeld, Vol. 11, Frankfurt-am-Main and New York 1986, pp. 263–342. Christof Dipper, *Deutsche Geschichte, 1648–1789*, Frankfurt-am-Main 1991, pp. 42–75. On the causes and effects of the hunger crisis in Berlin in the early 1770s see Helga Schultz, *Berlin 1650–1800. Sozialgeschichte einer Residenz*, Berlin, 1987, pp. 296–304.
10. Johann Peter Frank, *Akademische Rede vom Volkselend als Mutter der Krankheiten*. Reprint of the edition Pavia 1790, Leipzig 1960. Markus Pieper, 'Der Körper des Volkes und der gesunde Volkskörper. Johann Peter Frank, *System einer vollständigen medicinischen Police*', *Zeitschrift für Geschichtswissenschaft*, **46** (1998), pp. 101–19.

11. Ute Frevert, *Krankheit als politisches Problem 1770–1880. Soziale Unterschichten in Preußen zwischen medizinischer Polizei und staatlicher Sozialversicherung. (Kritische Studien zur Geschichtswissenschaft Band 62)*, Göttingen, 1984, pp. 21–83. Francisca Loetz, '"Medikalisierung" in Frankreich, Großbritannien und Deutschland, 1750–1850: Ansätze, Ergebnisse und Perspektiven der Forschung', in Wolfgang U. Eckart and Robert Jütte (eds), *Das europäische Gesundheitssystem: Gemeinsamkeiten und Unterschiede in historischer Perspektive.* Medizin, Gesellschaft und Geschichte, Beiheft 3, Stuttgart, 1994, pp. 123–61.

12. Münch, *Gesundheitswesen* (n. 7), pp. 27–47.

13. Otto Ulbricht, 'Die Welt des Bettlers um 1775. Johann Gottfried Kästner', *Historische Anthropologie*, 2 (1994), pp. 371–98. In my opinion, the author's criticism of the concept of social disciplining does not deal with its theoretical content adequately. See also Christoph Sachße and Florian Tennstedt, *Soziale Sicherheit und soziale Disziplinierung. Beiträge zu einer Geschichte der Sozialpolitik.* Frankfurt-am-Main, 1986; see the arguments of Martin Dinges and Robert Jütte in *Geschichte und Gesellschaft*, **17** (1991); Norbert Finzsch and Robert Jütte (eds), *Institutions of Confinement: Hospitals, Asylums, and Prisons in Western Europe and North America, 1500–1950*, Cambridge, 1996; Sachße and Tennstedt, *Geschichte der Armenfürsorge* (n. 2), Vol. I, pp. 368–79.

14. One of the few works that methodically demonstrates such differences by using empirical data is Norbert Finzsch, *Obrigkeit und Unterschichten. Zur Geschichte der rheinischen Unterschichten gegen Ende des 18. und zu Beginn des 19. Jahrhunderts*, Stuttgart, 1990.

15. Ulbricht, 'Die Welt eines Bettlers' (n. 13). Martin Dinges, 'Aushandeln von Armut in der Frühen Neuzeit: Selbsthilfepotential, Bürgervorstellungen und Verwaltungslogiken' *Werkstatt Geschichte*, **10** (1995) pp. 7–15; Finzsch, *Obrigkeit und Unterschichten* (n. 14), pp. 55–62.

16. See Robert Jütte, 'Health Care Provision and Poor Relief in Early Modern Hanseatic Towns', in Grell and Cunningham *Health Care and Poor Relief* (n. 4), pp. 108–28. Jütte includes the 18th century in his article, 'which saw the most important changes in health care provision in Germany before the rise of the modern welfare state at the end of the last century'; Frevert, *Krankheit als politisches Problem* (n. 11), pp. 84–115.

17. Jütte, *Poverty and Deviance* (n. 3), p. 109f. See also August Winkelmann, *Litteratur der öffentlichen Armen- und Krankenpflege in Deutschland*, Braunschweig, 1802.

18. Sachße and Tennstedt, *Geschichte der Armenfürsorge* (n. 2), Vol. I, p. 130f.

19. Würzburg and Bamberg serve as examples of reforms originating from central government. See Eva Brinkschulte, *Krankenhaus und Krankenkassen. Soziale und Ökonomische Faktoren der Entstehung des modernen Krankenhauses im frühen 19. Jahrhundert. Die Beispiele Würzburg und Bamberg. (Abhandlungen zur Geschichte der Medizin und der Naturwissenschaften, Heft 80)*, Husum, 1998. The example of reforms initiated by a patriotic society is included in Mary Lindemann's chapter below.

20. Quoted from *Allgemeines Landrecht für die Preußischen Staaten von 1794* (hereafter ALR), Textausgabe, with an introduction by Hans Hattenhauer and a bibliography by Günther Bernert, Frankfurt-am-Main and Berlin 1970. An important work is Reinhart Koselleck, *Preußen zwischen Reform und Revolution. Allgemeines Landrecht, Verwaltung und soziale Bewegung von 1791 bis*

1848. Industrielle Welt. Schriftenreihe des Arbeitskreises für moderne Sozialgeschichte, Vol. 7, 2nd edn, Stuttgart, 1975, especially pp. 23–149 on the *Allgemeines Landrecht.* On the older Prussian legislation, see Michael Doege, *Armut in Preußen und Bayern (1770–1840),* Miscellanea Bavarica Monacensia, ed. Karl Bosl und Richard Bauer, Bd. 157, Munich, 1991, pp. 163–75; see also Reinhold August Dorwart, *The Prussian Welfare State before 1740.* Cambridge, MA, 1971.

21. *ALR* (n. 20), para. 1. On legislative developments, see also Emminghaus, *Das Armenwesen* (n. 2), pp. 41–48.
22. Emminghaus, *Das Armenwesen* (n. 2), p. 53.
23. A special Rhenish practice of expulsion of unwanted poor people to the Netherlands came to the attention of the Berlin ministry of the interior in July 1852; see Fritz Dross, 'Die Versorgung von Armut und Krankheit in Hilden in der ersten Hälfte des 19. Jahrhunderts', in *Stadt und Gesundheit. Zur Entwicklung des Gesundheitswesens in Hilden,* Hildener Museumshefte, Band 7, Hilden 1998, pp. 5–36.
24. Münch, *Gesundheitswesen* (n. 7), p. 155.
25. Quoted in Bernd Wagner, ' "Um die Leiden der Menschen zu lindern, bedarf es nicht eitler Pracht." Zur Finanzierung der Krankenhauspflege in Preußen', in Alfons Labisch and Reinhard Spree (eds), *Allgemeine Krankenhäuser – Wer bezahlt? Wer wird behandelt? Patienten, Finanzierung und Träger Allgemeiner Krankenhäuser in den Städten des 19. Jahrhunderts,* (forthcoming). Cf. the examples from Bielefeld and Liegnitz in Frevert, *Krankheit als politisches Problem* (n. 16), p. 158.
26. For example, in Silesia in 1835. See Doege, *Armut* (n. 20), p. 36.
27. Quoted in Wagner, 'Um die Leiden der Menschen' (n. 25).
28. *ALR* (n. 26), II, 19, para. 12.
29. Ibid., II, 8, para. 355.
30. Wolfgang R. Krabbe, *Die deutsche Stadt im 19. und 20. Jahrhundert,* Göttingen, 1989, p. 8f.
31. *Ordnung für sämmtliche Städte der Preußischen Monarchie mit dazu gehöriger Instruktion, Behuf der Geschäftsführung der Stadtverordneten bei ihren ordnungsgemäßen Versammlungen. Vom 19ten November 1808,* para. 179, section c. *Sammlung der für die Königlichen Preußischen Staaten erschienenen Gesetze und Verordnungen von 1806 bis zum 27ten Oktober 1810,* Berlin, 1822, pp. 324–60.
32. Münch, *Gesundheitswesen* (n. 7), p. 150ff.
33. Schultz, *Berlin 1650–1800* (n. 9), p. 317.
34. In this context, Münch states that 'in the end the city physicians were more of an extension of the police authority than coordinators of general health care.' Münch, *Gesundheitswesen* (n. 7), p. 67.
35. Schultz, *Berlin 1650–1800* (n. 9), p. 315f.
36. On the discussion regarding the 'modernising' function of the state's intervention in municipal matters, see also Berthold Grzywatz, 'Residenziale Kommunaladministration im Zeitalter des Absolutismus. Die Konstituierung staatlich-städtischer Integration am Beispiel Berlins', *Zeitschrift für Geschichtswissenschaft,* **46** (1998), pp. 406–31.
37. See also Mary Lindemann's chapter in this volume.
38. Ludovica Scarpa, *Gemeinwohl und lokale Macht. Honoratorien und Armenwesen in der Berliner Luisenstadt im 19. Jahrhundert,* Munich, 1995.

39. Quoted in Sachße and Tennstedt, *Geschichte der Armenfürsorge* (n. 2), Vol. I, p. 152f.

40. Volker Hunecke, 'Überlegungen zur Geschichte der Armut im vorindustriellen Europa', *Geschichte und Gesellschaft*, **9** (1983), pp. 480–512 at p. 484.

41. See also Werner Conze, 'Arbeit', Otto Brunner, Werner Conze and Reinhart Koselleck (eds), *Geschichtliche Grundbegriffe. Historisches Lexikon zur politisch-sozialen Sprache in Deutschland*, Stuttgart, 1972, Vol. 1, pp. 154–215.

42. Christian E. Fischer, *Versuch einer Anleitung zur medizinischen Armenpraxis*, Göttingen, 1799, p. 41f.

43. C.W. Hufeland, 'Die Armenkrankenverpflegung zu Berlin, nebst dem Entwurfe einer Armenpharmakopöe', *Journal der practischen Heilkunde*, **XXIX** (1809).

44. Ibid.

45. See also A.F.H. Hecker, 'Welches sind die bequemsten und wohlfeilsten Mittel, kranken Armen in den Städten die nöthige Hülfe zu verschaffen?', *Beiträge zum Archiv der medizinischen Polizei und der Volksarzneikunde*, **V** (1795), pp. 31–72. For an 18th century discussion, see Isabelle von Bueltzingsloewen, *Machines à instruire, machines à guérir. Les hôpitaux universitaires et la médicalisation de la société allemande 1730–1850*, Lyons, 1997, pp. 87–100.

46. Bernd Wagner, 'Armut, Krankheit und Gesundheitswesen im vorindustriellen Bielefeld', *Jahresbericht des Historischen Vereins für die Grafschaft Ravensberg*, **77** (1988–89), p. 89.

47. Schultz, *Berlin 1650–1800* (n. 9), pp. 269–73 at pp. 296–319.

48. See also Arthur E. Imhof, 'Die Funktion des Krankenhauses in der Stadt des 18. Jahrhunderts', *Zeitschrift für Stadtgeschichte, Stadtsoziologie und Denkmalpflege*, **4** (1977), pp. 215–42; Münch, *Gesundheitswesen* (n. 7), p. 75. See also papers from a conference on the relationship between science and health care in the Charité during the 18th and 19th centuries edited by Eric J. Engstrom and Volker Hess in the *Jahrbuch für Universitätsgeschichte*, **3** (2000).

49. Theodor Philipp von der Hagen, 'Nachricht, von den berlinschen deutschen Armen-Anstalten', *Magazin für die Neue Historie und Geographie*, **XII**, Halle 1778, pp. 493–502. Quoted in Sachße and Tennstedt, *Geschichte der Armenfürsorge* (n. 2), Vol. I, p. 153.

50. Quoted in Münch, *Gesundheitswesen* (n. 7), p. 178.

51. Hufeland, *'Die Armenkrankenverpflegung'*, p. 9.

52. Schultz, *Berlin 1650–1800*, p. 270.

53. Hufeland, 'Die Armenkrankenverpflegung' (n. 43), p. 13. Münch, *Gesundheitswesen* (n. 7), p. 155.

54. See Mary Lindemann's chapter below; also von Bueltzingsloewen, *Machines à instruire* (n. 45), pp. 87–100.

55. Hufeland, 'Die Armenkrankenverpflegung' (n. 43), p. 10: The influence of this discussion and particularly the influence of Hufeland has, in my opinion, been ignored by Münch, *Gesundheitswesen* (n. 7), p. 177.

56. See also Bernd Sösemann (ed.), *Gemeingeist und Bürgersinn: Die preußischen Reformen*, Forschungen zur brandenburgischen und preußischen Geschichte, NF Beiheft 2, Berlin, 1993. Barbara Vogel (ed.), *Preußische Reformen 1807–1820*, Neue wissenschaftliche Bibliothek, Band 96, Königsstein and Taunus, 1980.

57. Wagner, 'Armut, Krankheit und Gesundheitswesen' (n. 46), describes corresponding developments in Bielefeld.

58. Hermann Beck, *The Origins of the Authoritarian Welfare State in Prussia*.

      Conservatives, Bureaucracy and the Social Question, 1815–1870, Ann Arbor, 1995, pp. 169–74.

59. See also Carl Jantke and Dietrich Hilger, *Die Eigentumslosen. Der deutsche Pauperismus und die Emanzipationskrise in Darstellungen und Deutungen der zeitgenössischen Literatur*, Orbis Academicus Geschichte der politischen Ideen in Dokumenten und Darstellungen, Freiburg and München, 1965; Lieselotte Dilcher, *Der deutsche Pauperismus und seine Literatur*, Frankfurt-am-Main, 1957.

60. See also, on the more recent discussion on pauperism, Günther Schulze, 'Armut und Armenpolitik in Deutschland im frühen 19. Jahrhundert', *Historisches Jahrbuch*, **115** (1995), pp. 388–410.

61. See also Beck, *Origins* (n. 58), pp. 31–122.

62. See the 'classic' definition according to the Brockhaus encyclopedia of 1846, quoted in Hans-Ulrich Wehler, *Deutsche Gesellschaftsgeschichte*, Vol. 2: *Von der Reformära bis zur industriellen und politischen 'Deutschen Doppelrevolution' 1815–1845/49*, **2**, Edition München 1989, 283. See also Wolfram Fischer, *Armut in der Geschichte. Erscheinungsformen und Lösungsversuche der 'Sozialen Frage' in Europa seit dem Mittelalter*, Göttingen, 1982. The quotation from the Brockhaus is on p. 62. See also the review in Beck, *Origins*, (n. 58), pp. 1–30, as well as Conze, 'Arbeit' (n. 4).

63. Quoted in Doege, *Armut* (n. 20), p. 56 and 212f.

64. In my opinion, this contradiction is ignored by Beck, *Origins* (n. 58). Thus proving that the Prussian ministerial bureaucracy did not follow liberal, but rather conservative patterns in its social policy is not very enlightening.

65. Ibid., pp. 149–68; Doege, *Armut* (n. 20), p. 210: 'The Ministry of Justice was practically flooded with complaints from municipalities about the poor relief obligations they were burdened with.'

66. Interior Minister Schuckmann called for a corresponding vote in May, 1824: See Doege, *Armut* (n. 20) p. 199f; Beck, *Origins* (n. 58), p. 152f.

67. 'Gesetz über die Aufnahme neu anziehender Personen', paras 4, 5, emphasis by FD. *Sammlung 1843*, pp. 5–7. See also the vote of Schuckmann of May 1824 in Doege, *Armut* (n. 20), p. 199f.

68. 'Gesetz über die Verpflichtung zur Armenpflege', para 1, Abs. 3. *Sammlung 1843*, 8–14.

69. Ibid., para. 2. See also Reskript des K. Min. of the Interior of 21 October 1843, quoted in W. G. von der Heyde, *Staats- und Orts- Angehörigkeits- und Armenverpflegungs-Verhältnisse, so wie polizeiliche Behandlung der Bettler, Landstreicher und Arbeitsscheuen. Geordnet durch die Gesetzgebung der Jahre 1842 und 1843, die darauf bezüglichen Ministerial-Rescripte und die aus der ältern Gesetzgebung noch zur Anwendung kommenden Vorschriften*, Magdeburg, 1844, p. 59. On the judicial and administrative interpretation of the three poor laws of 31 December 1842 and 6 January 1843, see also W. Dittmar, *Die Gesetze vom 31. Dezember 1842 und 6. Januar 1843 … nebst den dieselben ergänzenden und erläuternden Gesetzen, Verordnungen, Ministerial-Reskripten und Judikaten des Ober-Tribunals und des Gerichtshofes zur Entscheidung der Kompetenz-Konflikte …* , Magdeburg, 1862.

70. *Sammlung 1843* (n. 67), p. 19f.

71. Wilhelm Roscher, *System der Armenpflege und Armenpolitik*, Stuttgart, 1894. Quoted in Sachße and Tennstedt, *Geschichte der Armenfürsorge* (n. 2), Vol. I, p. 281.

72. Arno Pokiser, 'Armut und Armenfürsorge in Berlin 1800 bis 1850. Von den

Schwierigkeiten im Umgang mit neuen Phänomenen', in K. Wernicke (ed.), *Neue Streifzüge in die Berliner Kulturgeschichte. Von Arbeitern und Armen, Schriftstellern und Schützen, Spaßvögeln und Streithähnen, Vereinen und Verkehrswegen*, Berlin, 1995, pp. 19–86, quote at p. 21.

73. Quoted in Jürgen Reulecke, *Geschichte der Urbanisierung in Deutschland*, Frankfurt-am-Main, 1985, p. 37. See also Beck, *Origins* (n. 58), p. 163, on the sceptical stance of the Rhenish provincial parliament to the poverty laws of 1842.

74. See note 23 *supra*.

75. 'Städteordnung für die sechs östlichen Provinzen der preußischen Monarchie vom 30. Mai 1853', *Sammlung 1853*, pp. 261–90.

76. 'Gesetz zur Ergänzung der Gesetze vom 31. Dezember 1842 über die Verpflichtung zur Armenpflege und die Aufnahme neu anziehender Personen, vom 21, Mai 1855', *Sammlung 1855*, pp. 311–15.

77. Krabbe, *Die deutsche Stadt* (n. 30), pp. 99–107. See also Reulecke, *Urbanisierung* (n. 73), p. 212. The figures on the annual expenditures for poor relief are difficult to compare directly with each other because the degree to which old foundations and donations were incorporated into the (central) municipal welfare facilities varied greatly. The amounts spent by new, bourgeois, associations for private charity are likewise not immediately comparable between cities. Emminghaus, *Das Armenwesen* (n. 2), p. 62, presents the welfare expenditures for the Prussian districts in 1849, as well as their sources from the municipal budgets, foundations or private funds.

78. 'Gesetz über den Unterstützungswohnsitz vom 6. Juni 1870', *Bundes-Gesetzblatt des Norddeutschen Bundes 1870*, pp. 360–73.

79. 'Gesetz betr. die Ausführung des Bundesgesetzes über den Unterstützungswohnsitz vom 8. März 1871', *Sammlung 1871*, pp. 130–51.

80. von der Heyde, *Armenverpflegungs-Verhältnisse* (n. 69), p. 62ff.; Dittmar, *Die Gesetze* (n. 69), p. 301f.; Emminghaus, *Das Armenwesen*, (n. 2), p. 66f.

81. The *Allgemeine Kranken- und Sterbelade*, established in 1841 in Düsseldorf, had the goal of ensuring the members adequate pay during illness in return for minimal premiums. See Margaret Asmuth, *Gewerbliche Unterstützungskassen in Düsseldorf. Die Entwicklung der Krankenversicherung der Arbeitnehmern 1841 bis 1884/5*, Köln, 1984, p. 26. Frevert, *Krankheit als politisches Problem* (n. 11), pp. 151–61.

82. Annette Godefroid, 'Das Berliner Krankenkassenwesen im 19. Jahrhundert. Von der "Auflage" zur AOK', in Wernicke, *Neue Streifzüge*, (n. 72), pp. 87–108.

83. Joseph Bücheler, *Die Reform des Armen-Wesens mit Rücksicht auf den Entwurf der neuen Armen-Ordnung zu Düsseldorf.* Düsseldorf, 1851, p. 9f. Similar quotations abound. For a more sober account, see also Emminghaus, *Das Armenwesen* (n. 2), p. 22. This was one of the few points that aroused no comments during the debates on the two laws of 31 December, 1842; see Beck, *Origins* (n. 58), p. 157f.

84. See also von der Heyde, *Armenverpflegungs-Verhältnisse* (n. 69), p. 72f. and pp. 124–27.

85. Wagner, *Armut, Krankheit und Gesundheitswesen* (n. 46), pp. 83 and 100.

86. The welfare authorities in Cologne had a budget item for 'impoverished artisan masters' in the 1830s; see Gisela Mettele, *Bürgertum in Köln 1775–1870. Gemeinsinn und freie Association*, Stadt und Bürgertum, Volume 10, München, 1998, p. 134. On the social situation of craftsmen, see also Friedrich Lenger,

Zwischen Kleinbürgertum und Proletariat. Studien zur Sozialgeschichte der Düsseldorfer Handwerker 1816–1878, Kritische Studien zur Geschichtswissenschaft, Band 7, Göttingen, 1986.

87.   Quoted in Frevert, *Krankheit als politisches Problem* (n. 11), p. 16. On poor relief in Elberfeld and Barmen, see Bernd Weisbrod, 'Wohltätigkeit und "symbolische Gewalt" in der Frühindustrialisierung. Städtische Armut und Armenpolitik im Wuppertal', in Hans Mommsen and Winfried Schulze (eds), *Vom Elend der Handarbeit: Probleme historischer Unterschichtenforschung*, Stuttgart, 1981, pp. 334–57. On the situation in Berlin, see Scarpa, *Gemeinwohl* (n. 38), pp. 248–54.

88.   Frevert, *Krankheit als politisches Problem* (n. 11), p. 161. See also the Cabinet Directive of 9 August 1827 on the establishment of obligatory contributions for municipal servants' insurance in von der Heyde, *Armenverpflegungs-Verhältnisse* (n. 69), p. 124.

89.   'Allgemeine Gewerbeordnung vom 17. Januar 1845', *Sammlung 1845*, pp. 41–78, especially paras 168–70.

90.   'Verordnung, betreffend die Errichtung von Gewerberäthen und verschiedene Abänderungen der allgemeinen Gewerbeordnung vom 9. Februar 1849', *Sammlung 1849*, pp. 93–124, particularly paras 56–59.

91.   'Gesetz, betreffend die gewerblichen Unterstützungskassen vom 3. April 1854', *Sammlung 1854*, p. 138f.

92.   Quoted in Asmuth, *Gewerbliche Unterstützungskassen* (n. 81), p. 19. On the *Unterstützungskassen* in the Rhineland and Westphalia, see also Ludwig Puppke, *Sozialpolitik und soziale Anschauungen frühindustrieller Unternehmer in Rheinland-Westfalen*, Schriften zur rheinisch-westfälischen Wirtschaftsgeschichte; NF Band 13, Cologne, 1966, pp. 82–166.

93.   'Gewerbeordnung für den Norddeutschen Bund vom 21. Juni 1869', *Bundes-Gesetzblatt für den Norddeutschen Bund 1869*.

94.   On the development in membership in the commercial *Unterstützungskassen* and *Knappschaftskassen*, see Wolfram Fischer, *Materlialen zur Statistik des Deutschen Bundes 1815–1870*, Sozialgeschichtliches Arbeitsbuch I, p. 208f.; Johannes Frerich and Martin Frey, *Handbuch der Geschichte der Sozialpolitik in Deutschland*, Volume 1: *Von der vorindustriellen Zeit bis zum Ende des Dritten Reiches*, Munich and Vienna 1993, Tables 3 and 4, 57 and 64.

95.   See the chronological register of pertinent laws, directives, decrees, and so on from 1793 to 5 May 1861 in Dittmar, *Die Gesetze* (n. 69), pp. 442–47.

96.   See Beck, *Origins* (n. 58), pp. 201–9, fn. 30, which describes the motives of the Prussian Minister of Culture Altenstein, who had been concerned with this matter since 1828. 'One of the main tenets of the factory bill was to enforce school attendance.'

97.   The annual defence report of Lieutenant General Horn of 1828 ascertained an alarming fall in the number of raid-capable (*aushebungsfähig*) recruits in the Rhenish industrial areas. On the refutation of the Horn legend, see A.H.G. Meyer, 'Schule und Kinderarbeit. Das Verhältnis von Schul- und Sozialpolitik in der Entwicklung der preußischen Volksschule zu Beginn des 19. Jahrhunderts', Philosophy dissertation, Hamburg, 1971; Alfons Labisch, 'Die Montanindustrie in der Gewerbeaufsicht des Regierungsbezirks Düsseldorf', *L'Homme et la terre – Mens en aarde – Mensch und Erde. Actes du 13e Congrès Benelux d'Histoire des Sciences, Echternach 5.-7. October 1995*, Luxembourg, 1996, pp. 41–72, especially at p. 48f.

98.   See *Quellensammlung zur Geschichte der deutschen Sozialpolitik 1867 bis*

1914. Begründet von Peter Rassow im Auftrag der Historischen Kommission der Akademie der Wissenschaften und Literatur edited by Karl Erich Born, Hansjoachim Henning and Florian Tennstedt, I. Abt., Volume 3: Arbeiterschutz. Ed. Wolfgang Ayass, Stuttgart, Jena, New York 1996.

99. Barbara Dettke, *Die asiatische Hydra. Die Cholera von 1830/31 in Berlin und den preußischen Provinzen Posen, Preußen und Schlesien,* Veröffentlicheungen der Historischen Kommission zu Berlin, Volume 89, Berlin and New York, 1995; Olaf Briese, 'Das Jüste-milieu hat die Cholera. Metaphern und Mentalitäten im 19. Jahrhundert', *Zeitschrift für Geschichtswissenschaft,* **46** (1998), pp. 120–38.

100. See Alfons Labisch, 'Experimentelle Hygiene, Bakteriologie, Soziale Hygiene: Konzeptionen, Interventionen, soziale Träger – eine idealtypische Übersicht' in Jürgen Reulecke and Adelheid Gräfin zu Castell Rüdenhausen (eds), *Stadt und Gesundheit. Zum Wandel von 'Volksgesundheit' und kommunaler Gesundheits-politik im 19. und frühen 20. Jahrhundert,* Nassauer Gespräche der Freiherr-vom-Stein-Gesellschaft, Volume 3, Stuttgart, 1991, pp. 37–47. Alfons Labisch and Wolfgang Woelk, 'Geschichte der Gesundheitswissenschaften' in Klaus Hurrelmann and Ulrich Laaser (eds), *Handbuch Gesundheitswissenschaften,* new edn, Weinheim and Munich, 1998, pp. 49–89.

101. Dettke, *Die asiatische Hydra* (n. 99), p. 8. She compares the effect of the cholera epidemic of 1830–31 with the Silesian weavers' uprising of 1844, as the most important event during the *Vormärz* which ripped the Prussian bour-geois out of their *Biedermeier* lethargy and drew their attention to the social ills in their immediate vicinity.

102. Ibid., p. 178.

103. Ibid., p. 172f.

104. See the cabinet order of 8 August which regulates hygienic measures for the most common infectious diseases, *Sammlung 1835,* pp. 240–86.

105. See Alfons Labisch and Reinhard Spree, 'Die Kommunalisierung des Kranken-hauswesens in Deutschland während des 19. und 20. Jahrhunderts' in Josef Wysocki (ed.), *Kommunalisierung im Spannungsfeld von Regulierung und Deregulierung im 19. und 20. Jahrhundert,* Schriften des Vereins für Socialpolitik, Gesellschaft für Wirtschafts- und Sozialwissenschaften, NF. 240, Berlin, 1995, pp. 7–47.

106. See Thomas Küster, *Alte Armut und neues Bürgertum. Öffentliche und private Fürsorge in Münster von der Ära Fürstenberg bis zum Ersten Weltkrieg (1756–1914).* Studien zur Geschichte der Armenfürsorge und der Sozialpolitik in Münster, Volume 2, Quellen und Forschungen zur Geschichte der Stadt Münster, NF 17/2, Münster, 1995, pp. 149–153; Dieter Körschner, 'Der Kampf ums Cholerahospital in Bonn im Jahre 1832', in Manfred van Rey and Norbert Schloßmacher (eds), *Bonn und das Rheinland. Beiträge zur Geschichte und Kultur einer Region. FS für Dietrich Hörold,* Bonn, 1992, pp. 277–310. Bernd Wagner, *Das Bielefelder Krankenhaus im 19. Jahrhundert,* Master's thesis, Bielefeld 1988, 2. Aufl. Bielefeld 1994; idem, *Armut, Krankheit und Gesund-heitswesen* (n. 46). In Düsseldorf in 1832, Karl Heinrich Ebermaier, a hospital doctor, became an energetic supporter of improved communal hospitals after he studied the effects of cholera as an *Hilfsarbeiter* of the royal government in Berlin and Magdeburg in 1831. The report submitted by Privy Councillor Esse on his tours of the lunatic asylums and hospitals in the Rhine Province had special ramifications, being particularly critical of the municipal hospital in Düsseldorf. HStA Düsseldorf, Regierung Düsseldorf, 1616, pp. 181–92.

107. Instruction über das bei der Annäherung der Cholera, so wie über das bei dem Ausbruche derselben in den Königl. Preuß. Staaten zu beobachtende Verfahren. Berlin 1 Juni 1831. paras 13–15. See also paras 21–22, 40–41, 50 in *Beilage zum Amtsblatt der Regierung zu Düsseldorf Nr. 62*, Düsseldorf, 22. August 1831. On the appointment of the Intermediat-Kommission in Berlin and its 'technical department,' who produced the directive, see Dettke, *Die asiatische Hydra* (n. 99), pp. 74–76.

108. 'Regulativ über die sanitäts-polizeilichen Vorschriften bei den am häufigsten vorkommenden ansteckenden Krankheiten vom 8. August 1835', *Sammlung 1835*, pp. 239–286, paras 16, 24.

109. Ibid., para. 18 a).

110. Fischer, *Sozialgeschichtliches Arbeitsbuch I* (n. 3), p. 205. Further material is available in S. Neumann, 'Die Krankenanstalten im Preußischen Staate, nach den bisherigen vom statistischen Büreau über dieselben veröffentlichten Nachrichten', *Archiv für Landeskunde der Preußischen Monarchie*, 5 (1858), erstes Quartal, 345–88, as well as in Reinhard Spree, '*Quantitative Aspekte der Entwicklung des Krankenhauswesens im 19. und 20. Jahrhundert: Ein Bild innerer und :äußerer Verhältnisse*', in Alfons Labisch and Reinhard Spree (eds), '*Einem jeden Kranken in einem Hospitale sein eigenes Bett.' Zur Sozialgeschichte des Allgemeinen Krankenhauses in Deutschland im 19. Jahrhundert*, New York and Frankfurt: Campus, 1996, pp. 51–88; idem, 'Krankenhausentwicklung und Sozialpolitik in Deutschland während des 19. Jahrhunderts' in *Historische Zeitschrift*, 260 (1995), pp. 75–105.

111. Neumann, 'Die Krankenanstalten' (n. 110), p. 350.

112. Alfons Labisch, 'Stadt und Krankenhaus. Das Allgemeine Krankenhaus in der kommunalen Sozial- und Gesundheitspolitik des 19. Jahrhunderts' in Labisch and Spree (eds.), *Einem jeden Kranken* (n. 110), p. 253–96, especially pp. 268–74.

113. On the 'Elberfeld system,' see Sachße and Tennstedt, *Geschichte der Armenfürsorge* (n. 2), Vol. I, pp. 214–56; Florian Tennstedt, *Sozialgeschichte der Sozialpolitik*, Göttingen, 1981, pp. 95–100.

114. Scarpa, *Gemeinwohl* (n. 38) on the 'Prinzip Nachbarschaft', p. 329f.

115. Ibid., pp. 166–68, 335–37, as well as Christoph Sachße, 'Frühformen der Leistungsverwaltung: die kommunale Armenfürsorge im deutschen Kaiserreich', *Jahrbuch für europäische Verwaltungsgeschichte*, 5 (1993), pp. 1–20.

116. Erlaß über die Einführung der am 3. November errichteten Wohlthätigkeitsanstalten zum 1. Dezember 1811 vom 5. März 1811; J.J. Scotti, *Sammlung der Gesetze und Verordnungen, welche in den ehemaligen Herzogthümern Jülich, Cleve und Berg und in dem vormaligen Großherzogthum Berg über die Gegenstände der Landeshoheit, Verfassung, Verwaltung und Rechtspflege ergangen sind*. 4 Teile, Düsseldorf 1821/22, No. 3226, 1416; HStA Düsseldorf Großherzogtum Berg 4682–4684.

117. *Gesetz-Bulletin des Großherzogthums Berg / Bulletin des lois du Grand-Duche de Berg*, 2. Teil, No. 2, Düsseldorf 1810, Dekret No. 5, pp. 92–123. On the legal orientation of the welfare system on the French model in the Kingdom of Westphalia, see Susanne Grindel and Winfried Speitkamp (eds), *Armenfürsorge in Hessen-Kassel. Dokumente zur Vorgeschichte der Sozialpolitik zwischen Aufklärung und Industrialisierung*, Veröffentlichungen der Historischen Kommission für Hessen, Volume 62, Marburg, 1998, Dokumente 37–39, 76–86.

118. Calixte Hudemann-Simon, *L'Etat et les Pauvres. L'Assistance et la Lutte*

contre la Mendicité dans les Quatre Départements Rhénans, 1794–1814, Beiheft der Francia, Vol. 41, Sigmaringen, 1997; August von Pommer-Esche, 'Die französiche Gesetzgebung über das Armenwesen bis zur Trennung der Rheinprovinz von Frankreich', *Archiv für Landeskunde der Preußischen Monarchie* 6 (2) (1859) Quartal, 209–47; Rudolf Schwander, *Die Armenpolitik Frankreichs während der großen Revolution und die Weiterentwicklung der französischen Armengesetzgebung bis zur Gegenwart*, Straßburg, 1904.

119. Poor relief by the parishes was strongly supported by the ministry for spiritual matters. GStA PK Archiv I B, Min. d. Inn., Rep. 77 Tit. 223 e.

120. The *Bezirksregierung* reminded the ministry of the interior in July 1823: 'Es scheint, daß der Berichterstatter .. ein hohes Ministerium nicht genau über das Verhältniß unterrichtet habe. [...] Ew. Excellenz ersuchen wir, .. bei künftigen Beschwerden gegen unsere Verfügungen, uns vor allen Dingen ein hochgeneigtes Gehör schenken zu wollen': GStA PK HA I B, Min. d. Inn., Rep. 77 Tit. 223 e, Armensachen der Rheinprovinz 1818–1830 (no page numbers). The *Bezirksregierung* pleaded its case for municipal poor relief, as 'hier überall in den Fabrikgegenden die kirchlichen Gemeinden verschiedenen Bekenntnisses durch einander leben und fast in der Regel die eine dieser Gemeinden allen Reichthum des Orts in sich vereinigt, während die anderen aus den wenig bemittelten und dürftigen Miteinwohnern desselben Orts besteht': ibid.

121. Ibid.; StA Düsseldorf II 1611, Bl. 60; *Amtsblatt der Regierung zu Düsseldorf* Nr. 79, 12. November 1825, pp. 633–35; *Bilanz über Empfang und Ausgabe bey der Hauptverwaltung der allgemeinen Armen-Versorgungs-Anstalt zu Düsseldorf für das Jahr 1822*, Düsseldorf o. J. [1823], Vorwort; *Übersicht der Einnahme und Ausgabe in den Jahren 1825–1833*, Düsseldorf, 1834: *Die unterzeichnete Central-Armen-Verwaltung, nach Vorschrift des Dekrets vom 8ten November 1809 gebildet*.

122. On the welfare system of the city of Cologne under French rule (1794–1814), see Finzsch, *Obrigkeit und Unterschichten* (n. 14).

123. Ulrike Dorn, *Öffentliche Armenpflege in Köln 1794–1871. Zugleich ein Beitrag zur Geschichte der öffentlichrechtlichen Anstalt*, Rheinisches Archiv, Vol. 127, Cologne and Vienna, 1990.

124. Mettele, *Bürgertum in Köln* (n. 86), pp. 132–57.

125. The poverty administration took the magistracy by surprise in 1864, when it did not direct the surplus from the capital of the convents to general poor relief, but rather to reserves, which raised the municipal contribution to the poverty fund from 67 940 to 92 782 thaler! See Dorn, *Öffentliche Armenpflege* (n. 123), p. 162.

126. Weisbrod, 'Wohltätigkeit' (n. 87), p. 352.

127. A. Lammers, 'Stadt Elberfeld' in Emminghaus, *Das Armenwesen* (n. 2), pp. 89–97, cited at p. 89f.

128. *Verwaltungs-Bericht für das Jahr 1851 und Etat der Gemeinde Düsseldorf für das Jahr 1852*, vorgetragen vom Bürgermeister Hammers, Düsseldorf, 1852, p. 19; Otto Most, *Geschichte der Stadt Düsseldorf*, Vol. 2: *Von 1815 bis zur Einführung der Rheinischen Städteordnung (1856)*. Düsseldorf, 1921, page 387f.; StAD II 2209 contains the *Instruction für die Bezirks-Armen Commissionen der Bürgermeisterei Düsseldorf* of 25 August 1851; Bücheler, *Die Reform des Armen-Wesens* (n. 53).

129. *Bericht über die Verwaltung und den Stand der Gemeinde-Angelegenheiten der Stadt Düsseldorf für den Zeitraum vom 1. April 1877 bis 31. März 1878*, Düsseldorf 1878, pp. 75–83.

130. Küster, *Alte Armut* (n. 106), pp. 153–66.

131. Ibid., pp. 239–43.

132. Ibid., p. 245f.

133. Münch, *Gesundheitswesen* (n. 7), pp. 150–71; Scarpa, *Gemeinwohl* (n. 38); H. Schwabe, 'Das Armenwesen in Berlin', in Emminghaus, *Armenwesen* (n. 2), pp. 68–88.

134. Berthold Grzywatz, 'Armenfürsorge im 19. Jahrhundert. Die Grenzen der kommunalen Daseinsvorsorge', *Zeitschrift für Geschichtswissenschaft*, **47** (1999), pp. 583–614.

135. 'Städte-Ordnung für die sechs östlichen Provinzen der Preußischen Monarchie vom 30. Mai 1853', *Sammlung* 1853, pp. 261–90.

136. Scarpa, *Gemeinwohl* (n. 38), p. 335.

137. Grzywatz, 'Armenfürsorge' (n. 134), p. 602f.

138. Mettele, *Bürgertum in Köln* (n. 86), p. 139f. On the spatial distribution, see Pierre Aycoberry, *Köln zwischen Napoleon und Bismarck. Das Wachstum einer rheinischen Stadt*, Kölner Schriften zur Geschichte und Kultur, Volume 20, Cologne, 1996, p. 418.

139. See the comprehensive study of Meinolf Nitsch, *Private Wohltätigkeitsvereine im Kaiserreich. Die praktische Umsetzung der bürgerlichen Sozialreform in Berlin*, Veröffentlichungen der Historischen Kommission zu Berlin, Volume 98, Berlin and New York, 1999.

140. See also Jürgen Reulecke, 'Stadtbürgertum und bürgerliche Sozialreform im 19. Jahrhundert in Preußen' in Lothar Gall (ed.), *Stadt und Bürgertum im 19. Jahrhundert*, Munich, 1990, pp. 171–97; Christoph Sachße and Florian Tennstedt, *Geschichte der Armenfürsorge in Deutschland. Vol. 2: Fürsorge und Wohlfahrtspflege 1871–1929*, Stuttgart, 1988; Jürgen Reulecke (ed.), *Die Stadt als Dienstleistungszentrum. Beiträge zur Geschichte der 'Sozialstadt' in Deutschland im 19. und frühen 20. Jahrhundert*, St Katharinen, 1995; idem, *Geschichte der Urbanisierung* (n. 73), pp. 62–67, 118–31; Krabbe, *Die deutsche Stadt* (n. 30), pp. 99–128.

141. Rudolf Schwander, *Bericht über die Neuordnung der Hausarmenpflege der Stadt Straßburg, erstattet von Dr. Schwander*, Strasbourg, 1905. Quoted in Sachße and Tennstedt, *Geschichte der Armenfürsorge* (n. 2), Vol. I, p. 221.

142. Krabbe, *Die deutsche Stadt* (n. 30), p. 35.

143. Ibid., quoted from a decision of the Prussian *Oberverwaltungsgerichts* in Berlin of 15 February 1885.

144. Otto Most, 'Städtische Krankenanstalten im Lichte vergleichender Finanzstatistik' in *Zeitschrift für Soziale Medizin*, **5** (1910), pp. 213–36 and 334–58, especially p. 215.

145. See also the figures in Moritz Fürst, *Stellung und Aufgaben des Arztes in der öffentlichen Armenpflege*, Jena, 1903; also M. Fürst and F. Windscheid (eds), *Handbuch der Sozialen Medizin*, 8 vols, Jena, Vol. 1, pp. 116–19.

146. Reinhard Spree, 'Krankenhausentwicklung und Sozialpolitik', *Historische Zeitschrift*, **260** (1995), Table 1, p. 87; Alfons Labisch and Florian Tennstedt, 'Die allgemeinen Krankenhäuser der Städte und Religionsgemeinschaften Ende des 19. Jahrhunderts – Statistische und juristische Anmerkungen am Beispiel Preußens (1877–1903)' in Labisch and Spree, *Einem jeden Kranken* (n. 25), pp. 297–319.

147. Erwin Gatz, *Kirche und Krankenpflege im 19. Jahrhundert. Katholische Bewegung und karitativer Aufbruch in den preussischen Provinzen Rheinland und Westfalen*, Munich, 1971; Norbert Paul, 'Zwischen "christlichem Frauenamt" und

professioneller Krankenversorgung', *Medizinhistorisches Journal*, **33** (1998), pp. 143–60; Walter Klein, *Die ersten Krankenschwestern in Saarbrücken. Die Übernahme des Bürgerhospitals durch Kaiserswerther Diakonissen im Jahre 1841 und deren erste Zeit.* Master's thesis Saarbrücken 1993; Dominik Gross, '"Deprofessionalisierung" oder "Paraprofessionalisierung"? Die berufliche Entwicklung der Hebammen und ihr Stellenwert in der Geburtshilfe des 19. Jahrhunderts', *Sudhoffs Archiv*, **82** (1998), pp. 219–38.

148. See also Reulecke and Rüdenhausen, *Stadt und Gesundheit* (n. 100). A current discussion of the state of research can be found in Alfons Labisch and Jörg Vögele, 'Stadt und Gesundheit. Anmerkungen zur neueren sozial- und medizinhistorischen Diskussion in Deutschland', *Archiv für Sozialgeschichte*, **37** (1997), pp. 396–424.

149. Münch, *Gesundheitswesen* (n. 7), p. 67ff.

150. Max von Pettenkofer, 'Ueber den Werth der Gesundheit für eine Stadt. Zwei populäre Vorlesungen, gehalten am 26. und 29. März 1873 im Verein für Volksbildung in München' in idem, *Populäre Vorträge*, Zweites Heft, Braunschweig, 1876.

151. Jörg Vögele and Wolfgang Woelk (eds), *Stadt, Krankheit und Tod. Städtische Gesundheitsverhältnisse während der Epidemiologischen Transition*, Berlin, 2000. See also the excellent work on the Essen edited by Klaus Wisotzky and Michael Zimmermann, *Selbstverständlichkeiten. Strom, Wasser, Gas und andere Versorgungseinrichtungen: Die Vernetzung der Stadt um die Jahrhundertwende. Veröffentlichungen des Stadtarchivs Essen*, Volume 2, Essen, 1997.

152. Wolfgang R. Krabbe, 'Arbeitsmarktregulierung und Arbeiterschutz in den Städten des kaiserlichen Deutschland', *Jahrbuch für europäische Verwaltungsgeschichte*, **5** (1993), pp. 39–56.

153. Ralph Jessen, 'Polizei, Wohlfahrt und die Anfänge des modernen Sozialstaats in Preußen während des Kaiserreiches', *Geschichte und Gesellschaft*, **20** (1994), pp. 157–80.

154. Sachße, 'Frühformen' (n. 115); Christoph Sachße, *Mütterlichkeit als Beruf. Sozialarbeit, Sozialreform und Frauenbewegung 1871–1929*, Frankfurt-am-Main, 1986; Iris Schröder, 'Wohlfahrt, Frauenfrage und Geschlechterpolitik. Konzeptionen der Frauenbewegung zur kommunalen Sozialpolitik im Deutschen Kaiserreich 1871–1914'. *Geschichte und Gesellschaft*, **21** (1995), pp. 368–90; Nitsch, *Private Wohltätigkeitsvereine* (n. 139), pp. 469–511.

155. Sachße, 'Frühformen' (n. 118), 17; Nitsch thinks little of the cooperation between the associations in Berlin and the public welfare system there, see *Private Wohltätigkeitsvereine* (n. 154).

156. Basic works include: Gerhard A. Ritter, *Der Sozialstaat: Entstehung und Entwicklung im internationalen Vergleich*, 2nd edn, Munich, 1991, as well as the review of the first edition in 1989; see also Christoph Sachße, 'Der Wohlfahrtsstaat in historischer und vergleichender Perspektive' in *Geschichte und Gesellschaft*, **16** (1990), pp. 470–90; especially the *Quellensammlung zur Geschichte der deutschen Sozialpolitik 1867 bis 1914*; see also the assessment by Gerhard A. Ritter, 'Sozialpolitik im Zeitalter Bismarcks. Ein Bericht über neue Quelleneditionen und neue Literatur', *Historische Zeitschrift*, **265** (1997), pp. 683–720. Also, more recently, Florian Tennstedt, 'Peitsche und Zuckerbrot oder ein Reich mit Zuckerbrot? Der Deutsche Weg zum Wohlfahrtsstaat 1871– 1881', *Zeitschrift für Sozialreform*, **43** (1997), pp. 88–101.

157. *Quellensammlung Sozialpolitik*, I. Abt., Vol. 1: *Grundfragen staatlicher Sozialpolitik. Die Diskussion der Arbeiterfrage auf Regierungsseite vom*

preußischen Verfassungskonflikt bis zur Reichtagswahl von 1881. Revised by Florian Tennstedt and Heidi Winter with Wolfgang Ayass and Karl-Heinz Nickel, Stuttgart, Jena, New York 1994, p. 510f., fn. 8. Bismarck was more precise in this context in 1880: Tennstedt, 'Peitsche und Zuckerbrot', (n. 157), p. 96.

158. See also *Quellensammlung Sozialpolitik,* I. Abt., Volume 3: *Arbeiterschutz.* Revised by Wolfgang Ayass, Stuttgart, Jena and New York, 1996; *Quellensammlung Sozialpolitik,* II. Abt., Bd. 3: *Arbeiterschutz.* Revised by Wolfgang Ayass, Darmstadt 1998.

159. Ibid., Introduction, XXXIII. Wolfgang Ayass writes of 'the stubbornly maintained opposition of Bismarck to the expansion of protective regulations, which was founded in his personal attitudes. The material interests of the workers were more important than protective regulations. The workers' personal freedom to earn money should not be limited.'

160. *Reichs-Gesetzblatt 1871,* pp. 207–9; *Quellensammlung Sozialpolitik,* I. Abt., Vol. 2: *Von der Haftpflichtgesetzgebung zur ersten Unfallversicherungsvorlage,* revised by Florian Tennstedt and Heidi Winter with Heinz Domeinski, Stuttgart, Jena and New York, 1993, No. 13, pp. 47–49.

161. On the revealing conflicts between Lohmann, Karl Hofmann, the Prussian Trade Minister, and Bismarck, see *Quellensammlung Sozialpolitik,* I. Abt., Vol. 2: *Von der Haftpflichtgesetzgebung zur ersten Unfallversicherungsvorlage,* as well as Florian Tennstedt, 'Sozialreform als Mission. Anmerkungen zum politischen Handeln Theodor Lohmanns' in Jürgen Kocka, Hans-Jürgen Puhle and Klaus Tenfelde (eds), *Von der Arbeiterbewegung zum modernen Sozialstaat.* FS für Gerhard A. Ritter, Munich, 1994, pp. 538–59.

162. Ritter, 'Sozialpolitik im Zeitalter Bismarcks' (n. 156), p. 697; Florian Tennstedt and Heidi Winter, '"Der Staat hat wenig Liebe – activ wie passiv". Die Anfänge des Sozialstaats im Deutschen Reich von 1871. Teil 1', *Zeitschrift für Sozialreform,* **39** (1993), pp. 362–92.

163. This does not mean that the establishment of the Reich met with widespread scepticism or resistance. See Hans Fenske, 'Bürgertum und Staatsbewußtsein im Deutschen Reich' in *Historische Mitteilungen,* **11** (1998), pp. 23–45.

164. *Quellensammlung Sozialpolitik,* I. Abt., Vol. 1: Grundfragen, No. 94, 278f.

165. Florian Tennstedt, 'Vorgeschichte und Entstehung der Kaiserlichen Botschaft vom 17. November 1881' in *Zeitschrift für Sozialreform,* **27** (1981), pp. 663–710, quotation at p. 732f.

166. Unfallversicherungsgesetz vom 6. Juli 1884. *Reichs-Gesetzblatt 1884,* pages 69–111; *Quellensammlung Sozialpolitik,* II. Abt., Vol. 2, Teil 1: *Von der zweiten Unfallversicherungsvorlage bis zum Unfallversicherungsgesetz vom 6. Juli 1884.* Revised by Florian Tennstedt and Heidi Winter with Heinz Domeinski and Elmar Roeder. Stuttgart, Jena, New York 1995, No. 186, pp. 637–52.

167. Tennstedt and Winter, 'Der Staat hat wenig Liebe' (n. 162), p. 366.

168. Gesetz betr. die Krankenversicherung der Arbeiter vom 15. Juni 1883, *Reichs-Gesetzblatt 1883,* pp. 73–104.

169. Theodor Lohmann did that against Bismarck's will in his bill of February 1882, and he had thereby 'reckoned with – intentionally and against instructions' the law on accident insurance. Florian Tennstedt and Heidi Winter, '"Jeder Tag hat seine eigenen Sorgen, und es ist nicht weise, die Sorgen der Zukunft freiwillig auf die Gegenwart zu übernehmen." Die Anfänge des Sozialstaates im Deutschen Reich von 1871, Teil 2', *Zeitschrift für Sozialreform,* **41** (1995), pp. 671–706, cited at p. 681. See also *Quellensammlung Sozialpolitik,*

II. Abt., Vol. 2, Part 2, No. 41, 161–63 as well as the introduction, XXVI–XXIX.

170. A term used by Frevert, *Krankheit als politisches Problem* (n. 11), p.181.

171. Gesetz betr. die Invaliditäts- und Altersversicherung vom 22. Juni 1889, *Reichs-Gesetzblatt 1889*, pp. 97–144.

172. It goes without saying that this did not mean that the legislation in this area was finished. The opposite was the case: the health insurance was modified in laws of 10 April 1892, as well as of 30 June 1900, and of 25 May 1903. The accident insurance was amended in a law of 30 June, 1900; the retirement and invalidity insurance was amended 19 July, 1899, to name only the most important. In the Imperial Insurance Code of 19 July 1911, (*Reichs-Gesetzblatt 1911*, 509–860) all of these regulations were revoked and summarised in a uniform law package.

173. Heidi Winter and Florian Tennstedt comment on the general lack of a social reform programme on Bismarck's part in *Quellensammlung Sozialpolitik*, I. Abt., Vol. 1: Grundfragen, Introduction, XXXV, fn. 44.

174. Tennstedt and Winter, Introduction, page XXI in *Quellensammlung Sozialpolitik*, II. Abt, Vol. 2, Teil 1, Stuttgart, Jena, New York 1995. On Thomas Lohmann's expressed misgivings on the compulsory nature of the body, see also No. 115, p. 383f., as well as Wolfgang J. Mommsen, *Das Ringen um den nationalen Staat. Die Gründung und der innere Ausbau des Deutschen Reiches unter Otto von Bismarck 1850–1890*. Berlin, 1993, p. 648.

175. On the early development of an institutionalised procedure guaranteed by the state for the mediation of labour conflicts, see *Quellensammlung Sozialpolitik*, I. Abt., Vol. 4: *Arbeiterrecht*. Revised by Wolfgang Ayass, Karl-Heinz Nickel and Heidi Winter with Marek Czaplinski and Elmar Roeder, Darmstadt, 1997.

176. Florian Tennstedt, 'Die Selbstverwaltung der Krankenkassen im deutschen Kaiserreich', *Jahrbuch für europäische Verwaltungsgeschichte*, 5 (1993), pp. 83–100.

177. Wolfgang Schröder, 'Subjekt oder Objekt der Sozialpolitik? Zur Wirkung der Sozialgesetzgebung auf die Adressaten' in Lothar Machtan (ed.), *Bismarcks Sozialstaat. Beiträge zur Geschichte der Sozialpolitik und zur sozialpolitischen Geschichtsschreibung*, Frankfurt-am-Main and New York 1994, p. 134f.

178. In 1900, 46.3 per cent of those insured were with local health insurance associations, in 1905: 50 per cent, 1910: 52.3 per cent, 1914: 62.2 per cent. Quoted from *Quellensammlung Sozialpolitik*, edited by Karl Erich Born, Otto Brunner, Wolfgang Köllmann, Theodor Schieder and Joseph Vogt, *Einführungsband*, revised by Karl Erich Born, Hansjoachim Henning and Manfred Schick, Wiesbaden 1966, p. 148f. In 1888, approximately one-fifth of the 300 000 insured in Berlin belonged to the general (*allgemeinen*) insurance associations, and two-thirds to one of the local insurance associations: Godefroid, 'Das Berliner Krankenkassenwesen' (n. 82), p. 94.

179. Gesetz über die Abänderung des Gesetzes, betreffend die Krankenversicherung der Arbeiter, vom 15. Juni 1883, vom 10. April 1892, para. 75.

180. Furthermore, the local insurance companies conducted a 'systematic campaign against the independent insurance funds': Tennstedt 'Selbstverwaltung der Krankenkassen' (n. 176), p. 93. In 1911, the registered supplementary insurance funds were abolished and thereafter considered to be private insurance associations: Gesetz über die Aufhebung des Hilfskassengesetzes vom 20. Dezember 1911, *Reichs-Gesetzblatt 1911*, p. 985ff.

181. Not until 1908 did the loss of certain public rights, such as voting rights,

connected with the receipt of public support become commonly discussed: *Quellensammlung Sozialpolitik*, IV. Abt., Vol. 3, 2. Teil: *Das Jahr 1908*, revised by Hansjoachim Hennig and Uwe Sieg with Carsten Dams. Stuttgart, Jena and New York 1995, No. 30 and No. 44. The 'Gesetz betreffend die Einwirkung von Armenunterstützung auf öffentliche Rechte' of 15 March, 1909 (*Reichs-Gesetzblatt 1909*, p. 319) made it possible for receivers of public welfare support to vote.

182.   Hedwig Herold-Schmidt, 'Ärztliche Interessenvertretung im Kaiserreich 1871–1914' in Robert Jütte (ed.), *Geschichte der deutschen Ärzteschaft. Organisierte Berufs- und Gesundheitspolitik im 19. und 20. Jahrhundert*, Cologne, 1997, pp. 43–95. On the participation of doctors and medical civil servants in private charity associations, see Nitsch, *Private Wohltätigkeitsvereine* (n. 139), pp. 425–44. On the situation in Berlin, see Godefroid, 'Das Berliner Krankenkassenwesen' (n. 82).

183.   Gesetz über die Abänderung ... vom 10. April 1892, para. 2: 'Versicherungsgesetz für Angestellte vom 20. December 1911, *Reichs-Gesetzblatt 1911*, p. 989ff. See also *Quellensammlung Sozialpolitik*, IV. Abt., Vol. 3, 2. Teil: *Das Jahr 1908*.

184.   See also the Hausarbeitsgesetz vom 20. Dezember 1911, *Reichs-Gesetzblatt 1911*, pp. 976–85.; *Quellensammlung Sozialpolitik*, IV. Abt., Vol. 4, Teile 1 und 2: *Die Jahre 1911 bis 1914*. Revised by Karl Erich Born, Reiner Flik, Klaus Hess, Gabriele Ilg, Ulrich Kreutle and Dieter Lindenlaub, Stuttgart, Jena, New York and Darmstadt, 1993/1998.

185.   *Reichs-Gesetzblatt 1911*, pp. 509–860.

186.   Gesetz betreffend die Krankenversicherung der Arbeiter vom 15. Juni 1883, paragraph 21; Gesetz über die Abänderung ... vom 10. April 1892, para. 6a, para. 21. See also the regulations on the care of new mothers.

187.   Quoted in Gerd Hohorst, Jürgen Kocka, G.A. Ritter (eds), *Sozialgeschichtliches Arbeitsbuch*, Vol. II: *Materialien zur Statistik des Kaiserreichs 1870–1914*. 2nd edn, Munich 1978, p. 154

188.   Herold-Schmidt, 'Ärztliche Interessenvertretung' (n. 182), p. 88.

189.   See the figures presented by Adolf Buehl, *Vergleichende Armen-Finanzstatistik deutscher Städte. Ein Beitrag zur einheitlichen Gestaltung der Armenstatistik*, Hamburg, 1900.

190.   See Dietrich Milles, *Akuter Fall und gesichertes Wissen. Konstruktion der Berufskrankheiten in der deutschen Geschichte*, Bremen: Habil.-Schrift University, 1993. The exemplary case of a mason in Frankfurt-am-Main in 1899, and his difficulties in receiving his pension is described in Schröder, 'Subjekt oder Objekt' (n. 177), pp. 140–53.

191.   Invalidenversicherungsgesetz, *Reichs-Gesetzblatt 1899*, pp. 393–531.

192.   On treatments in sanatoriums and invalidity insurance, see *Quellensammlung Sozialpolitik*, IV. Abt., Vol. 3, Teil 1: *Das Jahr 1907*, No. 90, pp. 339–41.

193.   Schröder, 'Subjekt oder Objekt' (n. 177), p. 127 points to 17 per cent of men and 21 per cent of women. See also Reinhard Spree, *Soziale Ungleichheit vor Krankheit und Tod. Zur Sozialgeschichte des Gesundheitsbereichs im Deutschen Kaiserreich*, Göttingen, 1981. Jörg Vögele, *Urban Mortality Change in England and Germany, 1870–1913*, Liverpool, 1998.

194.   Spree, *Soziale Ungleichheit* (n. 193), Table 18, p. 184. On the development of health, accident and retirement insurance, see Hohorst et al., *Sozialgeschichtliches Arbeitsbuch* (n. 187), Vol. II, pp. 153–56. Frerich and Frey, *Handbuch der Geschichte der Sozialpolitik* (n. 94), Table 9–11, pp. 102–6; also *Quellensammlung Sozialpolitik, Einführungsband* (n. 192), pp. 147–53.

195. Schröder, 'Subjekt oder Objekt' (n. 177), p. 129.
196. See the four 'classic' mechanisms of social security (labour laws, social insurance, welfare, and care) and their differentiation in Sachße, 'Der Wohlfahrtsstaat' (n. 156), p. 482f.
197. Labisch, *Homo Hygienicus* (n. 6), especially p. 142ff.
198. Reulecke, *Geschichte der Urbanisierung* (n. 73), p. 201f. Fischer, *Sozialgeschichtliches Arbeitsbuch I* (n. 3), pp. 37–39. Hohorst et al., *Sozialgeschichtliches Arbeitsbuch* (n. 187), Vol. II, pp. 42–52.
199. Fürst, *Stellung und Aufgaben des Arztes in der öffentlichen Armenpflege* (n. 145), pp. 93–115; Fischer, *Sozialgeschichtliches Arbeitsbuch I* (n. 3), pp. 205–7; Hohorst et al., *Sozialgeschichtliches Arbeitsbuch* (n. 187), Vol. II, pp. 150–53.
200. An example can be found in Karl Stommel, 'Der Armenarzt Dr. Andreas Gottschalk, der erste Kölner Arbeiterführer 1848', *Annalen des Historischen Vereins für den Niederrhein*, **166** (1964), pp. 55–105.

CHAPTER FIVE

Health Care Provision and Poor Relief in the Electorate and Kingdom of Bavaria

Michael Stolberg

Bavaria was not a driving force in the historical development of poor relief and health care provision in Europe. Indeed, except for the Count of Rumford's poor reforms in the 1790s, the measures taken in Bavaria went largely unnoticed abroad.[1] From a comparative perspective, however, Bavaria presents some interesting features. Not only was Bavaria, unlike most other central and northern European states, a deeply Catholic country, its economic development also differed considerably from that of most of the other states treated in this volume. In Bavaria, poor relief and health care provision for the labouring poor became major issues of political debate and reform at a time when there was hardly any industrialisation to speak of, and before the emergence of any of the social and political problems and tensions which are commonly associated with industrialisation, urbanisation and the formation of an urban industrial proletariat. Nevertheless, from the 1770s, a wide range of measures were taken, which fundamentally reshaped the organisation of poor relief and created one of the most comprehensive systems of health care for the poor in contemporary Europe.

The economic and social background

Until it joined the new German Empire in 1870–71, the Electorate and, from 1806, Kingdom, of Bavaria was for centuries an independent state with considerable power and influence on the highly fragmented political map of central Europe. Its importance grew further in the aftermath of the Napoleonic Wars. Vast territorial gains, including large parts of Franconia and the former imperial cities of Nürnberg and Augsburg, almost doubled its surface area to 75 000 square kilometres, as much as modern Belgium and Holland taken together and second, among the German states, only to Prussia. The population rose from about 1 million in 1790 to well over 3 million in 1817.[2]

While the European economy was still largely dominated by agriculture and trade, Bavaria was quite prosperous. In the 18th and 19th centuries, however, its economic development increasingly lagged behind that of England, France, Holland or even Prussia.[3] Industrialisation was slow. During the period between 1815 and 1840 only 62 enterprises with more than 50 workers are known, and just three of these employed more than 200 people.[4] Things began to change more rapidly after 1850, but by 1870 there were still only about 1000 steam engines in Bavaria.[5] Proto-industrial activities were somewhat more widespread. Especially in areas with small average landholdings, like Franconia, home industries such as weaving, spinning, carving or basket-making provided an important supplement to the meagre incomes from agriculture. However, these home industries were largely wiped out, particularly in the textile sector, in the 1830s and 1840s, when lower tariffs and the ensuing competition from industrial mass production abroad prompted a partial re-agrarianisation of the economy. In the late 19th century, agriculture, and the small-scale local artisan activities linked to it, still provided the primary source of income for at least 75 per cent of the Bavarian population.

Urbanisation was slow, too. In 1792 Munich counted only some 40 000 inhabitants, and by 1840 the population had not even risen to 100 000 – no match for cities like London, Paris or Hamburg.[6] In 1880 still only 26 per cent of the Bavarian population lived in towns of over 2000 inhabitants, compared to 39 per cent in the German Empire.[7] Gradually, especially in the suburbs of Munich, Nürnberg and Augsburg, a steady influx of day labourers and servants created some of the problems commonly associated with industrial pauperism. But until the 1860s and 1870s there was virtually no new, industrial proletariat.

Poverty was nevertheless very widespread in 18th and 19th century Bavaria. Indeed, contemporary observers in the early 19th century described Bavaria as one of the countries with the largest numbers of beggars. Theirs was largely a 'traditional', pre-industrial kind of poverty, however. It was almost equally to be found in small market towns as in the few bigger cities, and its principal cause was population increase. The population grew relatively slowly in Bavaria, from 3.7 million in 1818 to 4.8 million in 1864 – much more slowly, than, for example, in Prussia, where it more than doubled over the same period, from 7.9 million to 16.9 million.[8] But it grew steadily, and it had already grown in the 18th century. Land therefore became increasingly scarce. In an economy dominated by agriculture this meant that more and more people depended on additional income from home industries, paid labour or artisan activities.[9] But Bavaria had already the highest known density of artisans in Europe.[10] While guild restrictions and concession procedures made access extremely difficult for newcomers, increasing foreign imports led home industries and existing small-scale artisan activities into a further decline.[11]

Detailed statistical data on the extent of poverty in Bavaria go back to the 1790s, but their validity and reliability remains somewhat dubious. Problems of definition – who was or should have been considered as 'poor'? – combine with inadequate registration and data collection procedures. Claims that, in 1794, far more than 6.3 per cent of the Bavarian population depended on public poor relief[12] are little more than an educated guess, although they may roughly indicate the magnitude of the problem. A tax census of 1812 reached similar conclusions. It showed that 43 500 of the 700 000 families (6.2 per cent) in the kingdom were on poor public relief, with a further 18.9 per cent earning incomes which placed them on the very fringe of poverty.[13] Figures on the officially registered poor were considerably lower in the 19th century: around 1850 they were in the region of 2.5 per cent.[14] These figures are unlikely to reflect the full extent of poverty, however, since they do not usually seem to have included migrating beggars, beneficiaries of individual private charity, or inmates of institutions. In fact, despite the relatively low percentage of registered paupers, 1151 communes were described as 'over-burdened' with paupers in the same period.[15] Furthermore, according to contemporary testimony, many – even among the very poor – avoided the dishonouring registration as a pauper, particularly since the support to which such registration entitled them was usually hardly sufficient for the most meagre living anyway.

Qualitative evidence supports the impression that poverty was a wide-spread phenomenon throughout Bavaria. Hundreds of medical topographies of individual Bavarian towns and districts described, in often very drastic terms, the appalling living conditions of large parts of the population.[16] The houses were crammed and unhealthy, the diet poor and in some places almost exclusively based on potatoes. The swollen bellies of presumably badly mal-nourished and/or worm-infested children were described in detail. According to these accounts, conditions were particularly difficult not in Munich, but in the smaller towns, to which the landless from the surrounding areas flocked. In 1816–17 and 1846–47 Bavaria again suffered the deadly toll of severe food shortages, thought to belong to a distant past. Infant mortality averaged 30 per cent in the first half of the 19th century, peaking to almost 50 per cent in some areas in bad years.[17]

The repression of beggary

As in most European states, measures against poverty in 17th and early 18th century Bavaria, focused primarily on the repression of beggary. As early as 1531, all public begging had been forbidden,[18] and innumerable mandates and ordinances against beggary were issued over the following centuries.[19] They either aimed at the complete abolition of beggary or, more commonly, restricted the permission to beg largely to those old and invalided people who were considered to be deserving. These had to wear a special badge, which entitled them to demand alms in a specific area. Regular police and so-called *Bettelvögte* were to arrest any offenders. Punishment was draconic, ranging from whipping and branding to forced military service and life imprisonment; foreigners had to leave the country. And these penalties did not just remain on paper. Some of the elderly or sick might get away with a warning, but others were whipped, even when they complained of physical or mental disorders.[20]

As the government repeatedly acknowledged, the regulations were nevertheless largely unsuccessful, and the question how to deal with the problem of beggary became a matter of intense public debate in the late 18th century. It seems that many among the middle and upper classes were no longer prepared to accept beggary as inevitable. Indeed, the inability to effectively cope with the problem was one of the principal complaints in a protest note which the Munich magistrate and the heads of various guilds presented to the Elector in 1778.[21]

Beggary was a cause of great concern for several reasons. First, beggary, it was claimed, bred disorder and crime; it was a threat to public security. Under the pretext of alms-seeking, beggars would slip through open doors and steal whatever they found. Organised gangs of beggars were said to split up districts among themselves, while others moved from town to town, extorting alms rather than begging for them. Beggar parents, it was affirmed, cruelly beat their children when they did not bring home enough money, or even blinded or mutilated them in order to attract the almsgivers' pity.[22] Even if they did not commit crimes, the younger, ablebodied beggars still offended enlightened ideas of an active, useful life and threatened to transmit the contagion of idleness to others, in particular to their own children. Thanks to their audacity they were also more successful in obtaining alms than the more timid, truly deserving poor, making the common haphazard giving of alms to whoever asked for them an inefficient, as well as unjust, method of distributing the available funds. Last but not least, beggary was quite simply perceived as a real nuisance – an aspect which historians would be unwise to neglect in favour of more fundamental and intellectually challenging ideological motives. Respectable citizens were described as literally beleaguered by hoards of beggars, at home as well as in the streets. They constantly had to change the side of the road, just to escape their demands or, alternatively, pull out their purse at every corner. Travellers on the country roads were followed over long distances by whining children and shepherds. Not even in the churches, thus the complaints ran, could peace and quiet be found, because the piety of the mass was disturbed by insistent demands for alms.[23]

This resentment of beggary among the upper classes increasingly combined with a deep dissatisfaction with the inefficacy of traditional repressive approaches. In 1778 Michael Adam Bergmann, a judge and high-ranking town official in Munich, summarised the argument in a treatise, which, together with the measures taken in Bamberg and Würzburg in the 1780s, may well have been the principal, though unacknowledged inspiration for the poor reforms which the Count of Rumford undertook a decade later.[24] Many beggars, Bergmann maintained, were truly in need. They simply had no choice, because towns and municipalities did not sufficiently provide for them, or refused any help, as in the case of unmarried mothers. If begging was to be eradicated, close police supervision and punishment had to go hand-in-hand with more adequate poor relief and a more efficient distribution of available funds – not to the most audacious, but to those most in need. At the same time, work opportunities had to be offered to the ablebodied, to invalidate their excuse that they had to beg for lack of alternative sources of income. Bergmann therefore proposed a more efficient organisation of alms distribution and he wanted poorhouses to provide work or shelter for those who needed it, to which a school and a hospital for the poor could be added. Only then would it finally be possible to deal rigorously with the lazy and idle as well.

Proclaiming his 'feeling of love for humanity',[25] Bergmann articulated a growing philanthropic current in late 18th century Bavaria. In the same year, 1778, the *Mildthätige Gesellschaft* ('Charitable Society') was founded, the first private relief organisation in Munich, which soon counted leading personalities among its members, including the sovereign himself.[26] In 1777 a manuscript memorandum to the Elector had similarly justified the demand for a poorhouse by pointing out that, without such an institution, 'our fellow human being, the pauper, staggers about at all hours in the cold and rigour of the winter time, in misery, with no roof and shelter, no bed and dress'. Even those who received support, it argued, often could not survive without begging, because the support was so meagre.[27]

If Bergmann's was a general demand for action, others called more specifically on the state to intervene on behalf of the poor. The one and true purpose of the state's existence, Joseph Maria Friedrich Piaggino, a *Hofkammerrat* from the Palatinate, declared, was to secure the welfare of the commonwealth, and this the state could achieve only if all its members were put into a position to contribute to this aim. The state; therefore, had an obligation to provide the poor with the necessities of life.[28] In practice Piaggino, like Bergmann and others before him,[29] suggested opening a work- and poorhouse. In 1778 he signed a contract with the Munich magistrate, designating him as the director of such a house.[30]

According to Piaggino's account, his project was, however, overturned, and his financial investments were lost, when Benjamin Thompson, Count of Rumford (1753–1814), was put in charge of fighting beggary in Bavaria. An American Protestant and military man, who had remained loyal to the English in the War of Independence, Rumford enjoyed the personal favour and protection of the Bavarian Elector Karl Theodor, who had entrusted him with a thorough reform of the Bavarian army.[31] When he had brought this task to its conclusion he submitted a proposal, in 1789, for an equally thorough reform of Bavarian poor policy, which the Elector accepted.[32]

Rumford's measures attracted much attention inside and outside Bavaria, and he has entered the history books as the man who 'banished beggary from Bavaria'.[33] His approach was far from original, however: as already indicated, the principles of his reforms were largely those which Bergmann and others had suggested before. Rumford applied the same threefold approach: securing alternative sources of relief for those beggars who were truly in need; offering work opportunities to those who lacked them; and forcing those to work, who did not want to.[34] Begging was totally forbidden and, shortly after, the giving of alms to beggars was made punishable as well.[35] The only significant novelty in Rumford's approach was that he saw the fight against beggary as an opportunity to demonstrate the usefulness of the army in times of peace.[36] In 1790, on New Years Day, a traditional day of almsgiving, he employed two regiments of cavalry throughout the whole country in a massive raid designed to pick up and arrest all beggars.[37] Special poor funds were created to provide for the truly deserving poor and to take the place of the arbitrary and correspondingly inefficient private distribution of alms. A commission of high-ranking officials was to supervise the new, hierarchical organisation now responsible for the administration of poor relief. For those able to work for their living, a public workhouse was established in Munich. It employed 500 to 600 workers in making uniforms for the Bavarian army, which thus assured the sale of the products.[38]

Predictably, one is tempted to say in retrospect, Rumford's ambitious project largely failed. Begging and almsgiving continued to be widespread phenomena in 19th century Bavaria, both in the towns and the countryside.[39] In 1816 about 150 to 200 beggars were still arrested every month in and around Munich alone.[40] Begging by poor students also seems to have been fairly common, and the government issued various ordinances against it.[41] In the 1840s the administration still routinely lamented that begging in churches and private houses continued to prevail.[42]

The reasons for this failure are not difficult to grasp. First, many beggars still had little choice; 1800 out of 2000 beggars arrested in Munich in 1790 had to be recognized as belonging to the deserving poor.[43] And, especially outside of Munich, public poor relief remained insufficient. Even those who loudly lamented the plight of beggary conceded that many districts had chosen the easy way out, handing out a sound thrashing on the behind rather than soup.[44]

Moreover, there was widespread resistance among citizens and even government officials against what they saw as excessive repression. Apparently, most Catholic Bavarians continued to perceive almsgiving not only as the pious duty of any true Christian but also, in a more magical sense, as a practice apt to draw divine benevolence on the giver. 'Many', as a local official put it in 1791, 'are of the opinion that alms giving is not meritorious, if it is not handed out personally. From this the nearly general rule [derives] that only in this manner will God's blessing remain on the house.'[45] Correspondingly, refusing alms carried a certain risk. Especially in smaller settlements, the large majority of people were said to fear fire and other disasters from the curse which the rejected beggar was likely put on their house – and one never knew which supernatural powers a stranger might possess.[46] In Munich the voluntary contributions to the poor fund soon proved insufficient. In some cases, angry citizens even rioted to prevent the police from arresting beggars.[47] Neither did the fines for almsgivers prove very helpful. Outraged, some of those who were fined reportedly withheld their voluntary contributions to the public poor funds and persuaded others to do the same.[48]

The workhouse idea, finally, did not gain the momentum in Bavaria which it achieved in some of the Protestant states.[49] Hopes for financial profits soon proved overoptimistic. Even Rumford's workhouse in Munich had to close in 1799, although the army had guaranteed a fairly reliable demand for its products.[50] Among the population, the workhouse seems to have been perceived and resented as just another kind of prison, which, in fact, some of them were. Maybe in reaction to this negative public perception, a clearer distinction emerged in the early 19th century, between *Zwangsarbeitshäusern*, or correction houses for forced labour, and the so-called *Armenbeschäftigungsanstalten*, institutions for the voluntary employment of the poor, which, in 1808, every local poor commission was ordered to establish.[51] Proposals to found rural, agricultural colonies to provide work for the poor and an education for their children seem to have remained largely on paper in Bavaria.[52]

Poor relief

For centuries the principal source of poor relief in Bavaria was, as far as we know, private almsgiving, supplemented by churches, monasteries and pious foundations which ran most of the hospitals and similar institutions for the aged or otherwise incapacitated, and also distributed alms to the poor. However, from the 17th century onwards, the public authorities and the state increasingly assumed first control, and eventually responsibility, for the provision of poor relief. In 1531, on the occasion of a severe famine, and again in 1627 and 1655, an explicit obligation was put on towns and communes to provide for their poor – a principle which was routinely confirmed in later poor laws.[53] On this basis, most towns and communes seem to have organised some kind of public poor relief, although much research still needs to be done in local archives to find out more details about practices outside the major towns.

Gradually, more specific structures for the administration of poor relief emerged. In 1599 the communes were ordered to carefully register all their paupers.[54] Many towns appointed so-called *Armenväter* or *Einsammler* and put them in charge of the distribution of the money which was collected for that purpose.[55] In Munich, in 1748, a special poor commission was established to organise alms collections and to make sure that they reached the worthy and deserving poor.[56] In government legislation, an ordinance in 1770 marks the shift from a system of poor relief based only on voluntary contributions to the establishment of a poor tax. From now on, towns and communes were entitled to raise tax-like contributions from all their inhabitants, with rates calculated according to the size of the respective land-holdings (Hoffuß).[57] Additional sources of income were created, from pecuniary fines and from various fees and taxes on weddings, gambling and music. In 1756 a new tax, the so-called *quarta pauperum*, channelled 25 per cent of all legacies left to the Church directly into the poor funds, exempting only those institutions which provided poor relief or education.[58]

As indicated above, following a mounting debate on new approaches to poor relief and the poor reforms in Bamberg and Würzburg, the Count of Rumford, from 1789, put a much more elaborate system into practice in Munich. Begging was totally prohibited, and the better-off citizens were urged to contribute to a central poor fund instead of haphazardly handing out individual alms. The givers' names, as well as the amount donated, were published in an unabashed attempt to increase the pressure.[59] A hierarchical network of commissions and subcommissions for each district and subdistrict was to ensure that the eligibility and needs of each individual were scrupulously assessed. Generally, the process included a medical examination of each poor person to establish work abilities and state of health, as well as an interrogation of landlords and neighbours about the person's moral qualities and economic circumstances.[60]

Direct private and clerical charity were no longer to play any role at all. This shift, from private and clerical charity to public poor relief, found a particularly apt expression in the ritual of alms distribution in Munich. While the traditional weekly collections for the poor in the churches were abolished,[61] the registered poor were to gratefully receive their weekly allowance every Wednesday morning from an official in the awe-inspiring surroundings of the town hall.[62] Even the traditional charitable distribution of soup to the poor by churches and monasteries or in private houses was forbidden. Instead, hundreds of portions of the famous – or notorious – Rumford soup were distributed in the workhouse.[63] Private and monastic soup donations were accepted as well, but they were collected and distributed centrally. When the result of mixing all this soup together was acknowledged as too disgusting even to feed the poorest, the old system was re-established, but now under police supervision.[64]

The government also called on smaller towns and villages to create work opportunities, such as spinning, and to provide school education in order to fight idleness,[65] but in practice Rumford's reforms remained largely limited to the capital. Only from 1799 did the strongly centralist, reformist and interventionist new government under Montgelas, take steps to create a national, state-run system of poor relief throughout the whole kingdom.[66] This was part of a massive and much more comprehensive political programme which, inspired by ideas of enlightened absolutism, was aimed at asserting state control in all areas of public life – in particular, against the rival powers of communal authorities and the Church.[67]

Local poor commissions were still to organise poor relief in every town and commune, but the ultimate control now lay with the ministry of the interior.[68] Responsibility for the administration of charitable endowments was similarly transferred from local magistrates to the government. In Munich, in 1803, the various endowments were even merged with the general poor fund.[69] In 1806 the government put all charitable endowments in the kingdom under the supervision of a special charity administration. This was justified as a means to increase their efficiency and to save administrative costs.[70]

The measures against the traditional role of Church institutions in providing poor relief were, in many ways, even more drastic although, for the most part, less direct and part of a longer tradition. In the 18th and early 19th centuries the Bavarian government made a consistent effort to reduce the wealth and power of the Church which, around 1750, owned about 56 per cent of the land in Bavaria and paid no regular taxes.[71] The Elector sought to impose taxation on the ecclesiastical institutions and took stricter measures against the increase of Church property. In 1754 older regulations against the accumulation of land in the 'dead hand' of the Church were revised and, from then on, all legacies of money, land or goods worth more than 2000 fl to ecclesiastical institutions were forbidden.[72] The power struggle with the Church culminated around 1800 in a massive and highly aggressive secularisation campaign, in the course of which most ecclesiastical property was confiscated and auctioned off or destroyed.

These anti-Church measures were part of a general trend towards the assertion of state control in Bavaria but, in part, they drew their principal ideological justification from the same enlightened ideas of an active, socially useful life which made beggary so offensive. Thus, lamenting the misdirection of legacies, Bergmann in his treatise of 1778, wondered whether providing for the poor might not be more pleasing to God, than when some bad-humoured monks or nuns sent Latin prayers to Heaven, which they often did not understand themselves.[73] Like ablebodied beggars, the inmates of convents and monasteries seemed to be outright parasites: they ate other people's bread without contributing to the common good.

The trend towards an increasing centralisation in the organisation of poor relief – though not towards state control – came to a fairly abrupt end in 1816. The first detailed and comprehensive poor law for the whole kingdom, issued in 1816, marked the return from a national poor relief system back to the traditional principle of local welfare provision by the towns and communes.[74] This was part of a more general trend in many areas of political life in post-Restoration Bavaria – away from radical reforms and highly centralised state intervention, and towards a more conservative approach and a certain respect for local autonomy. The move ran parallel with a gradual shift from mercantilist to liberal principles in economic policy, and a certain *rapprochement* between government and Church. In each commune an independent poor commission, a so-called *Armenpflegschaftsrat*, was established. Its task was to closely examine all those who claimed to need support, to register them and to secure food, clothes and shelter, when neither family nor private charity provided sufficiently. Furthermore, it was to set up houses for those who needed care, and in 1817 the local magistrates also regained responsibility for the administration of charitable endowments and communal funds.

This system remained the basis for public poor relief in Bavaria throughout the 19th century. Poor relief continued to be granted almost exclusively on the basis of *Heimatrecht*, which was acquired by birth, marriage or, exceptionally, through long years of work in one locality. Only in 1916 did Bavaria change to the principle of the *Unterstützungswohnsitz* which most other German states had adopted much earlier: every town was responsible for those poor who lived and worked within its confines.[75]

The most notable new development in Bavarian poor relief after 1816 was the growth of organised private charity. The above-mentioned *Mildthätige Gesellschaft* was, for a long time, the only private association in this field. In the first decades of the century, private charitable associations were permitted only under the closest supervision and control of the state administration. When the government assumed a more relaxed attitude, the citizens were quick to grasp this rare opportunity to play an active, responsible role in the kingdom's public life. In 1836 the first private soup kitchens were opened.[76] The 'St Vinzentiusverein' founded in 1845 attracted leading personalities from the Bavarian aristocracy, as well as scientists. By 1866, 1500 members were taking care of 971 paupers.[77] The most important of these private associations, however, was the *Johanniterverein*, founded in 1853 with the active encouragement and financial support of the king. By the end of 1854 the '*Verein*' and its hundreds of local branches already had 91 603 members, and their assets were worth more than 700 000 fl.[78] At about 560 000 fl, their financial contributions to the public poor funds at times surpassed those of the communes.[79] The local branches of the *Johanniterverein* were autonomous in their administration as well as in their activities. In addition to providing general poor relief in the form of money or soup, many of them also aimed at the moral and religious 'improvement' of the lower classes. They created saving schemes, nurseries and schools for the children of the poor, took care of poor orphans and so on.[80] By 1880, 582 private poor relief organisations in Bavaria spent almost 2 000 000 fl a year.[81]

Health care for the poor

Town physicians and town surgeons as well some private practitioners, probably provided free medical treatment to the poor in most larger towns in 17th and 18th century Bavaria, although the extent of this practice remains as unclear as the funds from which the medicines were paid for. Hospitals and similar institutions also offered some medical treatment to their inmates, and frequently physicians and surgeons received an annual allowance for this service. In Munich a *Stadtkrankenhaus* (town hospital) was established as early as 1743, explicitly designed for patients with acute curable and especially feverish diseases.[82] But all in all, the provision of health care did not play a prominent role in traditional Bavarian poor relief. Even in the Bavarian capital the various hospitals offered only space for about 200 patients, and the biggest of these institutions, the *Siechenhaus* in Gasteig, was described as a vermin-infested, 'long, moist, dark hall, filled with all kinds of exhalations, resembling more a crumbling cellar vault'.[83]

This situation changed dramatically in the late 18th and early 19th centuries. Within a few decades, the provision of curative health care for the acutely sick became a major feature of organised poor relief. Bergmann, in his treatise of 1778, had already lamented that the richly endowed hospitals in the large towns did not serve the truly poor. He painted the sad picture of a simple mason, carpenter or day labourer who fell sick, lacking food, care and medicine and whose wife and children might see no choice but to beg for a living.[84] Soon after, a more elaborate medical service for the poor was established in Munich as a major element of Rumford's poor reforms. Probably modelled on similar schemes recently set up in Hamburg and Mainz, the service involved more than two dozen physicians and surgeons, who were distributed over the various districts of the capital.[85] After a period of decline, the service was re-established in 1813.[86] The scheme later caused many problems and conflicts, principally because the government refused to grant any payment; eventually, work as a poor-doctor was made a prerequisite, instead, for permission to open a private practice in Munich. Not surprisingly, the physicians were accused of unduly preferring their paying patients and of being rather quick off the mark when it came to sending the poor patients into the general hospital.[87] But the service continued to provide basic health care for the poor over the next decades. By 1835–36 the doctors were writing an annual total of 16 300 prescriptions for medicines, baths and so on. The medicines alone cost, on average, 5400 to 7500 fl.[88] Some private doctors also set up special free polyclinics, for children or for eye and ear diseases,[89] and the homoeopathic doctors also ran a fairly extensive scheme of free treatment for the poor.[90]

Munich was a somewhat special case, however. With respect to the rest of the country, the poor reforms were, at first, only of secondary importance for the provision of health care. Here the measures taken as part of a comprehensive reform of the health care system in early 19th century Bavaria were much more incisive. Between 1803 and 1806 a district physician was appointed for each of the more than 200 rural and urban administrative districts, with a state salary. This so-called *Gerichtsarzt* had various tasks within the health administration and as a forensic expert, and he was expected to practise privately. But part of his job was also to give free medical treatment to all the registered poor in his district. District midwives were appointed as well, to assist poor women free of charge. This was the first time that the Bavarian state assumed direct financial responsibility for the provision of health care to the poor.[91]

Although the district physicians received no fees for treating the poor, the provision of free health care soon put considerable strain on local poor funds. The medicines still had to be paid for, and although physicians were repeatedly admonished to use the best possible economy in their prescriptions, and pharmacists were asked, and finally forced, to give a rebate of 33 per cent on medicines for the poor, drug expenditure rose dramatically. Some local poor commissions even became interested in homoeopathic remedies because of their cheaper price.[92] On top of that, the district physicians proved not only unwilling, but often truly unable, without unduly neglecting their other duties, to travel across their large districts in order to treat the poor. Over the next decades the central government increasingly acknowledged this problem. In the end, district physicians were held responsible only for the treatment of the poor in the very proximity of their place of residence.[93] As a result, many smaller towns without a resident district physician found that, in order to secure medical care for the poor they had to pay some allowance to other physicians, or to the semi-academic so-called *Landärzte* who had completed a three-year course at a special school. Alternatively, they had to pay on a case-by-case basis, including the very substantial travel fees. By 1848, according to a national survey, in many districts at least three or four physicians and surgeons received an annual allowance from the poor funds in return for providing free medical treatment of poor patients.[94] The provision of health care had become an integral part of poor relief outside the cities as well.

In-patient care for the curable sick among the poor expanded similarly. A national survey carried out in 1811 identified 25 Bavarian towns with at least one institution for the medical treatment of curable diseases, and there may have been a few more. But only ten of these treated more than 100 patients a year.[95] In some places, a few beds in the local poor house or similar institutions served a similar purpose, but most smaller towns and villages had no facilities for in-patient care whatsoever.

This situation changed dramatically over the following decades. Many older, multifunctional hospitals were transformed into institutions which aimed primarily if not exclusively, at the medical treatment of curable diseases. New ones were built. The biggest of them was the *Allgemeine Krankenhaus* in Munich, which treated more than 80 000 patients between 1813–14 and 1831–32.[96] But this expansion of facilities for in-patient care – all serving almost exclusively the lower sections of society was not limited to the larger cities such as Munich, Erlangen, Nürnberg or Augsburg. As early as 1785 an anonymous German pamphlet had demanded that the state, whatever the cost, establish a hospital for the curable sick in every district, with a room and a bed for every patient.[97] Along similar lines, the poor law of 1816 obliged smaller towns and communes to provide rooms and beds for the poor sick. Gradually at first, and then increasingly after 1850, a large number of hospitals was established in the smaller country and market towns as well. By 1869 there were 393 general hospitals in Bavaria, 155 of which were regional hospitals serving several towns or communes.[98] Even in fairly small towns like Landsberg, Miesbach, Kösching or Eggenfelden, several hundred patients were treated annually. In the 1860s, on average one out of every 30 Bavarians was hospitalised every year. In comparison, in the German Reich of 1877 the figure was not even one in a 100.[99] Furthermore, these Bavarian statistics do not cover the full range of in-patient facilities which were available for the curable sick. Many smaller towns and villages furnished at least one or two rooms, sometimes in institutions for the aged and invalided, and sometimes in local poorhouses, and similar buildings. For example, in the lower Bavarian district of Greding, which had a population of about 15 000, 45 towns and villages had created such facilities by 1861, each with one or two wardens to take care of the sick.[100]

Health insurance

An important feature of the massive expansion of in- and out-patient care for curable poor patients in 19th century Bavaria was that many measures and institutions did not exclusively target the officially recognised and registered poor. They aimed equally at providing medical care to the wider group of the labouring poor – that is, to those mostly single journeymen, servants, day labourers and, later, factory workers and railway construction workers, who managed to scrape a living under normal conditions, but worked away from home and thus lacked family support and the means to pay for adequate care and treatment when they fell ill. The Hamburg poor reform had already famously included in its health care provisions those at the very fringe of poverty but not on poor relief. Following this model, a poor reform proposal put forward in 1791 by the Society for Promoting Patriotic Industry in Nürnberg had also demanded health service for the labouring poor as well.[101] Making competent health care – or what contemporary élites considered as such – accessible to the journeymen, servants and day labourers and other labouring poor reflected the increasing recognition that health care was a basic human need, to which all men were entitled. But the provision of health care to these groups was justified most of all on the basis that timely, competent health care would prevent an initially benign, uncomplicated disease deteriorating and becoming chronic. Since chronic disease was in turn recognised as a major cause of poverty, health care for the labouring poor was, in this sense, an important prophylactic measure against long-term dependence on poor relief.

The original idea of financing medical services for journeymen and other unmarried workers from poor funds was soon discarded, however. Following the example set by the then still autonomous Catholic territories of Bamberg and Würzburg in the late 18th century, health care provision for this group was instead organised on the principle of collective insurance and, in this area, Bavaria was something of a vanguard force. Würzburg, under its bishop, Ludwig von Erthal, had established a so-called *Geselleninstitut* for journeymen, in 1786; a similar scheme applied to domestic servants in 1801. Bamberg soon followed with two similar institutions for artisans and domestic servants. In the case of the domestic servants, the employer initially had to pay the rates since, it was argued, he was spared the trouble of providing care in his own house.[102] The idea spread quickly. By 1811 *Gesellen-* and *Dienstboeninstitute* could be found in about two dozen Bavarian towns.[103] The new *Allgemeine Krankenhaus* in Munich had one from the outset,[104] and their number multiplied in the following years. After paying an entry fee and a relatively small weekly contribution into a common fund, the members were usually entitled to free care and treatment in case of disease, sometimes at home, but mostly in local general hospitals or in special rooms which were set up in old-style hospitals for the aged and incapacitated, or in poorhouses or similar institutions. As Reinhard Spree has recently shown, these funds soon proved an important source of income for the hospitals.[105]

In 1850 a government ordinance set the stage for a further expansion and generalisation of such insurance practices. Marking the only major exception to the prevailing criterion of *Heimatrecht*, towns and communes were from now on obliged, for a period of 90 days, to provide care and treatment also for those servants, day labourers, factory workers and such like who came from other places and would normally not have been entitled to poor relief. There was to be no compensation from the patient's home town either.[106] In order to allow the financially hard-pressed communes to retrieve the expenses they thus incurred, the Poor Relief and Health Care Provision Act of 1869 entitled them to do what some, in practice, seem to have been doing already: they could demand a compulsory weekly contribution from those journeymen, factory workers and the like, who had no right of domicile. And they could furthermore demand the same contribution even from those workers who did have right of domicile in the respective community, but did not live with their parents and had no house of their own. In return, all these workers were entitled to free medical care for a maximum of 90 days.[107] The 1869 act established, in other words, the framework for a general workers' health insurance – an insurance which was, however, financed exclusively by the workers themselves, without any contribution from the employers.[108] The large majority of town magistrates and communal councils seems to have made use of the new opportunity. When the German Reich under Bismarck, in 1883, introduced a much acclaimed general health insurance for workers, this had hardly any effect in Bavaria. The existing communal insurances were recognised and many continued to function until 1914. Only a few new ones were established.[109]

A parallel development was the creation of sick funds by factory owners and other employers, about which little is known so far. In 1854, 112 such schemes for factory workers existed, with 17 038 members, and there were a further 125 so-called *Hilfskassen* (relief funds), presumably for other dependent workers.[110] The poor law of 1869 then explicitly entitled the communes to oblige the owners of large factories within their territory to create a sick fund. The factory owners could, however, demand contributions to these sick funds from their workers.

Conclusion

In many ways, the history of general poor relief in Bavaria mirrors similar trends in other countries. Even the Count of Rumford's fame as a successful poor reformer seems to owe more to his self-fashioning as a man who – most famously in creating the soup associated with his name – applied modern scientific principles for the good of humanity, than to the novelty of his approach.

Until about 1750 government policy focused on the repression of beggary. Private almsgiving and clerical charity were of paramount importance. Public poor relief in the proper sense was primarily a local affair and, for all we know, was institutionalised only to a limited degree outside the larger cities. In the following period, the ultimate targets remained largely the same as those formulated at least from the 16th century: the eradication of beggary, the fight against idleness, and a more efficient distribution of available resources only to those who were truly in need. The methods and structures changed, however. Poor relief was increasingly institutionalised. Special poor commissions were established, usually from the ranks of the citizens, and often headed by officials. The deserving poor were to be carefully identified and registered, and the distribution of available funds was rationalised accordingly. The creation of work opportunities for the unemployed was moved to the forefront. For a while, the government assumed total responsibility, creating a state system of poor relief. From 1816 some of the responsibility was given back to the local authorities, but the government remained in control.

As to the ideological factors behind this process, clearly, in view of the backward economic development, the labour needs of industrial capitalism or the need to appease a growing urban proletariat, were of very limited importance in Bavaria, at least for the major reform period between 1780 and 1818. Only in the 1850s did the Bavarian debate on poor relief also give greater consideration to the collective plight of the labouring poor and to the dangers which they posed to public order.[111] Rather, among the urban élites in late 18th century Bavaria, a more secular, paternalistic philanthropy began to emerge as an important force. It combined with changing, enlightened perceptions of the state and its duties towards the citizens, which culminated in the law of 1808 which, for the first time in Bavarian history, established an individual right to poor relief.[112]

The influence of the strong Catholic tradition in Bavaria comes out as rather ambiguous. A 19th century commentator claimed that Protestant countries, due to their marked individualism, needed a much more extensive organised system of poor relief than Catholic countries, where the individual moral obligation of relatives, friends and employers remained powerful.[113] But many measures taken by the Bavarian government, rather than reflecting this tradition, were directed against it, against the predominance of the Catholic Church and against the popular appreciation of almsgiving as a means to acquire divine grace.[114] Indeed, the Catholic tradition in Bavaria probably found its most forceful expression not in the state measures but in the widespread misgivings and protests they caused, and their failure to eradicate beggary. In the 1830s many smaller towns still managed to raise sufficient voluntary contributions for the poor to have no need of a poor tax.[115] Furthermore, there also was a strong Catholic element in the development of private charitable associations, which in the course of the 19th century acquired an increasingly important role in the provision of poor relief.

In the creation of a comprehensive health care system for the registered poor, as well as for dependent labourers, Bavaria appears much more as a vanguard force. From as early as the early 19th century, hundreds of fully trained academic physicians, supported by a similar number of semi-academic *Landärzte*, made academic medicine accessible throughout the country, first for the registered poor only, but soon, with the expansion of in-patient care and the creation of insurance schemes, for a growing proportion of the labouring poor as well. With the exception of Munich, this development was initially only loosely linked to the poor reforms. Rather, its major roots must be sought in a fairly successful process of medical professionalisation and medicalisation. Among the medical profession in Bavaria there was a massive and highly successful drive to reshape and expand health care according to their own needs and desires. In particular, they demanded a decisive say within the health administration and the creation of salaried positions in the countryside. Leading physicians such as Adalbert Friedrich Marcus and Franz Xaver Häberl also played a decisive role in promoting the new hospital of the curative type and the insurance funds for journeymen and domestic servants, and they made no secret of the fact that the hospital, financed from poor funds and insurance contributions, provided them with welcome opportunities for research, teaching and prestige. At the same time, many among the enlightened élites came to accept that providing what they considered as competent health care not only helped secure, according to traditional populationist arguments, a large and healthy population as the fundamental basis of a sound economy and a powerful state, but was also a Christian and/ or philanthropic duty.[116] Poverty-associated epidemic crises in the 19th century, the petecchial typhus in 1816–17 and the cholera from the 1830s, added a further dimension: fast and professional health care for the poor would also reduce the risk that the contagion might spread to the other classes.[117] Only when a fairly extensive system of professional, academic or semi-academic health care had been established throughout the territory did the provision of in-patient and domiciliary health care for the poor increasingly become part of local poor relief as well, culminating in the creation of municipal insurance funds for the labouring poor.

Notes

1. Karl H. Metz, 'Staatsraison und Menschenfreundlichkeit. Formen und Wandlungen der Armenpflege im Ancien Régime Frankreichs, Deutschlands und Großbritanniens', *Vierteljahrschrift für Sozial- und Wirtschaftsgeschichte*, 72 (1985) pp. 1–26, see p. 16. According to J.R. Poynter, *Society and Pauperism. English Ideas on Poor Relief, 1795–1834*, London and Toronto, 1969, pp. 87–90, Rumford was, however, the most important foreign influence on English poor relief after 1795.
2. The Protestant minority also grew to about 25 per cent. For the general history of Bavaria in this period see Andreas Kraus (ed.), *Handbuch der bayerischen Geschichte*, Vol. 2, 2nd edn, Munich, 1983; and Max Spindler (ed.), *Handbuch der bayerischen Geschichte*, Vol. 4, Munich, 1974–75; geographically, I will limit my analysis to Bavaria in its changing configuration as a political entity. For the time before 1800, I will therefore not treat the situation in the independ-

ent Catholic territories of Bamberg, Würzburg and Passau or in the Imperial cities of Augsburg, Nürnberg and Regensburg. Some information can be found in Franz Xaver Bärlehner, 'Die Entwicklung der karitativen Wohlfahrtspflege in Bayern', Diss. phil. Erlangen. Nürnberg, 1927; Karl Geyer, 'Die öffentliche Armenpflege im kaiserlichen Hochstift Bamberg mit besonderer Berücksichtigung der Stadt Bamberg', Diss. phil., Bamberg, 1909; Rudolf Endres, 'Das Armenproblem im Zeitalter des Absolutismus', *Jahrbuch für fränkische Landesforschung* (1975), pp. 1003–20; Hofrat Lenz, *Historische Darstellung der freiwilligen Armen-Anstalten in Paßau*, Passau, 1804; *Unterricht an das Reichsstadt-Augsburgische Publikum die neue Armenanstalt betreffend* [Augsburg 1781]). I will also not deal, for the period after 1800, with the specific situation in the part of the Rhenopalatinate which belonged to Bavaria, but was geographically isolated from the main territory, and where, in many areas of political life, structures and regulations created by the French survived.

3. For an overview of Bavarian economic history see Eckart Schremmer, *Die Wirtschaft Bayerns. Vom hohen Mittelalter bis zum Beginn der Industrialisierung. Bergbau, Gewerbe, Handel*, Munich, 1970; and Spindler, *Handbuch* (n. 2), pp. 781–845.

4. Spindler, *Handbuch* (n. 2), p. 802.

5. Ibid., p. 805; the figure had risen from 132 in 1847.

6. Hubert Klebel, 'Das Pauperproblem in der Zeit des Spätmerkantilismus und beginnenden Liberalismus in Bayern. Eine sozial- und wirtschaftsgeschichtliche Untersuchung zur Entwicklung der Arbeitsverhältnisse und der staatlichen Wohlfahrtspolitik', Diss. oec., Munich 1955, p. 83, footnote.

7. Theodor Laves, 'Die bayerische Armenpflege von 1847 bis 1880', *Jahrbuch für Gesetzgebung, Verwaltung und Volkswirthschaft im Deutschen Reich*, **8** (1884), pp. 197–250 at p. 200.

8. Kraus, *Handbuch* (n. 2), pp. 463–64.

9. Spindler, *Handbuch* (n. 2), p. 754.

10. Klebel, 'Das Pauperproblem' (n. 6), pp. 63–67; Walter Demel, *Der bayerische Staatsabsolutismus 1806/08–1817. Staats- und gesellschaftspolitische Motivationen und Hintergründe der Reformära in der ersten Phase des Königreichs Bayern*, Munich, 1983, p. 72.

11. Spindler, *Handbuch* (n. 2), pp. 760–62.

12. Endres, 'Das Armenproblem' (n. 2), p. 1007; Angelika Baumann, ' "Armut muß verächtlich bleiben...". Verwaltete Armut und Lebenssituation verarmter Unterschichten um 1800 in Bayern', in Richard van Dülmen (ed.), *Kultur der einfachen Leute. Bayerisches Volksleben vom 16. bis 19. Jahrhundert*, Munich, 1983, pp. 151–79 at p. 155.

13. Demel, *Der bayerische Staatsabsolutismus* (n. 10), pp. 73–74; of course, the figures based on family counts are not directly comparable, because poor families may, on average, have been much smaller, due to the role of widowhood as a major cause of poverty.

14. Bayerisches Hauptstaatsarchiv München (HStAM) MA 62478, General-Uebersichts-Tabelle über den Stand des Armenwesens pro 1853/54, 16 May 1856.

15. Ibid.

16. Staatsarchiv Bamberg K3FIII 1481; Bayerische Staatsbibliothek, department of manuscripts, Cgm 6874; cf. Stolberg, Heilkunde.

17. Ferdinand Escherich, 'Die Kinder-Sterblichkeit im ersten Lebensjahre in Süd-Deutschland', *Aerztliches Intelligenz-Blatt*, **7** (1860), pp. 733–43. The principal

causes of death were those commonly linked to gastrointestinal infections, which tend to reflect poor food and hygiene, as well as regional patterns of breastfeeding.

18. HStAM GR Fasc. 39, N. 19, government ordinance, 27 March 1531.
19. Further ordinances and regulations were issued, for example, in 1594, 1599, 1606, 1614 (HStAM GR Fasc. 39, N. 19); later regulations are collected in Georg Karl Mayr (ed.), *Sammlung der churpfalz-baierischen allgemeinen und besonderen Landesverordnungen*, Vol. 5, Munich, 1797, see 721–730 (1748), 769–771 (1756), 779–780 (1760), 782–784 (1761), 910–912 (1775) Kreittmayr, 421–428 (1770); Döllinger, 494–510 (1780, 1790, 1793, 1799, 1801).
20. Baumann, '"Armut muß verächtlich bleiben ... "' (n. 12).
21. Joseph Maria Friedrich Piaggino, *Der Hofkammerrath Piaggino und der General Thompson oder das Münchner Armeninstitut*, Straßburg, 1791, p. 5; the Elector, at that time, resided in Zweibrücken and the citizenship wanted him and his court back in the old capital, Munich.
22. Lenz, *Historische Darstellung* (n. 2), p. 35; beggary ordinance of 27 July 1770, in Kreittmayr, (n. 19), 421–28; Benjamin Thompson, Count of Rumford, *Essays, Political, Economical, and Philosophical*, London, 1796, Vol.1, pp. 15–16.
23. Thompson, *Essays* (n. 22), pp. 14–15; Joseph Maria Friedrich Piaggino, *Sätze über die Pflichten eines Staats seine Armen zweckmäßig zu versorgen. Nebst der Errichtungsart einer allgemeinen Armenversorgungs-Anstalt.* nd, np, pp. 4–5.
24. Michael Adam Bergmann, *Gegründete Erörterung, daß alle Anstalten gegen den Bettel, außer einem Opus publicum nicht hinreichend, sohin alle diese Nebenanstalten der Aufmerksamkeit der Polizei nicht würdig seyn*, np, np, 1778. The treatise was published anonymously, but it is listed among Bergmann's works in Klement Alois Baader, *Das gelehrte Baiern*, Nürnberg and Sulzbach, 1804, Vol. 1, A–K, pp. 89–92.
25. Bergmann, *Gegründete Erörterung* (n. 24), p. 3.
26. Franz Xaver Peintinger, 'Wohlfahrtswesen und Wohlfahrtsrecht in München von 1808–1848', Diss. jur., Munich, 1952 (masch), p. 218.
27. HStAM GR Fasz. 38, N. 11, *Kurtzer Entwurf oder Beschreibung des zu errichten komenten armen Haus*, 1777.
28. Piaggino, *Sätze* (n. 23).
29. For example, in 1759, the Freiherr von Stubenrauch unsuccessfully proposed the creation of a workhouse to provide work opportunities for the poor in Munich (HStAM GR Fasz. 38, N. 10, 'Die vom Hofkammerrathe Freiherr v. Stubenrauch vorgeschlagene Armenmanufactur und Spinnstub betr., 1759–1778').
30. Piaggino, *Der Hofkammerrath* (n. 21); the contract is reprinted on pp. 41–58.
31. Benjamin Thompson, Count of Rumford, *Vollständiger Bericht und Abrechnung ueber den Erfolg der neu eingeführten Einrichtungen bey dem churpalzbaierischen Militär*, Munich, 1792.
32. Peintinger, 'Wohlfahrtswesen' (n. 26), p. 3.
33. T.L. Nichols, *Count Rumford. How he Banished Beggary from Bavaria*, London: Longmans, Green & Co., 1873.
34. Rumford's measures are described in detail by himself in Thompson, *Essays* (n. 22), pp. 3–184; see also *Abhandlung üdas Armenwesen von München*, Munich, 1814; Poynter, *Society and Pauperism* (n. 1), pp. 87–90.
35. Mayr, *Sammlung* (n. 19), pp. 196–97, ordinance of 6 April 1790; there was a

similar ordinance in 1756, which seems to have remained unenforced, however (HStAM GR Fasz. 40, N. 20, ordinance of 31 March 1756); the prohibition
against giving alms as well as asking for them, was repeatedly confirmed – for
example on 28 November 1816 the penalty was 1 to 5 fl.

36. Thompson, *Essays* (n. 22), p. 14; von Stubenrauch was more sceptical about
the use of the army to arrest beggars, because the local officials and the
general population distrusted and disliked the military, and also because it
would be a degrading task: HStAM GR Fasz. 38, N. 10, memorandum, 5 July
1778.

37. The first victim was unfortunate enough to ask Rumford himself for alms!

38. *Abhandlung* (n. 34), p. 31.

39. Spindler, *Handbuch* (n. 2), Vol. 4, p. 865.

40. HStAM GL Fasz. 2777, N. 1079, lists of arrested beggars.

41. Peintinger, 'Wohlfahrtswesen' (n. 26), p. 66; ordinances of 1796, 1823 and
1847. The penalties were not too drastic, however. After the eighth offence
only, the student could be dematriculated.

42. Ibid., p. 66.

43. *Abhandlung* (n. 34), p. 33.

44. Stiepen, *Erfahrungen und Gedanken über den Bettel. Ein Wort zur Zeit*,
Landshut, 1818.

45. HStAM GR fasz. 45, N. 26, letter to the Oberlandesregierung, 25 May 1791.

46. Ibid.

47. Friedrich Freiherr von Strauß, *Fortgesetzte Sammlung der im Gebiete der
inneren Staats-Verwaltung des Königreichs Bayern bestehenden Verordnungen
von 1835 bis 1852*, Neue Folge, Vol. 6, Munich, 1853, see 273, ordinance of
13 September 1793.

48. *Abhandlung* (n. 34), p. 37; between 1790 and 1796 the poor commission did
manage to raise about 230 000 fl in voluntary contributions however: ibid.,
Appendix D.

49. Cf., Christoph Sachße and Florian Tennstedt, *Geschichte der Armenfürsorge
in Deutschland. Vom Spätmittelalter bis zum Ersten Weltkrieg*, Stuttgart, 1980,
pp. 113–25; Augsburg had opened one in 1755: Bärlehner, 'Die Entwicklung'
(n. 3), p. 133.

50. Klebel, 'Das Pauperproblem' (n. 6), p. 133.

51. Koeniglich-Bayerisches Regierungsblatt 1808, coll. 593–602; in some areas
similar provision were already in force since 1804 (*Churpfalzbaierisches
Regierungsblatt* 1804, coll. 991–98). A special 'Armenbeschäftigungsanstalt'
was opened in Munich in 1804; it was followed by a 'Zwangsarbeitshaus' in
1806 for those unwilling to work as well as for those inmates of other charitable institutions who would not desist from begging: Klebel 'Das Pauperproblem'
(n. 6), pp. 128–33; Peintinger, 'Wohlfahrtswesen' (n. 26), pp. 67–71.

52. *Vorschlag durch Versorgung der Armen eine ansehnliche Renthe zu erlangen,
wie auch Bevölkerung und Benützung des Landes zu vermehren*, np, 1785;
Charlotte Koch, 'Wandlungen der Wohlfahrtspflege im Zeitalter der Aufklärung',
Diss. oec., Erlangen, 1933, pp. 243–47.

53. HStAM GR Fasz 39, N. 19, printed beggary ordinance of 1531; Emil Riedel,
*Das bayrische Gesetz über öffentliche Armen- und Krankenpflege vom 29.
April 1869*, Nördlingen: Beck, 1870, p. 3; Strauß, *Fortgesetzte Sammlung* (n.
47), 1784, pp. 948–54.

54. Riedel, *Das bayrische Gesetz* (n. 53), p. 2, footnote.

55. Bergmann, *Gegründete Erörterung* (n. 24); Riedel, *Das bayrische Gesetz* (n. 53), pp. 2–3; Bärlehner, 'Die Entwicklung' (n. 3).

56. Strauß, *Fortgesetzte Sammlung* (n. 47), pp. 721–30, beggary regulations for Munich and Au 2 January 1748.

57. Kreittmayr (n. 19), pp. 421–28, beggary ordinance of 27 July 1770; Klebel, 'Das Pauperproblem' (n. 6), p. 93, suggests that the Austrian cameralist Joseph von Sonnenfels may have been a strong influence here, with his demand to supplant individual alms with a public poor tax; in Munich such a tax was introduced in 1805.

58. Ludwig Hammermayer, 'Staatskirchliche Reformen und Salzburger Kongreß', in Andreas Kraus (ed.), *Handbuch der Bayerischen Geschichte*, 2nd edn, Munich, 1988, Vol. 2, pp. 1269–74; the 'quarta' was repeatedly confirmed and abolished only in 1840.

59. *Alphabetisches Verzeichnis der hiesigen Familien und ihrer monatlichen freyen Beyträge zu Unterstützung der Armenanstalt*, Munich, 1790.

60. *Abhandlung* (n. 34).

61. Strauß, *Fortgesetzte Sammlung* (n. 47), pp. 189–90, ordinance of 4 January 1790.

62. *Abhandlung* (n. 34), p. 41.

63. The soup had originally been introduced in the Bavarian correction houses: Peintinger, 'Wohlfahrtswesen' (note 26), p. 118. The composition could vary somewhat. In Passau, for example, to make 70 'Maß' of soup usually 16 pounds of potatoes, 10 pounds of peas and 9 pounds of barley were mixed with a pound and a half of salt, vinegar, some herbs and a pound of bone gelatine, but sometimes lung, calves' feet or intestines were also added. It was served with bread roasted in fat from bones: Lenz, (n. 2), pp. 48–50.

64. Lenz, *Historische Darstellung* (n. 2), pp. 55–56. In the early 19th century, after the workhouse and the monasteries had been closed, a soup kitchen, the *'Rumfordsche Suppenanstalt'*, was opened, which gave soup and bread to the needy for 1 kr each: Bärlehner 'Die Enstwicklung' (n. 2), p. 121.

65. Mayr, *Sammlung* (n. 19), pp. 198–99, ordinance of 25 May 1790.

66. This period is well covered in Riedel, *Das bayrische Gesetz* (n. 53) , pp. 2–12; Klebel, 'Das Pauperproblem' (n. 6); for developments in the other German states see Sachße and Tennstedt, *Gesichte der Armenfürsorge* (n. 49), pp. 85–132.

67. Klebel, 'Das Pauperproblem' (n. 6), pp. 74–87.

68. Riedel, *Das bayrische Gesetz* (n. 53), p. 5; the communes were encouraged to join forces in district poor commissions.

69. Peintinger, 'Wohlfahrtswesen' (n. 26), p. 126, ordinance of the *Landesdirektion* of 25 May 1803.

70. Koeniglich-Bayerisches Regierungsblatt 1807, coll. 49–53, ordinance of 29 December 1806; Anselm Martin, *Geschichtliche Darstellung der Kranken- und Versorgungsonstalten in München mit medizinisch- administrativen Bemerkungen ans dem Gebiete der Nosokomialpflege*, Munich, 1834, p. 5.

71. Hammermayer (n. 58); the Elector owned only about 15 per cent.

72. Ibid.; earlier laws in 1762, 1707 and 1730 had shown little effect.

73. Bergmann, *Gegründete Erörterung* (n. 24), p. 15.

74. Koeniglich-Baierisches Regierungs-Blatt 1816, coll. 779–816, 17 November 1816.

75. Spindler, *Handbuch* (n. 2), p. 866.

76. Peintinger, 'Wohlfahrtswesen' (n. 26), p. 120.

77. Ibid., p. 220.
78. *Hauptjahresbericht des St. Johannis-Vereines für freiwillige Armenpflege in Bayern vom Jahre 1854*, Munich, 1855.
79. HStAM MInn 62478, statistics on Bavarian poor relief, 1853–54; the poor funds' total income was 1.871.410 fl 16 1/4 kr, a figure which included income from property and contributions of food, clothes and so on.
80. *Hauptjahresbericht* (n. 78).
81. Laves, 'Die bayerische Armenpflege' (n. 7), p. 230; a little more than this sum was spent from charitable endowments, presumably primarily for institutional care.
82. Martin, *Geschichtliche Darstellung* (n. 70), p. 11.
83. Ibid., pp. 19 and 240 (cit.).
84. Bergmann, *Gegründelte Erörterung* (n. 24), p. 5.
85. Abhandlung (n. 34), pp. 10–20, pp. 46–47 and pp. 71–72; on Hamburg see Hildegard Urlaub, *Die Förderung der Armenpflege durch die Hamburgische Patriotische Gesellschaft zum Beginn des neunzehnten Jahrhunderts*, Berlin, 1932, pp. 42–44; and Mary Lindemann, 'Urban Growth and Medical Charity. Hamburg 1788–1815', in Jonathan Barry and Colin Jones (eds), *Medicine and Charity before the Welfare State*, London and New York, 1994, pp. 113–32; on Mainz see Friedrich Rösch, *Die Mainzer Armenreform vom Jahre 1786*, Berlin, 1929.
86. Georg Döllinger, *Sammlung der im Gebiete der inneren Staats-Verwaltung des Königreichs Bayern bestehenden Verordnungen*, Vol. 12, Munich, 1837, pp. 492–96, ordinance from the government of the Isarkreis 27 August 1813.
87. Ibid., pp. 50–51; HStAM MInn 61453, poor doctors; HStAM MInn RA 15626, medical services for the poor in Munich (1830s).
88. Peintinger, 'Wohlfahrtswesen' (n. 26), pp. 54–55; the figures declined to 6600 to 7000 prescriptions and drug expenses between 2800 and 4400 fl after 1840, when the doctors were obliged to keep to a limited positive list of permitted medicines.
89. Martin, *Geschichtliche Darstellung* (n. 70), p. 221; Peintinger, 'Wohlfahrtswesen' (n. 26), pp. 208–17. Between 1818 and 1838 Dr Reiner's clinic is said to have treated 12 800 eye and ear patients, mostly children; a special eye-clinic was founded by Schlagintweit, a paediatric clinic by Hauner, which eventually turned into today's university clinic,
90. Michael Stolberg, 'Die Homöopathie im Königreich Bayern (1800–1914)', *Studien und Quellen zur Geschichte der Homöopathie*, Vol. 5, Heidelberg, 1999; they also ran a hospital for poor patients, briefly in 1836–37, and, with a short interruption, on a permanent basis from the 1850s.
91. *Churpfalzbaierisches Regierungsblatt* 1803, coll. 912–916; ibid. 1804, coll. 196–198; *Koeniglich-Baierisches Regierungsblatt* 1806, coll. 165–166; ibid. 1808, coll. 2189–2210.
92. Stolberg, 'Die Homöopathie' (n. 90); for the long history of attempts to create special pharmacopoeas for the inexpensive medical treatment of the poor see Almuth Weidmann, *Die Arzneiversorgung der Armenzu Beginn der Industrialisierung im deutschen Sprachgebiet, besonderis in Hamburg*, Braunschweig, 1982.
93. Döllinger, *Sammlung* (n. 86), pp. 499–500, letter 25 March 1817 from the administration of the *Rezatkreis*, which, like many other ordinances, seems to have applied for the whole state.
94. HStAM MInn 61994, medical service in hospitals and poorhouses; a govern-

ment ordinance of 1839 had explicitly entitled the municipalities to make such payments: see Strauß, *Fortgesetzte Sammlung* (n. 47), p. 665.

95.   Bayerische Staatsbibliothek München, department of manuscripts, Cgm 6860, poor relief 1811/12.

96.   Martin, *Geschichtliche Darstellung* (n. 70), p. 19.

97.   *Vorschlag* (n. 52).

98.   Martin, *Geschichtliche Darstellung* (n. 70), pp. 57–63.

99.   Reinhard Spree, 'Krankenhausentwicklung und Sozialpolitik in Deutschland während des 19. Jahrhunderts', *Historische Zeitschrift*, **260** (1995), pp. 75–105 at p. 75.

100. Dr Hoffmann, 'Das Proletariat im kgl. Landgerichts-Bezirke Greding', *Aerztliches Intelligenz-Blatt*, **9** (1862), pp. 705–13.

101. *Plan einer neuen Anstalt zur zwekmäßigen [sic] Armen-Versorgung in Nürnberg, nach dem in Hamburg bereits ausgeführten Plane, auf Verlangen der Gesellschaft zur Beförderung vaterländischer Industrie bearbeitet von den Mitgliedern der dazu niedergesezten Committee*, Nürnberg, 1793.

102. Eva Brinkschulte, 'Die Institutionalisierung des modernen Krankhauses im Rahmen aufgeklärter Sozialpolitik. Die Beispiele Würzburg und Bamberg', in Alfons Labisch and Reinhard Spree (eds), *'Einem jeden Kranken in einem Hospitale sein eigenes Bett'. Zur Sozialgeschichte des Allgemeinen Krankenhauses in Deutschland im 19. Jahrhundert*, Frankfurt and New York, 1996, pp. 187–207; Franz Xaver Häberl, *Abhandlung über öffentliche Armen- und Kranken-Pflege*, Munich, 1813, pp. 170–71, footnote; Christian Pfeufer, *Geschichte des allgemeinen Krankenhauses zu Bamberg*, Bamberg, 1825; see also Spree, 'Krankenhausentwicklung und Sozialpolitik' (n. 99).

103. Bayerische Staatsbibliothek, Department of Manuscripts, Cgm 6858.

104. *Das neue öffentliche Krankenhaus zu München*, Munich, 1813, pp. 16–24. After a period of crisis, the Munich scheme was revitalised in 1832: Eugen Schirbel, 'Geschichte der sozialen Krankenversorgung vom Altertum bis zur Gegenwart' in *Auftrage des Hauptverbandes deutscher Krankenkassen e. V*, Berlin, 1929, p. 250.

105. Spree, 'Krankenhausentwicklung und Sozialpolitik' (n. 99).

106. Riedel, *Das bayrische Gesetz* (n. 53), p. 9, poor law, 25 July 1850.

107. Ibid.; for a detailed analysis of the 1869 act and its genesis see Horst Hesse, 'Die sogenannte Sozialgesetzgebung Bayerns Ende der sechziger Jahre des 19. Jahrhhunderts. Ein Beitrag zur Strukturanalyse der bürgerlichen Gesellschaft', PhD thesis, Munich, 1971; after that, their respective town of origin had to bear the costs – expenses for births and for the care of mentally ill had to be paid, from the start, by the commune of origin.

108. The communes could choose, instead, whether they wanted to create a separate fund from these contributions, or channel the money into the general municipal funds.

109. Ignaz Körbling, *Handbuch der öffentlichen Armenpflege im Königreiche Bayern*, 2nd edn, Munich: Abt, 1902, p. 4; Schirbel, 'Geschichte' (n. 104), p. 252.

110. HStAM MInn 62478, statistics on poor relief 1853–54.

111. Joh. Matth. Birkmeyer, *Zweckmäßige Vereinigung einer umfassenden öffentlichen Gesundheitsplfege und einer gut organisirten freiwilligen Armenpflege, das beste Mittel, der Noth der unteren Volksklassen kräftig und nachhaltig abzuhelfen*, Nürnberg, 1854, p. 17, for example, warned that the revolution had aimed more at changing the social conditions than the government; see also August Freiherr

von Holzschuher, *Die materielle Noth der untern Volksklassen und ihre Ursachen*, Augsburg, 1850.

112. Koeniglich-Baierisches Regierungs-Blatt 1808, col. 593.

113. Laves, 'Die bayerische Armenpflege' (n. 7), p. 199. Private, individual almsgiving was not limited to the Catholic countries, of course; see Robert Jütte, *Poverty and Deviance in Early Modern Europe*, Cambridge, 1994, pp. 139–42.

114. The same seems to be true for the poor reforms in the Habsburg Empire under Joseph II. Cf. Metz, 'Staatsraison und Menschenfreundlichkeit' (n. 1), pp. 14–15 *passim*.

115. Laves 'Die bayerische Armenpflege' (n. 7), p. 203; in Munich, the poor tax soon became the major source of income, however.

116. See Michael Stolberg, 'Heilkunde zwischen Staat und Bevölkerung. Angebot und Annahme medizinischer Versorgung in Oberfranken im frühen 19. Jahrhundert', unpublished medical dissertation, Munich, 1986, in particular pp. 11–38 and 320–51.

117. Cf. Döllinger, *Sammlung* (n. 86), pp. 496–99, Generalkommissariat of the Rezatkreis, 13 March 1817.

CHAPTER SIX

Urban Charity and the Relief of the Sick Poor in Northern Germany, 1750–1850[1]

Mary Lindemann

In 1793 the Göttingen Academy of Science posed the essay question: 'What are the most efficient and economical ways of distributing care to the sick poor in cities?' The eight essays submitted for consideration by the prize committee systematically reviewed the issues driving a debate on medicine and charity that had occupied the attention of the German learned public since the 1750s. The budgetary concerns raised and the ideological tools deployed to answer them would change little over the next century. The winner, Professor August Friedrich Hecker from Erfurt, offered a personal perspective:

> For over ten years, I have myself not merely observed but also actively participated in various plans for the sick poor in two of the most notable cities of our fatherland. [I] directed one such institution where annually an average of 500 sick poor received care. I am familiar both with schemes to supply assistance at home, the so-called *Krankenbesuchanstalten* [domiciliary care], that has recently been so praised in Hamburg, as with lazarettos and hospitals, from all their good and not-so-good sides ... and everything that I dare to present [here] ... results from my own experience and my own calculations.[2]

In a short disquisition Hecker then touched on all the major points of dispute. Did population size significantly affect care for the poor? Was assistance best provided in hospitals or at home? How could expenses be minimised? Might the Hamburg model be successfully implemented elsewhere? Was aid best provided by the state or by volunteers?

Broader 18th-century economic and intellectual currents influenced the debate, of course. A European-wide discussion of the serviceability of hospitals had arisen at the mid-century and these calls for hospital reform turned primarily on two premises. First, reformers stressed the need for new-style hospitals where, by 'privileging the role of the hospital', physicians would also 'extend authority over their patients as well as [over] their rivals'. Viewed as equally crucial was the renovation of existing hospitals to transform these 'burial pits of humankind' into what Jacques Tenon famously labelled the *machine à guerir.* Colin Jones and Laurence Brockliss have recently shown this particular 'Black Legend' to be a construct of enlightened critics who vastly exaggerated the insalubriousness of 18th century hospitals for their own purposes. Still, numerous plans in the second half of the century proposed redesigned and smaller hospitals or, even more radically, the dissolution of hospitals altogether.[3] While we know more about this movement in France than elsewhere, the exchange of ideas on the subject took place throughout western Europe and paralleled almost everywhere deliberations on how to improve traditional forms of charity.

By the time Hecker was writing in the early 1790s, the debate was, however, no longer an academic one. Several cities and territories had initiated poor relief reforms and were also experimenting with novel methods of distributing medical care to the sick poor. No programme received more attention than the one launched in Hamburg.

Most contemporaries regarded the poor relief established in Hamburg in 1788 – the General Poor Relief (GPR) (*Allgemeine Armenanstalt*) – as a model of its kind and the realisation of enlightened, humanitarian and rational principles. It is not my purpose here to review the story of the GPR (which I and others have done elsewhere), but to isolate the precepts that assumed special relevance for medical care and that then encouraged action elsewhere in northern Germany.

By the last third of the 18th century, knowledgeable observers had come to view extant systems of poor relief – generally some loose combination of parish maintenance, casual almsgiving and indoor relief – as deeply flawed and, indeed, even counterproductive. The discussion was by no means limited to Hamburg; rather, it crossed national boundaries. One can, for instance, demonstrate the strong influence of non-German writers, such as the Scot John Macfarlan on Johann Georg Büsch, one of the prime architects of medical relief in Hamburg. Much has been written about poor relief reform in the later 18th century, and it is not necessary to marshal that voluminous literature here. I want only to highlight three elements common to all endeavours at improvement: first, the universal wish to suppress mendicancy and vagabondage; second, the desire to reintegrate the pauper into the world of work; and, third and most important for our discussion here, the growing perception that the new poor *qualitatively* differed from their ancestors and were not merely more numerous. This third point in particular governed decisions about how to supply medical relief. It is also an important strand of continuity in a time of vast change.

Hamburg, as elsewhere in the 1770s and 1780s, buzzed with concern over what was perceived as a growing wave of impoverishment. The 1770s began the era of what is known in German history as *Pauperismus*, and although the term is generally connected with proto-industrialisation, industrialisation and proletarianisation, it can be as plausibly associated with population growth and the increase in numbers of those termed the labouring poor. While no-one in the period between 1750 and 1850 could apparently jettison the venerable dichotomy between the 'deserving' and the 'undeserving' or the 'blameless' and the 'culpable' poor, many began to recognise that poor relief's domain of action was changing. No longer were the traditional, shamefaced poor, widows and orphans the focal point of social welfare. Büsch, the most prolific publicist for poor relief reform in northern Germany (and perhaps overall in the Germanies), typically accepted the basic division into the culpable and non-culpable poor, but identified the 'primary root' of blameless impoverishment in 'that the common man earns too little to live on' and insisted that the needs of these creatures urgently demanded public notice and vigorous action. Macfarlan had argued some years earlier that 'the circumstances of the country, [and] of the rigour of the season' could result in an insufficiency of employment for 'the labouring part of society'.[4] Ludwig Gerhard Wagemann, in his *Göttingen Magazine for Industry and Poor Relief*, also enumerated the 'principal causes of impoverishment.' He argued that 'self-responsibility' (*die eigene Verschuldung*) accounted for only a limited degree of poverty and that, especially in cities, 'one can identify many cases in which it is doubtful whether one can ascribe guilt to individuals' for their distress. Wagemann believed that impoverished artisans, whose crafts were oversubscribed or had slipped out of fashion, formed the greatest source of those seeking assistance. Besides these, many people:

> ... frequently applied for relief having selected a livelihood which admittedly for a time provided adequate earnings. Many more, for instance, day-labourers, have [jobs] that ... depend on the whims of the well-to-do, and these [jobs] rise and fall with alterations in fashion. ... Such temporary positions may be lucrative while they last, and these are especially numerous in large cities.[5]

In short, Büsch, Macfarlan, and Wagemann were beginning to articulate a theory of structural poverty. This orientation would assume special significance for medical relief in the following decades.

As these men developed explanations for the origins of poverty that they linked to modernising economies with their unpredictable swings in fortune, they also reflected the ideological shifts shaking and transforming late 18th century society. While it is futile and probably wrongheaded to attempt to separate 'economic motives' from 'ideological motivations,' one can distinguish three factors at work recasting the world of charity and social welfare:

1. a redefinition of civic duty that increasingly emphasised volunteerism and patriotism (in the 18th century meaning of the latter word);
2. the rise of *Menschenfreundlichkeit*; and
3. the evolution of a service ethic that differed from *noblesse oblige* and inspired a new group of social philanthropists.

This last group were not social workers as we understand the term, but rather social theorists and activists (like Büsch) who devoted themselves to philanthropy as a civic duty *and* as a personal mission. Their motivation was by no means solely or even principally religious in nature, although it often remained Christian or deist in character. (There were similar trends identifiable among Jewish communities, however.)

These men spliced newer ideological strands into the older lines of cameralism, mercantilism and the medical police. The medical police, as defined by its most famous exponent, Johann Peter Frank, was:

> ... an art of defense, a model of protection of people and their animal helpers against the deleterious consequences of dwelling together in large numbers, but especially of promoting their physical well-being so that people will succumb as late as possible to their eventual fate from the many physical illnesses to which they are subject.[6]

Medical care preserved the health of a state's subjects (or citizens) and enhanced their own, and thus the state's, productive capacity. The late 18th century reformers conveniently, harmoniously and consciously built upon the foundations laid by their cameralist precursors.

Municipalities had, at least since the Middle Ages, always assumed responsibility for the poor. Parish poor relief (including medical provision) was as much a civic as an ecclesiastical undertaking even in Catholic communes and remained so in those that turned Protestant in the 16th century. In the 18th century, however, such civic commitments slowly floated loose of the older networks of communal obligations and became more deeply enmeshed with an emergent spirit of volunteerism that itself fed on the growing valuation of individual happiness as a social good. Philanthropic action could, of course, offer a way for some persons to climb the social ladder or to exert political power and patronage. Yet, the rhetoric and, for that matter, the reality of volunteerism accentuated choice. More and more people began to select involvement in the arena of public welfare rather than finance or government and viewed it as a means of personal fulfilment as well. This novel orientation toward civic action was one of the most important ideological characteristics of the poor relief reforms set into motion after 1750. It dominated until the middle of the 19th century when volunteerism began to fade as state responsibility (often at the level of the nation-state) grew and as professional social workers began to appear as the functionaries of welfare. In describing the Elberfeld system of the 1850s, August Lammers, for example, underscored its 'most striking feature' as 'the large number of persons who came forward voluntarily to take charge of the out-door poor'. It was a point upon which the Hamburg poor relief had prided itself equally.[7]

Menschenfreundlichkeit and *Patriotismus* were closely tied to poor relief reform as well as to improvements in other spheres, including education and penology. 'Humanitarianism' forms the most frequent translation for

Menschenfreundlichkeit, and the late 18th century reformers were indeed humanitarian in their opposition to slavery, cruel punishments, torture and the physical abuse of wives and children. Yet they also willingly accepted the need that cameralists had expressed for disciplining individuals whether they were children, prisoners or paupers. Even those most persuaded by structural interpretations of poverty were equally convinced that the poor (and, by extension, the labouring classes in general) lacked not only jobs but also tuition in frugality and prudence. Likewise, a citizen's patriotic conscience exhorted him to participate in poor relief either by monetary gifts or, even better, by volunteering to contribute time as well as money to assure the smooth functioning of such institutions. Active participation endowed bene-factors with the knowledge of having done their duty but also offered a deep and gratifying sense of individual pleasure.[8] Such moral satisfaction fostered an evolving service ethic that no longer arose principally from awareness of responsibility owed to Church and family as member of a parish or pater-familias. An interesting group of people emerged as social philanthropists: men like the Wagemann brothers in Göttingen, or Johann Arnold Günther and Johann Georg Büsch in Hamburg, or August Niemann in Kiel, and later women, like Amalie Sieveking in Hamburg. They constructed for themselves a fresh sphere of public life – social welfare service.

The problems presented by the burgeoning of what might be termed the *structural poor* typified most cities, although the dimensions soared in Hamburg as in other great and populous places. Hamburg was a commercial giant that depended on large-scale trade, transhipment, and a series of export indus-tries, such as sugar refining and calico printing, for its enviable prosperity. Its economy presented substantial employment opportunities – and even work at good wages – to tens of thousands, but it also proved tremulously sensitive to trade depressions which occurred with what seemed baffling capriciousness and puzzling frequency in the late 18th century. The chance of making one's fortune in Hamburg was great, but so, too, was the chance of sliding into more or less permanent impoverishment, especially for those clustered at the bottom of the occupational pyramid. By the 1770s Hamburg was no longer a major manufacturing centre and many trades which had thrived in the early 18th century (for example, velvet-weaving, silver and gold threadwork and ship-building) had gone under by the 1760s, to be replaced by more transient and temporary jobs, or ones totally dependent on trade or export.

The absence of an economic structure in which money flowed upwards from a manufacturing base had spawned a working class in Hamburg that depended in very real ways on the crumbs that tumbled from the tables of the rich. Büsch observed that:

> ... while in other countries and states the great machine of [monetary] circulation works up from the bottom, where the wealth of the better classes depends on the industry and ability ... of the lower [classes], so

is the working of the machinery in our state and in other cities like ours, completely topsy-turvy. The internal circulation moves almost exclusively from the top down. The little man can count on almost nothing for his sustenance except what is flung to him by his betters.[9]

In 1787 the Council of Elders (*Oberalten*), a governmental group responsible for parish affairs (including charity), likewise emphasised the structural bases of impoverishment, although, not surprisingly, their pronouncements also tended to moralise more directly about social breakdown, listing the causes of a much swollen destitution as:

> ... the decline and, in some cases, the total obliteration of several useful trades and manufactures ... the growing propensity among a large number of our inhabitants to indolence, folly, and improvidence; the lottery, whose unfortunate effects are perhaps nowhere so obvious as here; the shoddy quality of our schools where children learn with alacrity to be shiftless and slothful, but acquire nothing which could be serviceable to them in the future; and a misdirected sense of charity, which not only confirms our own wanton beggars in their indolence but which also ... entices outsiders to us.[10]

While Hamburg's economic situation was unique in northern Germany, the presence of structural poverty was not. It also appeared in Bremen, Lübeck, Altona, Kiel and Schleswig (the last three of which were Danish-governed but German in population and language).

If shifts in the composition of labour accounted for most of this unfavourable social situation, demographic trends played an equally decisive role. Hamburg was the third largest city in the Germanies and thus its problems quantitatively differed from those of small towns or even moderately-sized cities such as Lübeck, Bremen or Kiel. After reviewing attempts to reform charity in smaller cities (such as Bremen and Lübeck), Büsch insisted that these municipalities faced a less arduous task: 'an incomparably smaller mass of human beings to supervise'. In such 'modestly populated places ... one neighbour knows the other, one street the next, one parish the rest' and thus the whole system could be easily overseen.[11]

In 1787 Hamburg's population exceeded 100 000 or even 130 000 if those living outside the city walls were included. When the GPR investigated the numbers of poor (that is, those considered destitute and needing immediate assistance), it found 3903 families, or 7391 individuals – about 7 per cent of the population. This figure did *not*, moreover, include the 2000–3000 living in the city's poorhouses (the orphanage, almshouse, prison and hospitals). The extent of the labouring poor is, of course, unknown, but an indirect measure can be gained from the parish of St Michael, the least prosperous of the five metropolitan parishes. St Michael's inhabitants comprised 25.45 per cent of the city's population in 1764, but 31.49 per cent of the population in 1811. These figures imply that the least wealthy sector of the city's population was growing most rapidly.[12]

In Hamburg, as also in Kiel, innovative forms of medical care for the sick poor paved the way for the more general reforms of poor relief that occurred in 1788 and 1793 respectively. In Kiel medical relief was closely coupled to clinical education. Unlike the other towns considered here, Kiel had a university with a relatively active medical faculty. A plan submitted by the Society of Poor Relief Volunteers spearheaded the reorganisation of poor relief in 1793.[13] Yet a form of medical relief existed long before then. In 1785 Professor Georg Heinrich Weber opened a subscription drive to support a clinical institute (*Klinisches Institut*). Then, at the beginning of 1786, Weber produced the first of a series of printed reports recapitulating the initial eight months of the institute's existence during which its staff (he and his handpicked students) had treated 165 patients. The title of this foundation, a *clinical* institute, reflects its pedagogical mission. Weber explicitly sought 'not only to succour the sick poor', but also to educate young physicians and surgeons in their 'practical tasks and humanitarian (*menschenfreundliche*) burdens'.[14] Although Hamburg did not then have a university, the medical relief established there also endeavoured to train young physicians in physic and school them in humanitarianism; it was to be an apprenticeship in civics and medicine alike.

Medical relief in Kiel diverged somewhat, however, from the lines that the Hamburg relief would follow. In 1788 Weber proposed combining his clinical institute with 'a properly purpose-built hospital' for about six to eight patients. Hereafter, medical care for the sick poor in Kiel had two sides: a larger proportion of domiciliary care and a much more modest option of hospitalisation. Nonetheless, because the hospital was not ready to receive patients until the closing months of 1790, throughout 1789 and most of 1790 all medical relief remained domiciliary. The numbers cared for at home, rather than in institutions, were always much greater. The institute stood open to 'all inhabitants of our city who petition for assistance ... without having to submit to the strict investigation of their economic situation'. Thus not only the registered poor or the destitute were eligible. In fact the hospital planned for six classes of admissions. The first comprised the 'completely poor'; classes three, four and five admitted citizens of varying wealth and standing; class six existed for lying-in women. The second class, for the 'moderately poor' (*mittelarme*), deserves our special attention. The 'moderately poor' were people

> ... who are not in a position to pay for all the necessities of their maintenance [while ill], but can indeed contribute something. ... This category is intended for all local citizens who live in very modest circumstances.[15]

The list of those receiving medical assistance in Kiel during 1792 demonstrates the continued dominance of an at-home solution. Of the 380 recipients of aid, the hospital admitted only 31 and, of these, 17 came from the first and second classes – that is, the 'completely destitute' and the 'moderately poor'. The rules excluded servants entirely by relegating them to the benevolence of their masters and mistresses. They were not viewed as part of the new poor. Over the next years, this pattern shifted hardly at all.[16]

The establishment of the new poor relief in Kiel under the guidance of August Christian Niemann in 1793 linked the Weberian institute more intimately to broader social welfare. Weber promised the new organisation that he would be able to care for 200 patients in his institute (through visiting) and a further six each year in the projected hospital.[17]

Hamburg's medical relief enjoyed no formal ties with medical education at a university, so medical professors were not involved. Still the most ambitious charitable undertaking in Hamburg before the major reform of 1788 was, as in Kiel, an attempt to strike at illness, that 'pitiless destroyer' of the poor person's greatest asset – health. Until the end of the 1760s little formal medical care existed for the domiciled poor or, for that matter, for the labouring classes. City magistrates and parish relief administrators proffered temporary assistance in emergencies, but no system aided the sick poor on a regular basis – although they could, of course, be admitted to the *Pesthof* or another one of the city's many poorhouses. The charity of individual physicians and surgeons, who held special surgeries for the poor or who treated ophthalmic, dermatological or gynaecological complaints free of charge, could reduce these insufficiencies but not annul them. Traditionally, Hamburg had displayed more concern about separating the sick from the well. A 1714 plague edict, for instance, insisted that 'the preservation of the city' demanded the 'isolation of the poor, the sick, and the miserable' from the rest of human society and, especially in times of plague, dictated the 'removal of beggars, begging-Jews, and vagabonds, or other persons suspected of carrying disease' from the city.[18]

The direct tie between poverty and disease – or, rather, between disease and impoverishment – did not, however, escape comment. A *Report on the Care of the Sick Poor* from 1781 pointed out that 'if one let all our paupers recite the stories of their misfortunes, at least half of them would name an illness as the direct cause [of their misery].' Moreover, if one examined the history of their afflictions, it soon became apparent that the initial manifestation of the disease or injury had been mild and cure 'certain [*sic*] if this unhappy person had been able to obtain proper medical care promptly'. Nipping disease in the bud was supposed to curb poverty because 'all too often a complaint that appears trivial becomes deadly' without prompt attention. Experience seemed to demonstrate that most ailments could be successfully treated if not allowed to deteriorate into incurability. Cruelly victimised by such sequences of events was the labourer who thereby lost his ability to work, his health, and all too often his life.[19]

To snap the chains of illness and destitution, several physicians pledged to supply free medical care and medicines to the sick poor for a trial period of two years (1768–1770). The chief goal of medical relief was, explicitly, the prevention of impoverishment and not the care of the sick poor (although that, too, was achieved). The plan associated disease, illness and misfortunes on the one hand, with poverty on the other. For example, a typical family history (as the relief constructed it) might unfold with the family father – the sole breadwinner for his wife and several children – falling ill. He would then try a home remedy and, when that failed, take himself off to the 'next, best' apothecary or to some 'quack' or 'old wife' who promised to cure it. Instead of improving, he would sink ever deeper into illness and poverty. Finally, he would succumb 'to something that might have been remedied', leaving his wife a widow and his children orphans. The wife would then carry on as best she could until she, too, worn out by drudgery and worry, would follow her husband to the grave. She may even have already buried some of her children who, under more propitious circumstances, 'could have become useful members of the public'. A fate that was just as tragic and just as common awaited such families when the father lived on as a bedridden invalid for the remainder of his days. His illness would drag the entire family down with him into destitution.[20]

The demise of their first plan for medical care after only 18 months only temporarily discouraged Büsch and his friends. Ten years later, several of the same philanthropists and medical men founded a second Medical Relief (*Institut für Kranke Hausarmen*) on a much larger scale. This institution remained active until 1788 when the General Poor Relief incorporated it as the Medical Deputation. All three forms of medical relief functioned on the principles enunciated in 1768: 'to reduce the distress of suffering humanity'; 'to save the lives and [preserve] the health of thousands'; and especially, 'to return many upright and honest workers to the state'. The ten-year existence of the Medical Relief was a fertile period of experimentation that attracted the attention of philanthropists and magistrates almost everywhere.[21]

Medical care for the sick poor promised a panacea for the most intransigent problem of impoverishment. The first published report of the Medical Relief pointed out that, through its efforts, 'so many people ... have been cured, [people] we can return to the state as more useful and far healthier members [of society] than [they were] previously, and thereby [we have] stopped up many wellsprings of bitterest want'. Moreover, the Medical Relief reduced the burden on other charitable foundations as well as erasing economic losses due to sickness.[22]

While historians have shown great interest in the social control aspects of poor relief, they have neglected to appreciate the contemporary realisation that one was now dealing with a 'new' poor for whom the older forms of medical care, like the older forms of charity, were outmoded. It was no accident that the élite members of a pace-maker economy like Hamburg's were among the first to recognise what was needed.

The medical care offered by the GPR was almost invariably outdoor or domiciliary rather than institutional. Hospital admission applied only to incurables, although the Medical Deputation ran temporary wards for the isolation of scabies sufferers and for lying-in women. Like other enlightened reformers, Hamburg's improvers joined in the condemnation of old-style hospitals as 'gateways to death'. In Hamburg, the *Pesthof* bore the brunt of the attack. Critics portrayed it as an intensely overcrowded place, permeated with foetid air, and as a charnel house suitable only for the old, the moribund and the hopelessly insane. Yet more than a little evidence suggests that this 'house of horrors' served its purpose rather well and, at the very least, provided a modicum of shelter and morsels of sustenance that should not be quickly dismissed as valueless.[23]

Nonetheless, the supporters of large-scale visiting programmes rejected existing hospitals as proper sites for the medical treatment of the labouring poor. Only if the poor were 'dispensable' or 'extraneous' could these out-moded institutions be viewed as sufficient or appropriate. However, because the new poor were not expendable – and, indeed, had become increasingly critical to the state and to the economy – ancient hospitals, like 'archaic' methods of poor relief, no longer supplied timely answers to the modern problems of illness or poverty among the labouring classes. Thus, the *Pesthof*, and indoor relief more generally, evoked little enthusiasm in Hamburg's reformist circles. Like the old *Zuchthaus* (a combination of a workhouse and house of correction) and all other such 'primitive' structures, the hospital had become an unsuitable place for the working classes. These outdated institutions posed equally 'life-threatening' hazards to the physical, economic, social and moral well-being of thousands. The overwhelming emphasis on the labouring poor as the only proper recipients of relief meant that the greatest efforts were expended towards healing those who could be helped. Medical relief was to avoid expensive long-term care for the chronically ill or permanently incapacitated. In principle, then, both the Medical Relief and the Medical Deputation refused to accept invalids and incurables for treatment. In practice, however, the better funded Medical Deputation made provision for supportive care.[24]

The General Poor Relief consciously built on the experiences of the Medical Relief. Its greater resources, however, permitted it to venture beyond the relatively limited field of action that could be attempted by a handful of physicians and philanthropists. By the early 1790s medical relief had matured into an ambitiously conceived, far-reaching programme that sought to weed out one of the taproots of poverty – unpredictable illness. Free medical care unquestionably extricated some families from poverty and prevented others from becoming destitute through poor health. The policy implicitly (if never explicitly) acknowledged the 'honest worker's' prerogative of health, as well as his right to support and to employment. It reached beyond almsgiving and into the realm of rudimentary social security for the labouring classes that would develop more fully in the late 19th century – although not as a direct successor to medical relief.

Further proof of how decisive the notion of the labouring poor was to the GPR's vision can be found in its later decision to incorporate those who were not genuine paupers into the programme of medical care. The Relief's Medical Deputation was, like the earlier Medical Relief, a domiciliary service. Its scale of operations, however, was more impressive; it handled almost 50 000 cases from 1788 through 1801.[25] Most interesting is the extension of assistance to the so-called *non-registered* poor – a policy which made many members of the working classes eligible for free medical care. The 1788 *Instructions* to relief officers specified that medical aid applied not only to paupers but also to a wider group of people who would be able to earn their own living if they remained healthy, but would suffer a rapid deterioration of circumstances were they confronted with sudden, severe or crippling illness. Anyone thus struck down, and whose reserves were scanty or non-existent, could benefit. They would receive the same medical assistance enjoyed by the registered pauper, but with none of the disadvantages of being enrolled as indigent and dependent.[26] The numbers of the non-registered poor who applied for medical care under this paragraph rose rapidly. In 1788–89 they numbered only 526, about 12 per cent of all patients; by 1792 they numbered 1135 or about 30 per cent.

In some ways, this trend was cause for self-congratulation. Caspar Voght, for instance, postulated that 'the increase of the nonregistered poor treated among the sick shows how much this procedure contributes to the attainment of our goals of preventing destitution through timely intervention'. Nevertheless it swallowed up huge sums of money and the members of the Relief's governing council began to feel that false claimants were exploiting their goodwill. A period of more rigorous control from 1793 to 1795 (coinciding with a brief economic recession) drastically pruned back the numbers of the non-registered poor entitled to medical care. To reduce expenses, the Relief in 1793 instituted a programme of 'half-free' medical care for those who could not pay a physician but who could purchase medicines if provided at the low rates set in the *Paupers' Pharmacopia*. By early 1796 the Relief had abolished this experiment, fearing that it prevented people who truly required aid from seeking it. After 1796 the numbers of the non-registered poor shot up so steeply that by 1797–98 a full 36.57 per cent of those receiving medical care were *not* registered paupers and the numbers continued to climb thereafter. In the economically disastrous first decade of the 19th century, the total soon topped the 50 per cent level. Costs ascended precipitously as well, especially after the Relief established a lying-in ward for unmarried mothers in 1796. Yet even when financially hard-pressed, the Relief was extremely unwilling to abolish medical care for the non-registered poor.[28]

The years of war and occupation from 1799 to 1815 that practically destroyed the Relief caused significant alterations in attitudes towards the poor as well. After 1815 the Relief predicated its programme on alleviating *existing* distress and repudiated the prevention of poverty as an idle dream. The 1814 commission set up to reconstitute the GPR after years of inactivity rejected the older precepts of poor relief as 'faulty' and 'misconceived' and sought to curtail support. Nevertheless, the number of people (especially among the non-registered poor) who turned to the Relief for medical assistance from 1816 through 1824 skyrocketed, as did expenses. In 1817 of the 9089 persons who obtained medical care, 5454 (about 60 per cent) belonged to the non-registered poor; in 1821, of the 16 442 it was 11 301 (almost 70 per cent). Such statistics shocked the governing council which quickly attributed this 'paralysing' assault on its resources to excessive generosity and unwarranted leniency on its own part. As early as 1814 the council had begun to regard medical care as a creator of poverty rather than as a bulwark against it:

> It became customary for families which did not exactly live in comfort to request free medical care each time a member felt the least bit unwell ... [and] so the number of the 'ill' multiplied enormously. Soon these same people asked for monetary support [during their illnesses]. Thus many family fathers whom previously shame had deterred from turning to the Relief and who, despite having many dependents, really did not require aid, began to plead for assistance. A child fell sick and the father realised that it only cost him a trip to the relief officer to obtain medical aid ... . A second illness occurred and he [immediately] requested monetary support. Once he comes to know the relief officer, he approaches him once each winter seeking a bit of support for just a few months 'because he has so many children'. Then he seeks a prolongation, and thus we finally have a man as a registered pauper who perhaps never would have become one if he had had to request alms initially [instead of only medical care].[29]

The Relief claimed that the Medical Deputation was now frequently called upon to treat illnesses that sprang directly from immoral or dissolute behaviour: to maintain those whose dropsy had resulted from furious drinking bouts in taverns and whose consumption had been contracted in dance halls. Consequently, between 1824 and 1829, the Relief introduced a range of restrictions on medical care. In 1824 the Relief stipulated that those who benefited only from medical care must also submit to the embossing of their possessions with the stamp of the Relief as did the registered poor. They also had to name the Relief as their universal heir. In the revised instructions for relief officers circulated in 1829, the Relief announced that 'the non-registered poor are ineligible for monetary support during illness'.[30]

Nonetheless in Hamburg and in Kiel, as in other north German cities, medical care for the indigent and for the non-registered poor remained –

whether intentionally or not – a central pillar of relief programmes. Despite the sharp condemnation of Hamburg's 'imprudently generous policy' of medical care, such assistance consumed the largest portion of relief funds and efforts. Similar tendencies can be traced elsewhere – for example, in Bremen, which had reformed poor relief in 1829 along lines that one observer opined 'may be looked upon as a precursor of the English Poor Law of 1834' (that is, a workhouse test). Despite the harsh and seemingly uncompromising stance of the letter of the law, medical care continued to be allowed to the registered poor and others on a more lavish scale:

> The so-called medicine tickets that provide medical attendance and drugs gratis, are only to be given at once to those already on the list of Institute poor; they may however be given to others (valid for three days) after inquiry by the district deacon as to the real need for such help.[31]

By the mid-19th century, however, critics noted that 'it seems that this rule has by no means been strictly observed. Instead of making any previous inquiry, unconditional trust has been placed in the assertions of the claimants themselves.'[32]

Medical care for the sick poor and also for those members of the working class threatened by impoverishment in time of illness remained a central pillar of social policy well into the 19th century, despite a groundswell of criticism focused on reducing costs that seemed to be spiralling out of control everywhere. Thus, the sick poor, who were always considered among the most legitimate recipients of charity, continued to be viewed as such well into the 19th century, albeit under drastically altered conditions.

Contemporaries found much to admire in the Hamburg system and it was quickly emulated in many places – Altona, Braunschweig, Hanover and even smaller cities, like Schleswig. Locals tailored some aspects to fit specific conditions but the general outline prevailed. However, not everyone approved, and costs were not the only sticking point. Humanitarian and medical objections were raised as well.

In the 1780s two physicians, Dr Daniel Nootnagel and Dr Philipp G. Hensler, representing respectively the pro and con positions on domiciliary care, aired their opinions in print. These contributions subsequently reached a larger medical and philanthropic audience when reprinted in Scherf's *Supplement to the Archives of Medicine* among other places.[33]

Philipp Hensler had studied medicine at Göttingen, worked with Ernst Baldinger in his clinic, and received his doctorate there in 1762. Appointed *physicus* (medical officer) to the Danish areas of Altona, Pinneberg, and Rantzau soon after graduation, he accepted a professorship in 1789 at the university in Kiel. Hensler first published his views in 1785 and, despite praising the 'warm humanitarian spirit' that moved physicians and philanthropists to serve suffering humanity, he doubted whether the domiciliary system was – in its existing form – as beneficial as its advocates asserted. He acknowledged the 'celebrity' (*Rühmlichkeit*) of the Hamburg programme, but felt that costs incurred there were often 'excessive.' He related how in the immediately preceding years, three physicians of the Relief had died after contracting a putrid fever while engaged in their charitable pursuits. Two others had sickened but recovered. He rhetorically queried: 'Is not the life of the physician ... also precious?' While he conceded that a domiciliary form of care might be inexpensive, it was not therefore better. Almost everything could be provided more efficiently in a hospital: cleanliness, attendance, food, and medicines. Moreover, the 'purged air' of the hospital would also 'safeguard the physician's life'.

Daniel Nootnagel, who had worked for two years in Hamburg's domiciliary programme, rebutted Hensler's position point by point. He accepted that cleanliness could be better ensured in a hospital, but that promised only few benefits when arrayed against the many disadvantages of buildings – for example, the high costs of construction and maintenance, poor ventilation, the ease with which infections spread, and the problem of uncaring, unskilled and even venal attendants. The arguments advanced by Nootnagel, as well as the description of Hamburg's system in the preceding pages, has already revealed the purported advantages of visiting patients in their own homes. Nootnagel took up a theme raised by Hensler – that touching on the physician and his role – and turned it around. Hensler fretted about the physical safety of the medical man and felt that it was too much to expect even the most 'philanthropically inspired' man to jeopardise his life repeatedly, and perhaps needlessly, and be told that such was 'his duty'. Nootnagel, however, enumerated the medical as well as moral gains that visiting conferred on physicians and their patients.

> When the altruistic physician enters the humble, dilapidated, [and] filthy lodging of the poor man, when he clasps his hand and through the pressure of his grip says [to him]: I will be your support and your saviour, and when he visits him each day and spares himself no trouble to lighten his load ... in truth, this trust, which rarely can be achieved in a hospital, often accomplishes more than all of the medicines of both Indies.[34]

Yet, despite his strong preference for visiting, Nootnagel did not discount the value of hospitals entirely and, typically, recommended stepping out on a middle road. In addition to domiciliary care 'one must set up a small hospital into which [however] only those patients should be admitted who lack all attention and nursing [at home]'.[35]

By the end of the century, despite Hamburg's shining example, most cities opted for this middle way by erecting new buildings *and* maintaining, or even expanding, domiciliary care. The French-Swiss author, d'Apples Gaulis, writing in 1791, analysed conditions throughout Europe (although he seemed curiously ill-informed about German developments). After reviewing the domiciliary systems or *misericordes* found in France (and judging them 'at times useful' but nonetheless 'inadequate'), he strongly supported plans for renovating and simultaneously improving sprawling ancient hospitals such as the Hôtel-Dieu. He thus echoed the sentiments expressed in 1770 by the Dutch physician, Walther van Doevern, on the advantages of improved hospitals over domiciliary care.[36] A whole range of new general hospitals were built throughout the Germanies beginning with the great foundation in Vienna in 1784. By the early 19th century, the weight of opinion had turned decisively against domiciliary care. Johann Krünitz's bellwether *Encyclopedia* reprinted Hecker's article with its favourable position on hospitals and added that their advantages had been 'completely made clear' and that 'all discerning physicians recognise them'. Yet, even then, he could not disavow the reputation of the Hamburg programme nor deny that it had 'proven its virtues over a period of twenty years'.[37]

If the heyday of the classic domiciliary programme was so fleeting – at the most spanning 40 years from 1770 through 1810 – can it be considered important? By the turn of the 19th century, medical opinion clearly preferred hospitals. Yet medical inclinations alone did not dominate the course of charitable care for the sick poor. In fact, visiting care remained part – and in the northern German cities examined here, a substantial part – of all assistance for the poor well into the 19th century. Charitable organisations in Hamburg, Bremen and Kiel, for example, despite the harsher tone of their pronouncements, their growing concern about expense and their ever heavier emphasis on the depravity of the poor, still furnished a large share of relief in the form of medical aid *at home*. Furthermore, the many private charities that sprang up in the 19th century, and which were directed toward narrower groups of the destitute and the working classes, such as poor, married and pregnant women or impoverished and elderly servants, delivered their charity through voluntary visiting. Domiciliary programmes also helped promote the idea that medical relief was of special importance for the potential poor – that is, for the growing number of labourers whose livelihoods seemed more precarious than in the less economically fluid world that their grandparents and great-grandparents had supposedly inhabited. Finally, domiciliary care emphasised a factor that only increased in significance in the 19th century and that haunts us all today – cost. The great virtue of visiting was its thriftiness and, even if some of its critics tended to equate frugal with bad, the basic issues of how to dispense medical care to large populations without bankrupting the public purse, and the debate as to whether that support is best offered by the state or by private persons and groups, were here to stay.

Notes

1. This chapter presents material first published in my *Patriots and Paupers: Hamburg, 1712–1830* (New York, 1990) and expands that discussion to include other cities in northern Germany.
2. 'Beantwortung der von der K.[öniglichen] Societät der Wissenschaften in Göttingen aufgegebenen Preißfrage, 'Welche sind die bequemsten und wohlfeilsten Mittel, kranken Armen in den Städten die nöthige Hülfe zu verschaffen? Gekrönte Preißschrift vom Herrn Professor Hecker zu Erfurt. Nebst einem Nachtrag des Herrn Verfassers', *Scherfs Archiv der Medizinischen Polizey und der gemeinnützigen Arzneikunde*, **5** (n. 2) (1795), pp. 31–72, at p. 32.
3. Laurence Brockliss and Colin Jones, *The Medical World of Early Modern France*, Oxford, 1997, p. 675 and on the 'Black Legend', pp. 717–25; Dora Weiner, *The Citizen-Patient in Revolutionary and Imperial Paris*, Baltimore, 1993, pp. 36–76.
4. John Macfarlan, *Inquiries Concerning the Poor*, Edinburgh, 1782, pp. 295–96. See the extensive notes Büsch took on the work in Staatsarchiv Hamburg [hereafter StAHbg] Allgemeine Armenanstalt I [hereafter AAI], 1.
5. [Ludwig Gerhard Wagemann], 'Wagemann über vorzüglicher Ursachen des Verarmens, etc. (Fortsetzung)', *Göttingisches Magazin für Industrie und Armenpflege*, **1** (1795), p. 208.
6. [Johann Peter Frank], *A System of Complete Medical Police: Selections from Johann Peter Frank*, edited with an introduction by Erna Lesky, Baltimore, 1975, pp. 12–13.
7. A[rwed] Emminghaus (ed.), *Poor Relief in Different Parts of Europe, Being a Selection of Essays*, London, 1973, p. 94.
8. Roy Porter, 'The Gift Relation: Philanthropy and Provincial Hospitals in Eighteenth-Century England', in Lindsay Granshaw and Roy Porter (eds), *The Hospital in History*, London, 1987, pp. 149–78.
9. Johann Georg Büsch, 'Allgemeine Winke zur Verbesserung des Armenwesens', in idem, *Zwei kleine Schriften die im Werk begriffene Verbesserung des Armenwesens in dieser Stadt Hamburg betreffend* (Hamburg, 1786), unpaginated.
10. StAHbg, Senat Cl. VII Lit. Qd no. 3 vol. 12 fasc. 1.
11. Johann Georg Büsch, 'Vorschläge zur Verbesserung des Hamburgischen Armenwesens 1786', in StAHbg, AAI, p. 1.
12. *25ste Nachricht*, July 1799, p. 177; Hans Mauersberg, *Wirtschafts- und Sozialgeschichte zentraleuropäischen Städte in neuerer Zeit: Dargestellt am Beispielen von Basel, Frankfurt a.M., Hamburg, Hannover und München*, Göttingen, 1960, p. 43; Jonas Ludwig von Heß, *Hamburg, topographisch, politisch und historisch beschrieben*, 2nd edn, Hamburg, 1811, Vol. III, Appendix, Table I.
13. Wilhelm Seelig, 'Elbherzogthümer,' in Arwed Emminghaus (ed.), *Das Armenwesen und die Armengesetzgebung in europäischen Staaten*, Berlin, 1870, pp. 127–30.
14. August Christian Heinrich Niemann, *Ueber Armenversorgungsanastalten*, Altona and Hamburg, 1794; idem, *Ueber die Grundsätze der Armenpflege*, Kiel, 1794; idem, *Uebersicht der neuen Armenpflege in der Stadt Kiel Sr. Königl[ichen]. Hoheit des Kronprinzen Befehl vorgelegt von der Gesellschaft freiwilliger Armenfreunde in Auftrag derselben abgefasset von ihrem Wortführer*, Altona, 1798.
15. *Nachricht van dem hieselbst errichteten klinischen Institute zum Besten der*

Armen, Kiel, 1785; see also 'Vom dem klinischen Institut zum Besten der Armen zu Kiel', in *Schleswig-Holsteinische-Provincial-Berichte*, **1** (1787); 'Krankenanstalt in Kiel', *Göttingisches Magazin*, **3** (1793), pp. 343–59.

16. The series of printed reports continued with *5te Nachricht van dem Zustande des klinischen Instituts und der jetzt erweiterten Krankenanstalt überhaupt*, Kiel, 1791; the sixth through the twelfth reports appeared from 1792 to 1798 (Kiel); finally, *Kurze Geschichte der hiesigen Krankenanstalt als 13. Nachricht van dem Zustande derselben*, Kiel, 1804.

17. 'Krankenanstalt in Kiel', *Göttingisches Magazin*, **3** (1793), pp. 345–50; 'Darstellung der Armenanstalt in Kiel als Muster für Städte von ähnlicher Große, deren Bewohner gemeinsam genug haben sich zu diesem edlen Zweck zu vereinigen', *Göttingisches Magazin*, **5** (1802), pp. 101–36 'Vorschläge und vorläufige Einrichtung zur Verbesserung der Armenanstalt in Kiel', *Göttingisches Magazin*, **3** (1793), pp. 321–42; see also the various reports published by Weber listed in n. 14.

18. 'Etwas über die hamburgische Gesundheitspolizei aus einem Brief eines reisenden Arztes an seinen Freund L. in Thüringen. Hamburg, den 18. Juni 1805', *Hamburg und Altona*, **4**, (2) (1805), pp. 355–56. Quoted in Johann Klefeker, *Sammlung der Hamburgischen Gesetze und Verfassung in Bürger- und Kirchlichen, auch Cammer-Handlungs- und übrigen Policey-Angelegenheiten und Geschäften samt historischen Einleitungen*, 12 vols, Hamburg, 1765–73, Vol. 12, pp. 63–69.

19. 'Nachrichten von der Verfassung des medicinischen Armen-Instituts in dem ersten zweyjährigen Zeiträume vom 1sten Jul. 1779 bis zum 1sten Jul. 1781', pp. 19–20, an undated report signed by the directors von Axen, Prösch, and Oberdorffer in StaHbg, AAI, p. 106; and Georg Merkel, *Briefe über einige der merkwürdigsten Städte in Deutschland*, Leipzig, 1801, p. 300. The classic discussion of the advantages of a good medical police, including care for the sick poor, is, of course, Johann Peter Frank, *System einer vollständigen medicinischen Polizey*, 4 vols, Mannheim, 1779–88.

20. See announcement in *Hamburgische Adreß-Comptoir Nachrichten* [hereafter: *ACN*], 14 May 1768 and in the *Gemeinnützige Nachrichten aus dem Reiche der Wissenschaften und Künste*, 15 January 1768; 'Vereinigungs-Plan verschiedener Aerzte und Wundärzte zum Vortheil der hamburgischen kranken Hausarmen', in *Berliner Sammlungen zur Beförderung der Arzneywissenschaft, der Naturgeschichte, der Haushaltungskunst, Cameralwissenschaft und der dahin einschlagenden Litteratur*, **1** (1768), pp. 162–73; 'Senat-Protocoll (1768)', in StAHbg, Senat Cl. VIII; Senat Cl. VII Lit. Dd no. 4 Vol. 3, p. 175. On the new programme instituted in 1779, see *Plan zum Vortheil der hiesigen kranken Haus-Armen* (Hamburg, 1779, p. 2 (also in *ACN*, 20 and 27 May 1779).

21. 'Nachricht an das Publikum', *ACN*, 14 May 1768.

22. *Nachricht van der neuerrichteten medicinischen Anstalt für kranke Haus-Arme in Hamburg*, Hamburg, 1781 [hereafter: *Nachricht 1781*], pp. 16, 20; *Zweite Sammlung van der Nachrichten vom medicinischen Armen-Institut in Hamburg: Vom 1sten Juli 1781 bis January 1784*, Hamburg, 1784 [hereafter: *Nachricht 1784*], p. 40.

23. Heinz [Heinrich] Rodegra, *Vom Pesthof zum Allgemeinen Krankenhaus: Die Entwicklung des Krankenhauswesens in Hamburg zu Beginn des 19. Jahrhunderts*, Münster, 1977; J.J. Menuret, *Essai sur la ville d'Hambourg considérée dans ses rapports avec la santé, ou lettres sur l'histoire médico-topographique de cette ville*, Hamburg, 1797; Johann Jakob Rambach, *Versuch einer physisch-medicinischen Beschreibung von Hamburg*, Hamburg, 1801, pp. 411–12, 416–17.

24. 'Antrag der Medicinal Deputation, 1789,' StAHbg, AAI, 106; *Nachricht 1781*, pp. 20–22; 'Convention zwischen der Armen-Anstalt und dem Pesthof. Vom Jahr 1789'; 'Extractus Protocolli der Medicinal-Deputation,' 14 January 1789, StAHbg, AAI, p. 105; Johann Arnold Günther, *Argumente und Erfahrungen über Kranken-Besuch-Anstalten aus den 2jährigen Rechnungs-Abschlüssen, des Medicinal Departments der Hamburgischen Armenanstalt*, Hamburg, 1791, pp. 64–67; 'Übersichten und die Beschlüsse der Medizinaldeputation betr. die Behandlung langwieriger Kranken, 1789–1792', StAHbg, AAI, p. 107.

25. On the programmes and goals, see *6te Nachricht*, June 1790, p. 56; *9te Nachricht*, March 1791, pp. 85–108. On the types of care offered, see especially *15te Nachricht*, February 1794, pp. 222–23; *24ste Nachricht*, September 1798, p. 131. See also the deliberations of the Medical Deputation from 1788 to 1793 in StAHbg, AAI, p. 94 and the material covering the period 1789 to 1806 in StAHbg, AAI, p. 109. The total number of patients was 48 465. Sources: *21ste Nachricht*, February 1797, p. 67; *23ste Nachricht*, January 1798, p. 112; *25ste Nachricht*, July 1799, p. 170; *27ste Nachricht*, February 1800, p. 234; *28ste Nachricht* January 1801, p. 273; and *30ste Nachricht*, May 1803, pp. 353–52; and Paul Kollmann, 'Ueberblick über die Wirksamkeit der "Allgemeinen Armenanstalt" der Stadt Hamburg von 1788 bis 1870', *Statistik des Hamburgischen Staats*, **3** (1871), p. 128.

26. *Vollständige Einrichtungen der neuen Hamburgischen Armenanstalt, zum Besten dieser Anstalt herausgegeben vom Hamburgischen Armen Collegio*, Hamburg, 1788, pp. 99–100.

27. Caspar Voght writing in the supplement to the *14te Nachricht*, May 1793, pp. 207–8.

28. Deliberations on cost-cutting and the system of 'half-free' care can be found in StAHbg, AAI, p. 106; see also 'Anzeige und Ersuchen an die Herren Armen-Pfleger, die Ausgebung der Kranken-Zettel für solche Nicht-Eingezeichnete Arme betreffend, die zwar nicht die ganze Cur, aber doch die Arznei bezahlen können [March 1793]', supplement to *14te Nachricht*, May 1793, pp. 207–8; *22ste Nachricht*, June 1797, pp. 85–86; and the deliberations of the Medical Deputation from 1793 and 1796 in StAHbg, AAI, p. 94.

29. Quoted in Werner von Melle, *Die Entwicklung des öffentlichen Armenwesens in Hamburg*, Hamburg, 1883, pp. 141–42.

30. *38ste Nachricht*, July 1818, p. 270; *Nachricht an die Herren Armenpfleger über den Geschäftsgang bei der Armenfürsorge*, Hamburg, 1829, p. 64.

31. August Lammers, 'The Town of Bremen,' in Emminghaus, *Poor Relief* (n. 7), pp. 109, 111.

32. Ibid., p. 111.

33. 'Ueber Krankenbesuchanstalten von Dr. D. Nootnagel,' *Scherfs Archiv* 4 (2) (1786), pp. 60–81; 'Ueber Krankenanstalten von Doktor P.G. Hensler,' ibid., 47–60; Daniel Nootnagel, in *ACN* nos 23–24 (1780).

34. Philipp Gabriel Hensler, *Ueber Kranken-Anstalten*, Hamburg, 1785; idem, 'Vortheile der Krankenhäuser verglichen mit Krankenbesuchanstalten,' *Staatsanzeiger*, **7** (1785), pp. 272–83.

35. Nootnagel in *ACN*.

36. The title of the work was *Parallele entre les misericordes et les hôpitaux*, Lausanne, 1789. Parts were translated into German and appeared in *Scherfs Beyträge zum Archiv der medizinischen Polizey und der gemeinnützigen Armenpflege*, 3 (1), (1791), pp. 133–48.

37. 'Medicinal-Anstalten', in *D. Johann Georg Krünitz's ökonomisch-technologische*

Encyklopädie oder allgemeines System der Staats-, Stadt-, Haus-, und Landwirthschaft und der Kunstgeschichte in alphabetischer Ordnung, Vol. 86 (1802), p. 633, reprint of Hecker's article, pp. 607–32.

PART THREE

Russia and Scandinavia

CHAPTER SEVEN

Health Care and Poor Relief in Russia, 1700–1856

Hubertus Jahn

'Every 4th doctor in the world is Soviet.' This statement appeared on a poster in Moscow in the year 1973. With its plain statistical information it sent a strong and quite daring propaganda message. It claimed nothing less than the superiority of the Soviet health care system over those in other countries. Less than 20 years later, according to opinion polls, 61 per cent of the Soviet population believed in the healing powers of a certain Anatolii Kashpirovskii, a TV celebrity and charlatan who promised to treat everything from AIDS to radiation sickness through hypnosis and telepathic sessions.[1] What had happened? And why are these two anecdotes relevant for the discussion of the history of health care and poor relief in 18th and 19th century Russia?

The Soviet social welfare system was notorious for the discrepancies between aspiration and reality. Health care and poor relief were no exceptions. According to all official sources, poor people and beggars simply did not exist in the Soviet Union. In 1970, to take an example from official statistics, only 0.1 per cent of the entire population did not live on a salary, stipend or pension.[2] In reality, however, many of these payments were quite low, in many cases insufficient, and sometimes simply non-existent; an unknown number of people who were caught begging were convicted of social parasitism and sent to labour camps. The state of health care was likewise far from satisfactory. Even if every fourth doctor in the world was indeed Soviet in 1973, other problems certainly overshadowed this achievement – poorly trained hospital staff, chronic shortages of medicine and basic supplies, a lack of modern medical technology, a basic neglect of hygiene and enormous environmental problems. Life expectancy in the Soviet Union has consequently been considerably lower than in other industrialised countries. In 1980, for example, the average life expectancy of Soviet men was 82 years. Today, this figure needs to be corrected to somewhere around 57. Life expectancy for women is only somewhat higher.[3] It is little wonder that all kinds of non-conventional treatments such as traditional folk medicine and faith healing could survive and even flourish under such circumstances.

In order to understand the window-dressing of the Soviet state and the strong position of non-conventional medicine in Russia today, it is imperative to return to the era of Peter the Great, the generally acknowledged starting point of modern Russian history.[4] Under his reign, Western ideas of health care and poor relief first entered Russia on a wide scale. As part of a larger effort to modernise the country along the lines of Western European absolutism, Peter's goal was to bring reason and progress to a place, which, in the words of one of his correspondents, the philosopher Gottfried Wilhelm Leibniz, was a *tabula rasa* and thus perfectly suited for setting up a new order.[5] However, as the tsar and others were soon to learn, Russia was much too large, diverse, and poorly administered for the smooth introduction of such a new order. Moreover, native religious traditions, popular customs and such social structures as serfdom hindered innovation and change. Consequently, many of Peter's reforms were confined geographically to the main cities, especially to Moscow and, after its foundation in 1703, St Petersburg. That city in particular was to serve as a model for the rest of the country and as a showcase for the outside world. As most innovations in the fields of health care and poor relief thus remained restricted to St Petersburg and Moscow well into the 19th century, this study will concentrate on the capital cities. Unfortunately, very little is known about the situation in the provinces before the 1860s, as the basic research still remains to be done.

The central goal of Peter's reforms was to mobilise the entire population for the benefit of the state. He thus implemented mandatory civil and military service for the nobility, strengthened the system of serfdom, and placed tremendous financial and military demands on the peasantry. Logically enough, people were expected not to be idle, drunk and sick, but healthy and productive in order to contribute actively to the common good, to pay taxes and to fight in the army. Towards these ends, Peter issued numerous and often very specific decrees (*ukazy*), which in many ways resembled the German police ordinances (*Polizeiordnungen*) of that time. As judged from their frequent repetition and re-issuance, however, these decrees were clearly ineffective and most likely never even implemented.[6] An additional characteristic of Peter's highly personal style of government was his proclivity to take things, literally, into his own hands. Not only did he himself administer all kinds of medical and dental treatments to all those who were careless enough to complain about pains in the tsar's presence, he also sent Russians abroad to study medicine and, during his own travels through Western Europe, invited foreign doctors to come to Russia and practise there. In 1706 a general military hospital and surgical school was thus opened in Moscow under the directorship of Nicholas Bidloo from Leiden University. Soon afterwards, in 1715 and 1717, the first two hospitals in St Petersburg were founded – one for the navy, the other for the army. From the very outset, therefore, health care in Russia was closely connected with the military and the state. In addition, Peter created a state office charged with medical administration, placed under the direction of an archiater or chief imperial physician. The medical chancery (*meditsinskaia kantseliariia*), as it was soon called, supervised all military and civilian doctors and pharmacists until it was abolished by Catherine the Great in 1763 and replaced by a so-called medical collegium (*meditsinskaia kollegiia*).[7]

While medical institutions in the capital cities could be created fairly easily and staffed with foreign specialists, poor relief faced altogether more difficult obstacles. As Richard Hellie has noted, early modern Russians were 'only on the threshold of dealing with the problem of poverty in any fashion and had hardly intellectualized the problem at all'.[8] Indeed, the role of religion was particularly important in Russian society, for Muscovy lacked a secular culture of literature, philosophy, art or law. In this highly traditional society, moreover, begging and almsgiving had themselves longstanding traditions which, even more importantly, fulfilled a central religious function. For Russian Orthodox Christians, the aspiration to salvation retained a central importance and, in this quest for redemption, the giving of alms played an important role. As an expression of piety and thanks, beggars were expected to pray for the souls of their benefactors. In the Orthodox world, this general Christian idea had also become a central issue of moral theology, founded on the sermons of the Byzantine Church father John Chrysostom, which had been disseminated in Russia for many centuries through numerous religious anthologies.[9] As a result, beggars were a constituent part of everyday religious practice, even enjoying special protection in early Russian law codes such as the 12th century *Russkaia pravda* (Russian justice) or the 16th century *Domostroi* (household-rule). Monasteries set aside special quarters for them, and, during the reign of Peter's father, a group of beggars even resided permanently in the Moscow Kremlin and in the palace of the Moscow patriarch. By the time of Peter's ascendancy to the throne in 1682, this world of religious traditions and age-old customs was coming under serious attack.[10]

Early on in his reign, Peter declared war against this customary phenomenon. In 1691, and again in 1694, Peter issued a decree against 'idle people' in Moscow, who 'by binding up their hands and also their legs' or 'by covering and screwing up their eyes, as if they are blind and lame, beg for alms in Christ's name by sham and cunning, but upon examination they are all healthy'.[11] All these people were to be rounded up and sent back to their village of birth or, in the case of serfs, to their lords. Should they return to Moscow and be caught a second time, they were to be beaten with the knout and exiled to Siberia. Subsequent decrees were still more specific: beggars were thus prohibited from moving around the country and relegated to almshouses, where they were also to be officially registered.

Obviously paraphrasing Western European legislation, a 1718 decree spelled out the basic precepts for future regulations of poverty and begging.[12] It called for a distinction between the deserving and the undeserving poor. Healthy beggars or those not registered in an almshouse were to be whipped 'mercilessly', and, if caught a second time, beaten in public with the knout and then sent to forced labour in exile. Begging women and children were to be assigned to a *shpingauz* (spinning house) where they were to earn their keep through spinning and weaving. This decree did not just punish the poor, it also introduced penalties of up to five rubles for those lords whose serfs were found begging. However, this measure was hardly sufficient to stem the waves of runaways. Serfdom was widespread in Russia until its abolition in 1861, and, as a result of absolutist politics, it expanded considerably under Peter and his successors. With more and more peasants being enserfed in the 18th and early 19th centuries, and with rising burdens of corvée and rents, the problem of rural poverty and of runaways thus became rampant. Consequently, many beggars were runaway serfs, whose masters were still legally responsible for them. Until the 20th century, however, the state did not concern itself with the causes of rural poverty and hence of migratory begging.

To enforce the new laws, new institutions of policing were also required, and these too followed a Western, primarily central European, model. These institutions, and not the Church, were made responsible not only for the suppression of begging but also for the administration of poor relief. As specified in special statutes from 1718 and 1721, their tasks ranged widely: the cleanliness of streets, the regulation of commerce, the supervision of visitors, the arrest of beggars and people who were simply 'hanging out', and, finally, the setting up of orphanages, prisons and workhouses (or *tsukhtgauzy*, as they were called then). The role of the Church was reduced to that of a paymaster and a provider of charitable infrastructures. Since 1701, monasteries in particular had been obliged to finance almshouses and to take care of disabled soldiers as well as illegitimate and abandoned children. Churches were required to set up extra offertory boxes in order to collect money for the support of almshouses. To ensure that donations reached their destination, decrees from 1718 and 1720 prohibited the non-institutional giving of alms. People who nonetheless gave money to beggars in the streets were to pay fines of five to ten rubles. Personal piety was thus regulated as a matter of public order and socioeconomic expediency.[13]

Despite these general decrees, it should be noted that Peter did not intend to create a state system of poor relief. Instead, he expected local authorities such as landlords, village communes and cities to organise charity on their own initiative. However, unlike western Europe, where magistrates had been setting up such secular institutions of poor relief as the 'common box' or the *gemeiner Kasten* on a local level since the 16th century, Russia had no traditions of civic responsibility or independent local government. Most of Peter's decrees, therefore, remained what Richard Stites has called an 'administrative utopia'.[14] Very few of the institutions mentioned in the decrees actually existed in reality, and those that were founded were far from sufficient. St Petersburg, for example, had only four almshouses by 1734. According to a contemporary source, 20 such houses would have been needed to accommodate all the poor eligible for charity in the capital.[15]

The problem was not simply an institutional or a financial one. The whole concept of secular and institutionalised poor relief was alien to most Russians, including those who were in charge of implementing it. What should they make of institutions which they had never seen before and which bore such strange Germanic names like *shpingauz* (spinning house) or *tsukhtgauz* (workhouse)? For that matter, how could they determine who was actually a truly poor and needy person and who was an impostor and false beggar? No such differences had existed before, and the traditional Russian words *nishchii* and *ubogii* had always been used interchangeably for both 'poor person' and 'beggar'. As a consequence, Peter's legislation also initiated a prolonged struggle over the semantic content of these words, which were constantly defined and redefined. Beggars and poor people were thus associated with various characteristics or different kinds of behaviour and, in the process, placed in all sorts of newly invented categories. The 'Spiritual Regulation' of 1721, for example, which abolished the patriarchate and placed the Church under the administration of the state, likened beggars to indolent rogues, vandals, thieves, arsonists and even spies.[16] Other legal sources attempted to define so-called 'real' beggars or the poor as the old and the sick, but such categories of deserving and undeserving poor were, of course, expandable. During the reign of Peter's daughter Elizabeth, beggars even gained an aesthetic meaning. After an encounter with an old beggar woman, whose face was disfigured by scars or pockmarks and described as 'utterly offensive', the empress decreed in 1758 that such people were not to show themselves anymore in the imperial capital.[17] Although this took place while Bartolomeo Rastrelli was embellishing St Petersburg with Italian rococo palaces, Elizabeth's decree did not only address the aesthetic quality of beggars in an imperial city. It also reflected the contemporary obsession with smallpox, one of the most prevalent and dangerous scourges of the era, that was to become a major issue of public health during the reign of Catherine the Great.

While Peter had largely relied on the knout for implementing reason and order, Catherine the Great propagated enlightened education and the prescriptions of German cameralist thought to achieve domestic reforms. Born in Stettin and brought up in the small world of northern German courts, she was able to observe firsthand the political and social ramifications of Lutheran ethics and Pietist edification.[18] In addition, she had been an avid reader since her early years, with a particular interest in French philosophical works. Thus, when she ascended the Russian throne in 1762, she was familiar with many of Voltaire's writings and had read a number of historical and dramatic works, as well as Montesquieu's *Esprit des lois*.[19] The latter in particular was to influence Catherine's so-called 'Great Instruction' of 1767, a 'compendium of the general principles on which good government and an orderly society should be based'.[20] Intended as a guideline for a commission in charge of drawing up a new code of law – a project which was never completed – the 'Great Instruction' served as an inspiration for administrative and social reforms in later years. In particular, its first supplement was full of practical advice for the implementation of a well-ordered police state, both in the cities and in the provinces. It relied almost exclusively on the work of German cameralists – particularly the *Institutions politiques* of Jakob Friedrich von Bielfeld – and it described the numerous tasks of the police, ranging from traffic control to the welfare of the sick and destitute.[21]

Consequently, under Catherine's reign the Russian state systematically organised health care and poor relief for the first time – at least in St Petersburg and Moscow. Instead of issuing repetitive and unrealistic decrees, Catherine created actual institutions which were sometimes run with moderate success. As a result of the secularisation of Church property and the closure of numerous monasteries in 1764, the involvement of the state in charity had also become necessary. Indeed, this policy had the largely unintended by-product of eliminating all the charitable obligations which Peter had laid on the Church, such as the maintenance of almshouses, for example.

The 'Statute on Provincial Administration of 1775' set out the legal framework for Catherine's new charitable institutions in the form of so-called 'social welfare boards'. These bodies, which were to be organised in every province, included representatives of the nobility, the urban estates and the free peasants. Chaired and *de facto* dominated by the provincial governors, they received a one-off endowment from the state treasury and were then to manage their finances independently – a strategy which generally ensured minimal compliance. Their funding came mostly from private donations, interest earned on their capital, and from certain obligatory payments contributed by local towns. This laid the sole foundation for medical and charitable aid in the Russian Empire. The social welfare boards thus ran schools, hospitals, orphanages, almshouses, insane asylums, workhouses and foundling homes. Between 1803 and 1862 the number of such institutions increased from 389 to 769 – a tiny number in a country the size of Russia. Quantity, moreover, did not mean quality. The reputation of the social welfare boards' institutions was terrible, to say the least. They were poorly run and constantly overcrowded, mortality rates were extremely high, and public support for, and participation on, the boards was hardly enthusiastic. Indeed, the boards often served the window-dressing function familiar from the aforementioned Soviet poster: often a governor responsible for the operation of a board would not even attend its meetings; indeed, protocols of meetings, which never took place, were sometimes simply invented and then sent to the members of the board to be signed.[22]

Despite such major shortcomings, public health was one of Catherine's general concerns. Although she had a pretty low opinion of professional physicians, was rather sceptical of medicine, and preferred for herself to rely on such natural treatments as fresh air, mild exercise and dietary moderation, Catherine also understood the dangers of diseases such as bubonic plague and smallpox. The latter in particular was a constant source of concern, although she herself was fortunate enough to never come down with it, and the reasons for her anxiety were of a more personal and political nature. Since Catherine had come to power in a *coup d'état*, in which her husband and predecessor had lost his life, her dynastic position was not always secure. Her personal fitness and the health of her only son and successor to the throne, the Grand Duke Paul, were thus necessary for her reign. When small-pox cost the lives of members of the Austrian Habsburgs in 1767 and also killed increasing numbers of people in St Petersburg court circles, including the fiancée of her closest adviser, Nikita Panin, Catherine, quite progres-sively, decided to have herself and her son inoculated. Through the offices of the Russian ambassador in London, she invited one of the leading British specialists on variolation, Dr Thomas Dimsdale, to come to Russia and se-cretly administer the inoculations. The treatment was successful in both cases, and, in the true spirit of the times, it was soon promulgated as an act of enlightenment – a means of liberating the population not only from disease but also from superstition and ignorance. As Catherine herself hastened to explain, 'My objective was, through my example, to save the multitude of my subjects from death, who, not knowing the value of this technique, frightened of it, were left in danger.'[23] Inoculation against smallpox became a minor success story. Special clinics were opened in the capitals, but also in provin-cial towns as far away as Irkutsk in Siberia. If one is to believe the statistics of the time, some 2 million people had been inoculated by the year 1800.

Right from the beginning of her reign, Catherine had conceptualised public health in terms of a politics of population growth. One of her first steps was to reform the state medical administration with the founding of a special *Collegium* in 1763 to supervise the medical profession. Its tasks included the training of medical doctors as well as the assignment of at least one doctor to each Russian province. On a more pragmatic level, Catherine founded Rus-sia's first public hospital in 1763, which she financed out of her own purse. Paul's Hospital, as it was called, was a small wooden house with 25 beds, located in the outskirts of Moscow and offering free treatment to poor pa-tients of both sexes. A public hospital in St Petersburg, with 60 beds and a ward for psychiatric patients, followed in 1779.[24]

Meanwhile, a terrible plague epidemic had ravaged Moscow and triggered a major riot in 1771, during which many people, including the archbishop, had been killed. As a direct result of this event, which had utterly shocked Catherine, efforts were made to expand medical education and to hire more foreign physicians. Measures to enforce public hygiene were also taken: vagrant beggars from out of town were prohibited from entering Moscow, as they might pick up the disease and distribute it in the rest of the country. Cemeteries and slaughterhouses were to be relocated to places outside the city limits. Finally, and symbolic of progress in more than one sense, so-called *ubogie doma* were abolished. These were open pits covered by shacks into which unclean corpses had traditionally been thrown – a category which included unidentified people found dead on the road and those who had committed suicide. Since these pits were covered with dirt only once a year, they did indeed pose a considerable health hazard. In addition, they were perceived as symbols and remnants of a superstitious Muscovite past.[25]

Progress had a different face, and it also had a name: in Catherine's Russian it was called *vospitanie*; in German *Erziehung* or 'education' – in the broadest sense of the word. The driving force behind this concept was Ivan Ivanovich Betskoi, the illegitimate son of a nobleman. Having lived in Western Europe for most of his life, Betskoi had met some of the leading writers of the Enlightenment and had familiarised himself with institutions of welfare and learning. When he returned to Russia in 1762, he drew up several proposals for the improvement of Russia's schooling and health care systems, which all appealed to Catherine's self-image as an enlightened monarch and to her interest in the latest philosophic trends. He thus won her financial and political support for a number of social projects. The most ambitious – and if compared to western European approaches, the most progressive – project was the establishment of imperial foundling homes in Moscow and St Petersburg. Of course, the idea of foundling homes as such was not new, but Betskoi and Catherine intended to use these institutions as more than just depositories for abandoned children; they wanted them to become 'incubators of an entirely new type of individual'. As David Ransel has put it, the foundling homes 'were to inculcate enlightened morality, the work ethic, civic-mindedness, and respect for constituted authority, and thus to create from unwanted children the educated, urban estate that Russia then lacked'.[26] A third estate made up of educated town-dwellers, artisans, bureaucratic specialists and different kinds of professionals was indeed missing in Russia and, in a combination of welfare and social engineering, the foundling home population was thus to fill that gap. Following Locke's conception of the subject, the foundlings were to be raised with the enlightened principles of *vospitanie* from the cradle through their school years in a controlled institutional environment. With the educational stress laid on moral training and patriotic sentiment, they were to become solid and honourable citizens, who would serve the state and pass on their civic attitudes and moral values to their children. Reality looked quite different. The mortality rates in the foundling homes were extremely high, due mostly to open admission. Of the 42 674 children admitted to the Moscow home between 1764 and 1798, only 5500 or 12.9 per cent survived. In later years, these numbers hardly changed. As late as 1912, 7000 out of 9770 children in both houses died.[27]

While a third estate did not emerge from Betskoi's educational system, a small circle of people nevertheless propagated civic and ethical standards in 18th century Russia. Most of them were freemasons, whom Catherine largely tolerated in the early years of her reign but whom she increasingly suppressed after the outbreak of the French Revolution as a potentially subversive force. Russian freemasons usually belonged to the service nobility which had evolved as a result of Peter's reforms. Detached from old Muscovite clan structures and traditions, this new social group aspired to Western ways of life, shared certain career experiences and developed its own corporate values. Typical Enlightenment ideas concerning human dignity, pedagogy, rational social organisation and mutual benefit proved crucial in the shaping of their world-view and helped them fashion a new social identity. The Russian freemason set a dual task for himself. On the one hand, he himself was to cultivate the highest moral standards and thus improve his moral personality. On the other hand, he had to stand up for the dignity of other human beings. Because this task conflicted with the system of serfdom, Russian freemasons generally, though with several notable exceptions, emphasised the spiritual sphere rather than social or political reform. Consequently, many became involved in the publication of uplifting literature which promoted poor relief and philanthropic attitudes as a constituent part of an enlightened aristocratic persona.[28]

The most influential of these writers and publishers was Nikolai Novikov who edited and published several journals in the 1770s and later managed the Moscow University Press. The first to put philanthropic theory into practice, Novikov launched the first private charitable initiative in Russia. In 1777 he founded the journal *Utrennyi svet* ('The Morninglight') with the specific purpose of collecting donations from its readers in support of two schools for poor children and orphans.[29] The schools were indeed opened in St Petersburg, and the journal began to report regularly on the progress and scholarly achievements of the students as well as on the noble motives of the donors. Novikov did not stop there. Once he had moved to Moscow, he founded the Society of Learned Friends (*Druzheskoe uchenoe obshchestvo*) which, apart from distributing useful literature, gave stipends to needy students and occasionally provided relief to the city's poor.[30]

Novikov's initiatives were truly exceptional for their time. Private charity on a larger scale developed in Russia only under Catherine's grandson, tsar Alexander I, in the first quarter of the 19th century. It would be plagued, however, by the controlling hand of the state, which was suspicious of independent initiative. Right at the beginning of his reign, Alexander proclaimed his humanitarian spirit in a edict which elaborated concepts of rational philanthropy and recommended the visiting of poor people by so-called guardians. In fact, the new tsar had been extremely impressed by the example of the Hamburg Charitable Society (*Hamburger Armenanstalt*), which had introduced a system of guardians and had allegedly eradicated begging in Hamburg. After a consultation with the Hamburg Society's co-founder and director, Caspar von Voght, Alexander decreed the creation of similar organisations in Russia. The first one to be established in 1804 was a Medical-Philanthropic Committee in St Petersburg, consisting of well-established physicians who offered free medical care and medication to poor people at home and in a number of out-patient clinics. A year later, a Committee for the Care of the Poor was opened, which sent out guardians to the city's needy.[31]

Finally, in 1816, the tsar founded the Imperial Philanthropic Society (*Imperatorskoe chelovekoliubivoe Obshchestvo*), which became the most famous charitable organization in Russia and survived until the fall of the Romanov dynasty in 1917. Financed in part through annual grants of the tsar, which in Alexander's time amounted to 150 000 rubles, the Philanthropic Society also created a system of membership fees and private donations. It was thus a hybrid institution, combining state and private initiative. In the first ten years of its existence, the Imperial Philanthropic Society opened branches in Moscow, Kazan, Ufa, Voronezh and Slutsk (near Minsk) and cared for an average of 4039 poor people per year. This number soon soared to 25 358 in the decade from 1836 to 1846 and reached 37 773 in the year 1857. Apart from its activities in poor relief, the Society also published a journal which helped disseminate the ideas of private charity and organised philanthropy. For the first time, Russian readers could learn about foreign charitable institutions, about famous philanthropists and progressive social projects such as Robert Owen's New Lanark community. Other features included information about benefactors and their philanthropic projects as well as heart-rending descriptions of the living conditions of poor families written in the style of sentimental literature. The civic spirit and the masonic influences evident in the pages of the journal also caused its downfall in the reactionary last years of Alexander's reign and led to its closure in 1826 after the accession of Nicholas I to the throne.[32]

Largely as a result of the Decembrist revolt of 1825, which had been planned in secret circles of young noblemen who propagated civil rights and popular sovereignty, Nicholas I was highly suspicious of any unofficial initiative or voluntary association. Nevertheless, between 1826 and 1855, the charters of some 20 new charitable associations received official approval and, in addition, several private philanthropic enterprises were established. In 1833, for example, Anatolii Demidov, the son of a rich industrialist family, opened a house of industry in St Petersburg, which offered work to needy people and ran a network of soup kitchens in various parts of the city.[33] In 1846 the St Petersburg Society for Visiting the Poor (*Obshchestvo poseshcheniia bednykh*) began its short-lived, but highly successful, operations. Planned simply as an intermediary between philanthropists and poor people, this association soon had 250 members drawn from the better circles of Petersburg society, a staff of voluntary physicians, a store which sold goods produced by the poor themselves, and an information office which contained the files of some 8000 needy people who had been investigated by members of the society and found to be deserving. Such examples of social organisation and initiative, however, only provoked the suspicions of the government. As a direct consequence of the revolutionary events in Europe in 1848, Nicholas revoked the Society's autonomous status and placed it under the auspices of the Imperial Philanthropic Society.[34]

Although an important act of civic engagement, neither the private donations of money, food and clothing, nor the pious visits to the poor in their homes solved the problem of poverty. Beggars, for example, were hardly reached by such charitable efforts, for they often did not have a home where they could be visited. Furthermore, Peter's decrees and Catherine's statutes had put them under the responsibility of the police. Accordingly, beggars were usually arrested and thrown into police prisons until it was decided whether they were eligible for an almshouse or if they were to be sent into a workhouse or to forced labour in Siberia. At a time when philanthropy was a much discussed topic among well-to-do Russians, this policy could suddenly seem inappropriate. It was tsar Nicholas himself, who, after a visit to a St Petersburg prison in 1834, criticised the confinement of simple beggars together with all sorts of criminals. On his order, the president of the Prison Guardian Society (*Obshchestvo Popechitel'noe o tiur'makh*), a charitable organisation in charge of the improvement of prison conditions, developed a plan for coping with beggars in the capital. His solution to the problem was to create a special committee, which was subsequently founded in 1837 and funded by donations and regular payments from the city authorities. Named the Supreme Committee for the Differentiation and the Care of Beggars in St Petersburg (*Vysochaishe uchrezhdennyi Komitet dlia razbora i prizreniia nishchikh v S.-Peterburge*), it was followed by a similar institution in Moscow a year later and it survived until 1903, when it was taken over by the St. Petersburg city government.[35]

The main task of the beggars' committee, as it was usually called, was the elimination of begging in the capital. In practice, it served as a reception area for all beggars arrested by the police and for everyone else who sought relief. The committee would then classify beggars according to four categories: the deserving poor who were unable to work; the deserving poor who were able to work; lazy and depraved people who professionally asked for alms; and, finally, people who had taken to begging temporarily because of some unhappy circumstance such as the loss of their passport or money. Beggars of the first category were to be transferred to the Imperial Philanthropic Society or to institutions of the social welfare boards. Those in the second category received help in finding work. People in the third category were handed back to the police to be punished as usual, and those of the fourth category were helped to get new documents or some money. Additional regulations applied for people from different social groups, such as retired state officials or the widows of soldiers.[36] Apart from the principal task of sorting beggars and transferring them to other institutions, the committee soon developed its own infrastructure: it opened hospitals for children and for adults, an orphanage, artisanal schools for poor children of both sexes, two almshouses and a dacha outside the city for poor and sick children. In the first 50 years of its existence, the committee dealt with the cases of 123 340 beggars.[37]

The main task of the committee was never fulfilled. It neither eliminated begging in St Petersburg nor, for that matter, provided a successful model for the rest of the Empire. Instead, it worked like a 'revolving door for transients and mendicants', to adopt Adele Lindenmeyr's expression.[38] By the second half of the 19th century, the committee was hopelessly overburdened. The abolition of serfdom in 1861, growing rural impoverishment and the beginnings of industrialisation each caused major social dislocations and led to a sharp increase of beggars and transients all over the country. Between 1882 and 1897 the number of beggars delivered to the committee almost tripled, from approximately 3000 to between 8000 and 10 000. By 1909 the number had risen to 17 595. By this time as well, the resources of the committee were simply overloaded. In 1897, for example, only 15 per cent of delivered beggars remained in the care of the committee; 52 per cent, or 4119 individuals, were merely released back into the city streets.[39]

In comparison to western, central and northern Europe, the historiography about health care and poor relief in Russia is at a very early stage. Basic information not only about the provinces but also about the capital cities is lacking. With the opening of former Soviet archives since 1991 and, more importantly, the opening of historical imagination with the end of the Soviet period, it is to be hoped that scholars will also ask new questions. However, despite these limitations, several conclusions and observations can be drawn.

In many respects, Russia poses an exceptional case in the European context. The expansion of serfdom in the 18th century, and its survival through to 1861, encouraged both the government and élite social groups to overlook such problems as rural poverty and a largely absent health care system (not to mention a basic system of primary education). It was assumed that patriarchy expressed itself through a benign paternalism – that serf owners had the best interests of their serfs at heart. Russia's aristocracy, particularly in the period under consideration, also differed in important ways from its Western counterparts. Lacking independent traditions and power bases, the gentry achieved social status through state service, yet, by the late 18th century, was also modelling itself on an idealised Western aristocracy. In this respect, the interest in charity can be seen not only as a simple expression of moral concern but also as an attempt to fashion a suitable public identity for itself apart from the state. However, in comparison to the West, private initiative was minimal in Russia, partly because of the official estate system and the absence of strong industrial and commercial classes. It was only in the late 19th and early 20th centuries that the middle classes (both industrial and professional) achieved a numerical significance and began to form what could perhaps be called a civil society. Indeed, since the era of Peter the Great, the absolutist state had assumed the role of moderniser. Even in the 19th century, when the state combated the emergence of an independent public sphere, such as in private charity, it remained the major force behind socioeconomic change.

Notes

1. See Murray Feshbach and Alfred Friendly, *Ecocide in the USSR. Health and Nature Under Siege*, New York, 1992, pp. 181–82.

2. Gordon Livermore and Fred Schulze (eds), *The USSR Today: Perspectives from the Soviet Press*, 5th edn, Columbus, Ohio, 1981, p. 33.

3. Feshbach and Friendly *Ecocide* (n. 1), p. 4; see also Michael Specter, 'Russia's Declining Health: Rising Illness, Shorter Lives', *The New York Times*, International Section, 19 February 1995, pp. 1–4.

4. For the most authoritative recent study of Peter's times, see Lindsey Hughes, *Russia in the Age of Peter the Great*, New Haven and London, 1998.

5. Dietrich Geyer, 'Peter und St. Petersburg', *Jahrbücher für Geschichte Osteuropas*, **10** (1962), pp. 181–200 at p. 191.

6. For the ineffectiveness and the repetition of decrees, see Christoph Schmidt, *Sozialkontrolle in Moskau: Justiz, Kriminalität und Leibeigenschaft, 1649–1785*, Stuttgart, 1996, p. 401.

7. Hughes, *Russia in the Age of Peter the Great* (n. 4), pp. 313–15; John T. Alexander, *Catherine the Great: Life and Legend*, New York and Oxford, 1989, pp. 81–82.

8. Richard Hellie, *Slavery in Russia, 1450–1725*, Chicago, p. 316.

9. G.P. Fedotov, *The Russian Religious Mind*, 2 vols, Cambridge, MA, 1966, Vol. 2, pp. 36–37.

10. See *Pravda russkaia*, 3 vols, Moscow and Leningrad, 1940–63, Vol. 2, pp. 707, 714–15; *Domostroi, po Konshinskomu spisku i podobnym*, Moscow, 1908, part 2, pp. 8–9, 39, 42–43, 51; I. Zabelin, *Domashnii byt russkikh tsarei v XVI i XVII st.*, part 1, 4th edn, Moscow 1918, pp. 391–92.

11. English quote after Adele Lindenmeyr, *Poverty is not a Vice: Charity, Society, and the State in Imperial Russia*, Princeton, NJ, 1996, p. 30.

12. 'O poimke nishchikh i ob otsylke ikh, po nakazaniiu, v prezhniia mesta', *Polnoe sobranie zakonov rossiiskoi imperii. Sobranie pervoe. 1649–1825* (hereafter *PSZ*), no. 3213; for Western European inspirations, see Robert Jütte, *Poverty and Deviance in Early Modern Europe*, Cambridge, 1994, pp. 171–77.

13. 'Punkty, dannye S. Peterburgskomu General-Politsiimeisteru', *PSZ*, no. 3203; 'O nepropuske v Sanktpeterburg, kogda shlagbaumy opushcheny, bez fonarei, o ezde izvoshchikam na vznuzdannykh loshadiakh i o neproshenii po ulitsam i pri tserkvakh milostyni,' ibid., no. 3676; 'Reglament ili Ustav Glavnago Magistrata,'

ibid., no. 3708. For the increasing role of the state in functions formerly associated with the Church, see Marc Raeff, *The Well-Ordered Police State: Social
and Institutional Change through Law in the Germanies and Russia, 1600–
1800*, New Haven and London, 1983, pp. 16–17.

14.   Richard Stites, *Revolutionary Dreams: Utopian Vision and Experimental Life in
the Russian Revolution*, New York, 1989.

15.   'O merakh k presecheniiu brodiazhestva nishchikh i ob uchrezhdenii dlia
soderzhaniia ikh pri tserkvakh bogadelen', *PSZ*, no. 6406.

16.   'Reglament ili Ustav Dukhovnoi Kollegii', *PSZ*, no. 3718; see also Lindenmeyr,
Poverty is not a Vice (n. 11), pp. 30–31.

17.   'O smotrenii za nishchimi, chtoby onye po ulitsam ne shatalis', ob otsylke
onykh v ikh vedomstva i zhilishcha', *PSZ*, no. 9992; 'O vospreshchenii uvechnym
khodit' v S.-Peterburge dlia prosheniia milostyni,' ibid., no. 10824.

18.   For Catherine's years in Germany and their impact on her, see Claus Scharf,
Katharina II., Deutschland und die Deutschen, Mainz, 1995, pp. 78–118.

19.   Isabel de Madariaga, *Russia in the Age of Catherine the Great*, New Haven and
London, 1981, pp. 7–9.

20.   Ibid., p. 151.

21.   Scharf, *Katharina II* (n. 18), pp. 124–25; see also Robert E. Jones, *Provincial
Development in Russia: Catherine II and Jakob Sievers*, New Brunswick, pp.
21–23.

22.   Lindenmeyr, *Poverty is not a Vice* (n. 11), pp. 34–36.

23.   Alexander, *Catherine the Great* (n. 7), pp. 144–47.

24.   Ibid., pp. 79–81.

25.   Ibid., pp. 154–60.

26.   David L. Ransel, *Mothers of Misery: Child Abandonment in Russia*, Princeton,
NJ, 1988, p. 31.

27.   Ibid., pp. 48, 307.

28.   Marc Raeff, *Origins of the Russian Intelligentsia. The Eighteenth-Century No-
bility*, New York, 1966, p.160; Douglas Smith, 'Freemasonry and the Public in
Eighteenth-Century Russia', in Jane Burbank and David Ransel (eds), *Imperial
Russia: New Histories for the Empire*, Bloomington, 1998, pp. 281–304.

29.   W. Gareth Jones, 'The *Morning Light* Charity Schools, 1777–80', *Slavonic and
East European Review*, **56** (1978), pp. 47–67.

30.   Lindenmeyr, *Poverty is not a Vice* (n. 11), p. 99–102; B.I. Krasnobaev, 'Eine
Gesellschaft gelehrter Freunde am Ende des 18. Jahrhunderts. "Drueskoe uenoe
obšestvo"', in Éva Balázs et al. (eds), *Beförderer der Aufklärung in Mittel- und
Osteuropa. Freimaurer, Gesellschaften, Clubs*, Berlin, 1979, pp. 257–70.

31.   Lindenmeyr, *Poverty is not a Vice* (n. 11), pp. 104–105.

32.   Ibid., pp. 106–9, 114–15.

33.   'Desiatiletie Demidovskago Doma Prizreniia Trudiashchikhsia, s 1833 po 1843
god', *Zhurnal ministerstva vnutrennikh del*, 1843, part 2, pp. 134–40.

34.   Lindenmeyr, *Poverty is not a Vice* (n. 11), pp. 115–18.

35.   For a general history of the Petersburg committee, see *Vysochaishe uchrezhdennyi
komitet dlia razbora i prizreniia nishchikh v S.-Peterburge. Ocherk deiatel'nosti
za piat'desiat let. 1837–1887*, St Petersburg, 1887.

36.   'Pravila dlia rukovodstva Komitetu o razbore nishchikh i izyskaniia sposobov k
iskoreneniiu nishchenstva', in Rossiiskii gosudarstvennyi istoricheskii arkhiv
(Russian State Historical Archive, St Petersburg), f. 1341, op. 38, d. 490, ll.
3–9.

37.   *Vysochaishe uchrezhdennyi komitet* (n. 35), pp. 22–23.

38. Lindenmeyr, *Poverty is not a Vice* (n. 11), p. 41.

39. *Otchet vysochaishe utverzhdennago Komiteta dlia razbora i prizreniia nishchikh v S.-Peterburge za 1872–1897 goda*, St Petersburg, 1884–99); *Statisticheskii ezhegodnik S.-Peterburga za 1909*, St Petersburg, 1917, pp. 73–74.

CHAPTER EIGHT

Health Care Provision and Poor Relief in Enlightenment and 19th Century Denmark

Gerda Bonderup

The background

The Enlightenment in Denmark started late. After a few false starts between 1710 and 1730 it began properly around 1750 and is marked by the king encouraging free debate about agricultural conditions. It ended more or less with the last reform changes in 1814. In this period the Danish intellectuals generally followed their north European counterparts concerning issues such as social recruitment, education, professional and leisure pursuits. The intellectuals moved in the spheres of the aristocracy and the (higher) bourgeoisie. They often came from a similar cultural and educational background and shared the same curiosity and intellectual interests. Many of them were, or became, clergymen, military or civil officials or academics. They were often in opposition, not so much to the feudal élite of the time as to the old doctrines and prejudices, as well as to the established Church. They were infatuated by the emerging science, the new philosophy and political science. Often encouraged by the king, as well as on their own initiative, the intellectuals discussed the economic, technical, social and political problems of society as these were described in the new 'media' such as newspapers and (scientific) periodicals. Thus they acquired an audience which was enthusiastic as well as enlightened. Their socioideological topics concerned the benefit of all in general and the education of society in particular, both with respect to knowledge and especially to the new 'civic' virtues such as honesty, decency, industry, cleanliness, moderation, modesty and so on. In their spare time they often met in clubs and associations.

The physicians in particular were on a level with their north European colleagues, because their education was largely similar, built on the models of Palermo, Edinburgh, Paris, Leiden and the like. The Danish physicians went on research trips, familiarised themselves with international literature and even contributed to it and participated in international conferences.

The national(istic) development in Denmark has only little, if any, influence on our chosen topic, since trail-blazing classes which focused on political goals began only in the 1830s.

Nor was the industrialisation of Denmark of any great importance to our theme because, lacking natural resources, Denmark was not part of the first industrialisation wave. It has long been held that industrialisation began in the 1870s at the earliest, but in reality it was probably not until the 1890s. In plain figures it can be said that during the first 25 years after 1870, industry's share of the gross national product started to climb from 4 per cent to slightly under 8 per cent. Not until the turn of the century did the net investments of the gross national product reach 10 per cent.[1]

However, population explosions and urbanisation were certainly well-known phenomena in Denmark. The total population in Denmark increased from 750 000 in the mid 18th century to 2.5 million around 1900. Copenhagen and the provincial towns accounted for 20 per cent of the total population up until 1850, and the capital alone accounted for 10 per cent. Then, as development progressed, the percentages for the towns alone nearly doubled during the next 50 years. The population in Copenhagen, for example, climbed from 138 000 to 240 000. It is important to bear in mind that Denmark was actually made up of three parts: the capital of Copenhagen, the provincial towns and the rural districts. Copenhagen was the seat for the reigning double monarchy of Denmark–Norway until 1814 and later for the monarchy of Denmark. It was the centre of the government, the administration, the army and trade. Although it attracted many people, there was not nearly enough work for everyone. Erecting buildings outside the city ramparts was prohibited until 1850, which caused some heavy slum areas to emerge during the urbanisation process.

The development within the poor relief system

Looking at the socioeconomic conditions in Denmark in general, we find that 5–10 per cent of the population were comfortably off, approximately 10 per cent had reasonable living conditions, while the 'rest' generally had to live near the starvation point. Depending on circumstances, 2–8 per cent of the latter were on some kind of poor relief. Until the 18th century the undeserving poor lived primarily by begging but eventually this created so much disorder that the conditions for the poor had to be reappraised. This gave rise both to intervention by the authorities as well as intensified private charity.

In 1708 no less than three poor laws were passed, applying to the rural districts, the provincial towns and Copenhagen respectively. Some of the regulations were the same in all three laws: namely, the prohibition of all mendicity and the classification of the poor into three classes – those who were unable to sustain themselves at all, orphans, and those who were able to undertake a certain amount of work. The old distinction between deserving and undeserving poor was maintained, as the two first-mentioned classes made up the deserving poor, and this classification has marked the debate concerning social security up until the present day. The necessary aid was to be procured by donations, collections in the churches and 'voluntary' collections where one would pledge a fixed annual amount.

The regulations applying to the rural districts and the provincial towns can be seen as one, whereas the regulations applying to Copenhagen were somewhat different because they had to be made to conform to the special conditions in the capital. In the countryside the chief constable and the rural dean were put in charge of the collections and the distribution of the aid. In the towns these tasks were to be carried out by the chief constable and the minister. In the countryside subdivisions consisting of the minister and some of the 'best and finest' parishioners were to be established – an early example of the principle of local democracy which we encounter many times during the period of absolutism. They were to make sure that the poor received their due and that they led respectable lives. The books were to be checked every year by the authorities.

Actual practice, however, generally turned out somewhat differently: in the rural areas the community decided who was to feed the poor for a specific period of time, so that thus the poor were passed from household to household. Clothing and other necessities were procured through gifts and money from the collection plates. Often the small towns also resorted to this type of public assistance, while the larger towns kept to the statutory parish division with the minister and distinguished citizens as the relieving officers.[2]

Those who continued their begging were now assigned to do forced labour on the fortress in Copenhagen. However, despite the country's small size, Denmark's roads were in poor condition making the transportation of people a long and costly affair. This meant that the rules had to be modified so that the beggars could be assigned to the nearest garrison or simply be expelled from the parish. In the event, only Zealand used the fortress in Copenhagen. As the ideas from mercantilism – and especially from its variation, cameralism – reached Denmark, a group of enterprising citizens began to establish textile manufactures to occupy the tramps and beggars caught by the new 'beggar kings' employed by the poor relief system. These new workhouses, which also housed other criminals carrying out forced labour, were established in several locations during the 1730s and 1740s. Although they were supposed to break even economically, they suffered large deficits. As it was still too costly for the distant parishes to transport the beggars to the workhouses, they never became a success and begging continued. The situation was exacerbated when it was decided that those who gave charity to beggars would also be punished. Nor did the ordinary poor relief suffice. People failed to honour their pledges, the ministers did not collect sufficient funds and, overall, there was never enough money.

As Copenhagen had the worst problems, the legislation in the capital had to be more precise. As early as 1708, and maybe even before then, we can see the outline of a system which, from 1788, was to become known as the 'Hamburg system', with its outdoor and indoor relief. A Public Assistance Committee ('Poor Committee') was created, consisting of five officials, served by five additional officials who were to distribute the poor relief to the poor every Wednesday. Two relieving officers from each parish were to investigate the needs of the poor. Resources from the poorboxes, interest on tied-up money contracted years ago, other private donations and the state lottery(!) were to supply these needs. After a while a poverty tax also became necessary. Such outdoor relief helped those who had their own homes – homes that had themselves often been donated.

Indoor relief was granted in the town's few social institutions. The sick and the weak were admitted here and given food and medical attention. Their condition dictated which 'nursing homes' they could be admitted to. The capacity was expanded with a large hospital, the General Hospital in 1768, which had an estimated capacity of 1200 new beds and catered for the lower social orders. In time, more than 2000 poor were packed into the hospital – first, a sick room was added, then an entire ward.

Despite the precise legislation for Copenhagen and despite the ingenuity of the magistrate and the Poor Committee, there was not enough money to go round. Urbanisation continued and eventually there were more beggars on Zealand than there was room in the hospitals in Copenhagen. Until the 1850s the burgeoning population had to live inside the city ramparts because the military needed several kilometres of unbuilt-up land for training. Thus, the slum areas expanded as buildings had to be heightened and built deeper into the mews.

By the middle of the 18th century the economic situation improved, the Enlightenment had penetrated, and a young philanthropic and religiously inspired prince had convinced his mentally disordered father that *he* should inherit the crown instead of the heir presumptive. All this combined to lead to the great reform period which began in the 1780s. 'The Public Weal' was written in capitals, and a concern with human rights prompted public demand for agrarian reforms and the abolition of serfdom – and especially a reorganisation of the old village communalism. Also on the agenda were reforms within the educational system and the poor relief system. A large-scale investigation was commissioned and, in 1787, a Public Assistance Committee was founded whose members included ministers and representatives from central and local government. A leading lay official, the Lord Lieutenant of Zealand, was appointed as chairman of the committee which was to investigate the entire poor relief system. It was said that the main reason for the failure of poor relief was the principle of voluntarism concerning the subscription.

The establishment of the committee resulted initially in two laws applying to Copenhagen and, a few years later, two further laws applying to the provincial towns and the rural districts. However, the ideas had not changed in the interim. The classification of the poor into three classes was maintained, and responsibility in both the country and the towns still lay with the ministers and their helpers as before. The three main changes were:

1. instead of the voluntary pledges, a poor tax was implemented;
2. the administration was provided with a fixed framework; and
3. the people in the third category were to be offered work.

This latter point resulted in the creation of a number of workhouses which, unlike the other workhouses, did not require the poor to live on the premises.

The Poor Committee of 1787 created a body of legislation for the capital that closely resembled that of the Hamburg system. The old division of the town on the basis of the parishes was now changed into a division of 12 (later 13) main districts with the necessary number of subdistricts to ensure that each subdistrict had only 15 poor families. This was estimated to be the number of families which a relieving officer, chosen by the Poor Committee, could take regular care of. This included keeping an eye on them, encouraging them to industriousness, order, domesticity and cleanliness, as well as educating them in the importance of well-prepared food, order and modesty to a healthy body and explaining that weakness and disease came from poor food, filth, laziness and strong, bitter coffee.

The members of the Poor Committee were recruited from the central administration, the magistracy, the elected town councillors and the ordinary citizens, and there was also a representative from the Protestant Church and the Catholic Church. All in all, it amounted to 24 people who founded boards to deal with various administrative tasks such as the poor relief itself, assignment of work, education, nursing and policing the poor. Next followed more than 200 paragraphs of detailed orders and prohibitions.

After the period of great economic difficulty (from 1815), and under the influence of Malthus, poor relief conditions were tightened all over the country. Consequently, no-one under the poor relief system was allowed to marry, nor, after the new Constitution of 1849, were they allowed to vote for parliament until they had paid back all the aid they had received. The considerable problems concerning poor relief for those who had lived outside their borough for a short period of time, will not be dealt with here.[3]

Thus the humanitarian tendencies of the Enlightenment were not reflected in the public poor relief system. If anything, rational and economic thought had influenced the poor relief system for more than 100 years. However, humanitarian ideas did express themselves in private charity – individual as well as collective. Individual charity in Catholic times had been a normal way of receiving indulgence for one's sins and it continued after the Reformation in the shape of testamentary gifts and donations of various sizes. Charity for beggars, however, was prohibited and money for that purpose was collected through church poorboxes. Collective charity in the shape of associations, whose members collected money, was also common. A well-known type of association in Denmark, as well as in the rest of Europe, from the mid-18th century was the 'patriotic association'.

As the bourgeoisie became more influential in Denmark, decency, humanity and mercy, combined with modesty, cleanliness and 'mission' work, formed a more important part of their morals. The establishment of societies – the society movement – gave the bourgeoisie the opportunity to practise these and other civic virtues, leading to a significant increase in the number of philanthropic societies during the 19th century. Their work was different from individual charity – which was often solely based on compassion – because their remits were broader and more rational. Their aim primarily had a general social focus, sometimes expressed in the words 'Help them to help themselves'. Such philanthropy had a very strong indirect impact on education, where modern subjects were pursued and emphasis placed on the passions. For instance, philanthropists wanted to support the poor daughters of officials and establish a reformatory for poor girls. The establishment of associations directed towards improving the conditions of neglected children continued into the 19th century, partly because the bourgeoisie had become aware of the fact that a sheltered childhood was a precondition for making the child a useful citizen. Around 1900 in Copenhagen more than 35 per cent of the philanthropic expenses were targeted on children in need.[4] In addition to the children, the philanthropists concentrated their efforts on poor working-class families, especially after the cholera epidemic of the mid-19th century.

In addition, there was the spontaneous philanthropy which emerged in crisis situations. One example was the association which provided healthy, nourishing and free food for the needy during the cholera epidemic.

The development of the health services

In the wake of mercantilism, various investigations into the population's size and general well-being had proved a clear connection between poverty and disease.[5] Inspired by the theses of the German philosophers and physicians and their work in German and French teaching hospitals, Danish physicians and the government started to work together on drawing up the concept of 'sanitary policing', which consisted of four main aspects:

1. the establishment of a maternity hospital with a nursing home attached to it;

2. the building of a hospital;
3. the establishment of a network of physicians throughout the country;
4. the improved training of surgeons.

But first, we must look at the general conditions before the mid-18th century. At this time, nothing even resembling a health care system existed – there was a fragmentary treatment system and a few regulations. There were three groups of healers. The first group consisted of university-educated physicians, with an almost exclusively theoretical training and without any practical experience. Nevertheless, they were the only ones with the authority to practise and prescribe internal medicine. Half of them lived in the capital and mainly worked as physicians to the court and as university professors with a private practice in town. The second group comprised the remaining physicians, who worked across the country as public health officers. After the Reformation they had taken over health care from the Church. For many years they were paid by a canonicate. All in all there were approximately 20 physicians in Denmark around 1750.

The third group consisted of artisans trained as surgeons, who were mainly specially trained barbers only allowed to perform external medical treatment (that is, wounds and fractures). Even though their number exceeded that of the physicians there were still only a few. They were principally employed in the army and in the merchant fleet and, in their occasional spare time, they worked as surgeons in private practice. These surgeons were town-based and were therefore only accessible to townspeople – though only very few of them. In the country, as well as in the towns, people tended to use their own treatments. Sometimes they would take the advice of their friends or turn to the folk healers, some of whom had obtained a licence to perform certain medical procedures such as hernia operations. Folk healers were found both in the towns and in the country.

The first result of the government's and the doctors' endeavours in the mid-18th century was the founding of a maternity hospital, where unmarried women could give birth anonymously and free of charge. At the beginning of the 18th century, King Frederik IV had been appalled by the awful behaviour of people who abandoned their infants in the streets of Copenhagen and imposed the death penalty for such an offence. At the same time the country was ravaged by the plague, increasing the number of orphans and, as a result, the king ordered the building of an orphanage. But neither the threat of capital punishment nor the orphanage could stop people from abandoning their children or committing infanticide. Thus, in 1750 a hospital was founded for single pregnant girls. The girls were granted total anonymity and a few 'good' midwives were connected to the institution. However, the founding of this hospital was criticised, especially by the Church, because it allegedly legitimised fornication. Worse still, the girls generally succeeded in avoiding

Church discipline, which usually meant that the girl had to confess her sins in church and state the name of the child's father. Eventually, mercantilism combined with humanitarian attitudes succeeded in defeating the Church.

From as early as 1760 the maternity hospital was to serve a variety of purposes. First, of course, unmarried girls no longer had to deliver their children clandestinely without physical or psychological support – a lack of support which had often resulted in infanticide. The child could then be handed over to the newly established nursing home which took care of organising the child's upbringing, thus saving a potentially useful citizen. Finally, the maternity hospital was used to train doctors in obstetrics and to train midwives.

The next step was the founding of the first somatic therapeutic hospital in Copenhagen (1757). Approximately ten years earlier several physicians had begun to agitate for, and write about, the need for such a hospital in order for them to become 'methodically better at learning and practising medicine'. However, they only had the teaching aspect in mind. At the demise of the Crown in 1746, A.G. Moltke, Lord High Steward, mentor and *de facto* prime minister had already made the young king, who in contemporary sources is characterised as a man with a kind heart, aware that the University of Copenhagen needed a hospital like all the other university towns in Europe. In his kindness the king laid the foundation stone and, a few years later, appointed a committee which was given the task of considering the old and weak part of the population which was no longer able to work or sustain themselves in other ways. This was interesting because it resembled normal indoor relief. According to the above-mentioned sources the most probable reason for this was that the king grew tired of state business and therefore did not familiarise himself adequately with the situation. The committee consisted of officials, surgeons and one physician.[6] They drafted plans and a charter, resulting in a treatment hospital for poor and destitute patients – a beautiful synthesis of their thoughts that moved the hearts of the leading figures of the establishment.

The small, damp, congested houses in the slums of Copenhagen were not suitable for nursing, but in the new hospital the poor and servants could receive medical treatment and care with nutritious food, fresh air and a regular daily routine. The hospital had 150–300 beds, and the charter was fully in accordance with the spirit of that time. Investigations into the age of the patients reveal that nearly half the patients were between 15 and 29 years of age, even though this age group only formed 30 per cent of the total population.[7] The chronically sick were excluded from treatment; only the very best among the young and fit were admitted.

At the beginning of the 19th century the provincial towns were directed to found similar hospitals to take care of their poor, but now especially for those with syphilis, because a new epidemic had broken out. However, only six hospitals had been built by the time the state went bankrupt towards the end of the Napoleonic Wars and, in the mid-19th century there existed only approximately 30 hospitals, only a few of which had more than 20 beds, and many of them only between five and ten.

A wide-mesh net of public health officers was spread all over the country. From the 1770s the physicians were supported by 20 district surgeons whose number doubled five times in the course of the next 100 years and who supervised the chemists, midwives and folk healers, as well as the quality of the food. The physicians solely carried out administrative work and lived in the larger cities. Both the physician and the district medical officer were paid an annual salary by the state. This salary was very low and was meant to be supplemented by their private practice to keep up their professional skills. Therefore it was required of the district medical officers that they treat anyone, rich or poor. In return, they would receive maintenance and free travel which were to be paid for by the patients themselves or from the poor relief, depending on the circumstances.

The training of physicians and surgeons gradually converged. During the 1780s the Surgical Academy (*Kongelig Chirurgisk Academie*) was founded. Here, potential surgeons had to take courses on anatomy and internal medicine. From 1838 onwards, the education of physicians and surgeons was harmonised: they were all required to attend university where the surgical subjects were given a higher priority.

This was the medical situation around 1850: all in all there were close to 500 physicians. Nearly 20 per cent of them were employed in the army. One-quarter of the remaining physicians were employed as civic district medical officers, while three-quarters worked as private physicians (50 years later the number of physicians in private practice had increased fivefold!). Copenhagen alone employed 200, due to the fact that it housed both the royal court, the rich bourgeoisie and most of the army and navy.

The doctor–inhabitant ratio was 1:600 for Copenhagen; however, under normal conditions, such a ratio was purely theoretical, because only the civic health inspectors had dealings with the poor. The city's 13 units of poor relief employed their own health inspectors to take care of approximately 10 000 inhabitants. Only in the event of an epidemic did the remaining physicians assist, on the basis of the Hippocratic oath.

The superior body of the health care system was the General Board of Health, established in 1803 to replace its antiquated predecessor. The Board was directly controlled by the central government and was located in Copenhagen. Its membership comprised physicians and surgeons whose tasks were to supervise the health inspectors and hospitals. They advised on all medical questions, on charges against folk healers, as well as in medico-legal matters. They announced and submitted recommendations for the posts for medical officers and supervised the collection and publishing of the health inspectors' abbreviated medical reports.[8] Until then, the university-trained physicians had monopolised these tasks in their forum, the *Collegium Medicum*, with the exception of the annual reports which were not published until 1803. A small number of surgeons were allowed to participate as observers in some of the negotiations to create the General Board of Health. Ever since the founding of the Surgical Academy there had been conflicts between the physicians and the surgeons, often unwittingly provoked by the central government which was not always able to keep medical and surgical matters apart. At the beginning of the 19th century one case concerning the application of a French dentist brought matters to a head. Eventually, the old system was remodelled into the new General Board of Health.

Laws to regulate the health care system were only issued sporadically in the case of an acute situation, as when the plague raged in Copenhagen at the beginning of the 18th century. At that time, a more general law was passed, which applied to the entire rural population (1782), while the towns followed the regulations from the plague laws of Elsinore (1710) and Copenhagen (1711). The most important aspect in this connection was that all treatment was free of charge. The money was to be collected by means of a land tax which obviously did not apply to the landless poor. The General Board of Health had to be notified immediately about the outbreak of an epidemic.

Another law concerned the 'folk healers', the quacks. A serious misdiagnosis by a certain folk healer was brought to the attention of the bishop and later to the county medical officer and an elaborate case containing revealing evidence was initiated. These officials had the Lord Lieutenant on their side, and he suggested corporal punishment. They were backed by the General Board of Health which proposed to implement a law against folk healers with high penalties and imprisonment on bread and water for both the folk healer and his patient. However, the political leaders felt that the experts were taking matters too far, claiming that the patient had been punished enough, especially since the treatment had gone wrong. In the event, the folk healer had to pay a penalty of 20 rigsdaler (a day labourer's approximate salary for 100 days of work) or be imprisoned for eight days on bread and water. Should he commit the same offence again the punishment would be twice as hard.

The folk healer could also choose to attempt to prove his abilities in front of the medical officer and the Lord Lieutenant. If they approved him he had to apply for a partial licence from the central government. The government in the capital was well aware of the fact that there were not enough physicians and that there were many skilled folk healers who had often been certified by the priests and Lord Lieutenants. They also emphasised that the services of the folk healers were less costly than the services of the authorised physicians. This was important for the poor relief system which these officials worked with on different levels. However, the General Board of Health which was presented with each application often dismissed them. The political leaders gave the local administration the final say in the matter because they had a better knowledge of the conditions and needs.[9]

This, then, was the foundation of the health care system – the first attempt to systematically improve the general state of health. It was a tremendous step up from the conditions of that time. However, neither the king nor the doctors were satisfied: the system had to be extended and supplemented by regulations and local bodies for sanitary policing and, at the beginning of the 19th century, a commission was appointed to achieve these goals. The economic tendencies in this period were still positive and the commission sent out a survey to all the physicians in the country. They were to give information about the conditions in their field of responsibility centred around 16 care issues taken from the Danish edition of *System einer Medizinischen Polizey* by Johann Peter Frank.[10] The answers certainly leave the historian some wonderful source material but they rendered the commission breathless. Denmark's involvement in the Napoleonic Wars, which led to the bombardment of Copenhagen and the bankruptcy of the state in 1813, put a stop to the work. Only a few urgent matters such as quarantine boards and the supervision of high-risk jobs had been completed.

In fact, all ideas about improving the health care system were put on hold, as the intellectuals were busy with politics. A brief and rude awakening came with the cholera threat in 1831, which resulted in action to draw up regulations concerning the implementation of the previously suggested sanitary police to fight the possible outbreak. This law, along with that of Prussia the first of its kind in Europe, became the foundation for the local Board of Health and contained all the key regulations for the later sanitary policy. However, as the cholera epidemic passed Denmark by, the concern was only brief. The concern re-emerged in the mid-19th century in response to a new threatened epidemic, but this time more violently and for many reasons.

Public health, the Constitution and cholera: 1850–1900

First, the political movement, mainly sustained by the intellectuals, had reached its goal – the free Constitution of 1849. This created a parliament based on universal suffrage – though excluding people receiving poor relief. Energies could now be concentrated on other matters.

Second, the young progressives in the world of medicine had moved from the contagious theory to the miasmatic theory, where the crucial points were hygiene and moderation. They now rose to the highest positions and were able to influence non-physicians in their circles. For years they had produced accounts of the monstrous conditions which the poor part of the population had to endure. One of their leading figures, Carl Emil Fenger, had become a member of parliament. Inspired by the British trade policy the government had asked the parliament to consider abolishing the very costly quarantine regulations. Fenger was appointed spokesman at the following debate as well as to the committee. After a few years of fierce discussions, in which the General Board of Health despite everything – and, more specifically, despite their belief in miasmas – did not dare take responsibility, it was agreed, in 1852, to abolish the quarantine with the proviso that the funds saved were to be spent on hygiene improvements. It proved difficult to get started, but the third reason, the cholera epidemic, helped emphatically. It attacked Denmark during the following year and glaringly highlighted social conditions in general and the conditions for the poor in particular. It revealed the wretched homes and the poor living conditions as well as the poor water and poor hygiene – problems which the physicians had often tried to call attention to, but in vain. Finally things were happening.

The most important task was to bring the sick to (provisional) hospitals and move the healthy citizens from the slums to a light, airy, and obviously clean environment. Physicians and volunteer middle-class citizens went from door to door to look after the sick, offering them advice on how to keep the house and themselves clean. Here it should be emphasised that the rules of the 1799 law, only permitting the relieving officers to supervise approximately 15 families, had obviously not worked, because already with the first threat of cholera in 1831 the newspapers in the capital contained advertisements encouraging voluntary citizens to help the physicians inspect the homes of the poor. These advertisements could also be seen in 1853 and this reaching-out on the part of the prestigious and generally prosperous middle-class citizens gave the poor trust in those responsible. Another 'project' was to collect charitable donations. One could almost read symbolism into the fact that the spontaneous private donations in support of the cholera patients corresponded to the total donations of the city, which came to a total of 15 per cent of the town's total tax revenue.[11]

I will elaborate on two of the improvements provoked by the cholera epidemic – the building of a public hospital and private housing. The most important hospital became the Community Hospital in Copenhagen, built in 1857 with a capacity of more than 800 beds – twice the total capacity of all the hospitals in Copenhagen at that time. The cholera epidemic had revealed the great shortage of hospital beds. Cholera patients had been admitted to the hospitals and had mainly been placed in the ward of the previously mentioned General Hospital. From there the epidemic had spread explosively to the rest of the poor. The physicians employed there wrote to the General Board of Health asking them to start an investigation into the hospital's suitability as a main hospital for the capital. Vigorously supported by terrifying descriptions in newspapers and pamphlets, the case was the subject of numerous discussions in the Assembly of Citizens and a committee was immediately set up by the minister of the interior. Two years later the decision was made to build a new hospital.

The hospital was quite obviously needed since, shortly after it was established, all the beds were occupied, causing speculation in medical circles and throughout the city as to whether they had been too generous in offering hospital treatment. On the other hand, in the long run, it was cheaper to treat (and cure) patients in a hospital free of charge than to let them – and possibly also their families – become a burden on the poor relief system. However, the voices expressing opinions about educating the poor with special reference to 'helping them to help themselves' became louder especially in the Assembly of Citizens during the 1860s and 1870s. It also became apparent that many people were admitted to the hospitals with only minor ailments such as swollen or broken fingers and boils, which caused them to be unable to work for a short period of time but were not sufficiently serious to confine them to bed. Subsequently, limiting the number of admissions in return for partly polyclinical/out-patient treatment was encouraged, as was the founding of (private) sick benefit associations. Such measures decreased the use of hospitalisation which was then only used when no other form of care could be found. Similar opinions were also heard from the provincial towns. Despite a substantial increase in population, both in the provincial towns and in the capital, the number of patients did not increase between 1810 and 1830.[12] This was a different way of thinking from that which had prevailed approximately 100 years before when the filth of the slums initiated the building of the first hospital.

Another important aspect of the public health care system was the council of Copenhagen's decision to separate poor relief from sick relief, placing the hospital system under another department of the magistracy. However, free treatment still meant losing one's civil rights. On the other hand, new wards were established in the new hospital – wards of a much higher standard for paying patients and for which there was a great demand because the good reputation of the physicians had further improved due to scientific and technical advances. All this led to a serious reorganisation of the health care system. Expressed in numbers, this development meant that the poor relief system's share of the city budget in 1865 dropped from 20 per cent to 15 per cent in 1880, while the hospital's share remained at approximately 8 per cent.[13]

After the poor housing conditions had been brought to light by the cholera epidemic, the physicians of Copenhagen took charge of constructing community housing. In the first phase of the epidemic they had established an association of doctors to fight it. Large sums had been collected for their work and these proved large enough to finance the construction work. In total 250 homes were built. They were let cheaply but not free of charge on the grounds that free housing would not teach the population to become hardworking citizens. Other kinds of private social housing emerged in the 1870s and 1880s, usually in the shape of newly established (workers') associations under the guidance of physicians, solicitors and politicians. The important aspect of these new associations was that they not only aimed at improving the workers' material conditions, including health, but also hoped – as explained by a leading physician – to raise their self esteem, their affection for their homes and families, their sense of decency, their respect for private ownership and their civic spirit.[14] All in all, approximately 3000 homes were built by different associations which retained a so-called 'human control' of the people living there in order to promote their health and morality. To a certain degree it can be argued that the above-mentioned moral virtues have subsequently become social values which are accepted as the norm.

The cholera epidemic had also proved that voluntary help for the needy was no longer enough. Until then, the clear 'liberal' opinion prevailed that help for the needy, over and above statutory poor relief, was a task to be carried out by private persons. This idea manifested itself in individual and collective philanthropic charity, as we have seen. However, it was now obvious that the relief measures had to be extended and made more efficient through more direct help from the state. The era of the night-watchman state, or rather the night-watchman community, was over, as far as hygiene and a number of other social arrangements were concerned.

The state mainly attended to tasks such as a more restrictive housing policy, the establishment of waterworks and sewerage, the building of a large hospital, and not least a statement of sanitary regulations requiring the local councils to establish health commissions and define their tasks. The philanthropy dedicated to the battle against hunger, unhealthy housing, infant mortality, drinking, prostitution and sick benefit continued within the private framework with a clear accentuation of the principle 'help them to help themselves'. During the 1860s and 1870s organised philanthropic work was at its height, both in scope as well as in self-awareness. By way of comparison it might be mentioned that in 1876 the collections of the philanthropists amounted to 2.5 times as much as the total expenditure of the poor relief system that year.

The philanthropists reached their highest goal when the state supported this principle by establishing health insurance in 1892. Until then, a number of private associations existed, but far from enough. To increase the number of insured the state now offered a grant for those sick benefit associations which were willing to take on people of limited means. The notion 'limited means' was carefully defined by the annual income – it is revealing that only 20 per cent of the population did *not* qualify as being citizens 'of limited means'. Whereas Bismarck chartered the sick benefit associations in Germany, in Denmark this took place voluntarily. This was the beginning of the state's intervention in social conditions. Later came old age provision, accident insurance and so on. One would have thought that the aims of the philanthropic associations would have clashed with the aims of the socialist labour movement, which believed that the state should take over the social work. This would have created a problem for the associations because they would either have to deny that it was the state's role to solve social problems, thus defending the social squalor that charity had to work in, or aim at making themselves redundant by allowing the state to take over the social tasks which charity currently performed. As it turned out, there was still room for the philanthropists. Historical research has subsequently seen the state's growing commitment to social affairs as the beginning of the approaching welfare state.

Conclusion

Without knowing a great deal about development in other countries, it is nevertheless my impression that Denmark generally followed the north European course in connection with the establishment and development of health care provision and poor relief.

A certain paternalistic line can be found in the Danish health services, whether it be public or private. The character of this line was influenced by the changes in society and how these changes were viewed by those responsible. During the Enlightenment political leaders and physicians were driven by the cameralist notion that there was a need to promote and preserve a large and healthy population. They saw themselves as responsible for caring for the poor and especially for the young fit groups among them who, when sick, were immediately admitted for treatment at the new hospitals. The Napoleonic Wars and the bankruptcy of the state brought about a significant economic depression, and the theories of Malthus became prominent – namely, that the individual should be able to sustain himself and should only be given a helping hand at the outset. Consequently, poor relief was drastically cut back, and private poor relief increased significantly, whereas the health care system remained unchanged.

When the cholera attacked Denmark, those committed to charitable giving helped with funds, expertise and physical work without paying any heed to the costs. After the epidemic, a certain degree of help was still given and the state and private benefactors shared the responsibility. However, those who received poor relief had to live up to the norms of the bourgeoisie. These can be described as certain educational, even disciplining, tendencies on the part of the paternalists, but the poor were readily convinced of the good in these virtues because of the bourgeoisie's efforts during the cholera epidemic.

Finally, I will point to a few typically Danish circumstances. Inspired by theories of professionalisation being discussed internationally a few years ago, I studied the cooperation and conflict between physicians and the political leaders.[15] Surprisingly, there appears always to have been a clear cooperation between the two. Thus, cooperation on the basis of compromise was the actual prime mover behind the establishment of the first therapeutic hospital. On the few occasions when the political leaders did not comply with the wishes of the physicians it was due to the physicians' officiousness; consequently there was a positive outcome for the local population and the normally well-functioning local government, as with the folk healers discussed above.

Even though these were times of absolutism the central government responded to local needs. Interestingly, the absolute administrative machine basically kept operating even after the death of absolutism. Therefore, when local Boards of Health were established as from 1857, the chief constable and the health inspector were *ex-officio* members and the remaining members were chosen from the local notables. This composition was a complete replica of the composition of the statutory Board of Guardians from 1803, and of other committees in absolute times. It can be said that the principle of local democracy had long ago been incorporated into the Danish political system – long before the free constitution of 1849.

There was also cooperation in times of crisis, despite the differences between social classes. Thus, the cholera epidemic had a harmonising effect on various opposites, was conducive for trust, and had a cumulative effect on everyone's sense of social responsibility. In an emergency everyone pulled together and the potential of voluntary helpers from the higher bourgeoisie could be mobilised. Together with the physicians they visited the wretched homes of the poor to detect the cholera patients. They inspected the state of cleanliness and donated food and clothing. And afterwards they all – both the authorities and the population – had learned from the enormous problems disclosed by the cholera epidemic. We saw a solution to some of these problems in the form of the building of a hospital and the founding of the local Boards of Health.

In recent years the Danish debate has focused on the question whether Danish society was a society of conflict or consensus. Conflict researchers inspired by Karl Marx, then by Charles Tilly and finally by Michel Foucault, have focused on the very few disturbances in Denmark throughout the centuries,[16] while others – including myself – point to the fact that the element of consensus dominates the course of Danish history.[17] This fact can be seen in crisis times, which are profound indicators of the fundamental character of a society. This more peaceful approach has been created by the authorities' understanding and pragmatic, yet sometimes regulating, attitude in absolute times. However, it should be emphasised that Denmark was not a harmonious and idyllic country, if we bear in mind that the debates in 'healthy' times sometimes had numerous spearheads – but that is another story.

188 HEALTH CARE AND POOR RELIEF

Notes

1. Hans C. Johansen, *Industriens vækst og vilkår 1870–1973*, Copenhagen 1988, pp. 21, 44ff.
2. Harald Jørgensen, 'Det offentlige Fattigvæsen i Danmark 1708–1770', in Karl-Gustaf Andersson (ed.), *Oppdaginga av Fattigdommen*, Copenhagen, 1982.
3. Harald Jørgensen, *Studier over det offentlige fattigvæsens historiske udvikling i Danmark i det 19. århundrede*, Copenhagen, 1940/1979.
4. Tyge Krogh, 'Filantropibegrebet mellem næstekærlighed, liberal politik og solidaritet', *Den jyske Historiker*, **67** (1994), p. 7ff; also Anne Løkke, 'Premierede plejemødre', *Den jyske Historiker*, **67** (1994), p. 38ff.
5. For the more general development see George Rosen, *From Medical Police to Social Medicine: Essays on the History of Health Care*, New York, 1974.
6. G. Tryde, *Det kongelige Frederiks Hospitals Oprettelse*, Copenhagen, 1945.
7. Signild Vallgårda, 'Hospitals and the Poor in Denmark 1750–1880', *Scandinavian Journal of History*, **13** (1988), p. 98.
8. These reports were published annually as supplement volumes to *Bibliothek for Læger*, and constitute excellent source material.
9. Gerda Bonderup, 'De "kloge" folk og det danske samfund', *Historisk Tidsskrift*, **I** (1997), pp. 275–303.
10. Rasmus Frankenau, *Det offentlige Sundhedspolitie under en oplyst Regjering*, Copenhagen, 1801.
11. Gerda Bonderup, *Cholera Morbro'r og Danmark*, Aarhus, 1994.
12. For this section on hospitals I rely on Signild Vallgårda, *Sjukhus och fattigpolitik*, Copenhagen, 1985.
13. *Staden Københavns Regnskab og Beretning om Kommunens anliggender* for the years 1865 and 1880, p. 3.
14. Emil Hornemann, 'Danske Arbejderboliger', *Hygiejniske Meddelelser*, new series 1 (1876), p. 40.
15. Gerda Bonderup, 'Konsensus i Danmark? Staten og lægerne i 1700– og 1800–tallet', *Historie* (1994), pp. 90–102.
16. For example, Jens Engberg, *Dansk guldalder eller Oprøret i tugt-, rasp- og forbedringshuset 1817*, Copenhagen, 1973; and Flemming Mikkelsen (ed.), *Protest og oprør*, Aarhus, 1986.
17. Most recently, Claus Bjørn, *Dengang Danmark blev moderne*, Copenhagen, 1998.

CHAPTER NINE

Ideology or Pragmatism?
Health Care Provision and Poor Relief
in Norway in the 19th Century

Øivind Larsen

What is specific to Norway?

Comparisons of health care and poor relief in Norway with other European
countries may easily resemble repeated descriptions of the same processes, as
the countries involved show substantial similarities in social development.
Solutions had to be local – a fact that explains differences which do not
necessarily call for special historical attention, if they do not reflect important
underlying ideologies. Therefore, for the case of Norway, it seems sensible to
line up some parts of the background which are specific for Norway, before the
main traits of the efforts to solve health and poverty problems are highlighted.
Thus some political facts may serve as an appropriate starting point.

A nation on its own

Any textbook of political history will describe how the country of Norway
was released from the longstanding ties to Denmark in 1814, and how the
nation entered into a union with Sweden with a relative independence which
lasted until 1905. In the years preceding 1905, mutual dissatisfaction with the
development led the two countries to the brink of a war, which was only
avoided through tough negotiations that rendered Norway a sovereign status.

This quite special situation implies that the country of Norway changed
itself from a status which in fact was, despite all metaphors, that of a Danish
province, through a forced political marriage with Stockholm, into a modern,
independent state in the course of 90 years. This period covers the 19th
century, when profound political, social and scientific changes took place all
over Europe. In the case of Norway, not only had a modern society to be
established just like in neighbouring countries, but a significant delay in this
process also had to be compensated for.

Health care and poor relief are parts of the infrastructure of a modern
society. In Norway this obvious fact is particularly important, because all

sorts of infrastructure had to be reinforced or built up anew in the 19th century. The establishment of an independent civil administration required substantial efforts, as did the modernisation of business, trades and industry. Health and poverty were only minor elements in the overall picture which faced the politicians of the new country, and only minor aspects of the problems which caused them concern and demanded their attention. In fact, doing anything useful about health and poverty was dependent on establishing a decent economy and a well-functioning state. There were priorities to be made all the time.

The demographic background

In the case of Norway, the rapid growth of the population, which was a consequence of the obviously universal process of the demographic transition, took place in a period which by and large covered the 19th century. A sharp decline in the mortality rates could be noted as early as 1815. The birth rates were still high, and did not fall markedly until around 1890. In 1815 the resident population numbered 885 431. In 1910, less than a century later, 2 391 782 inhabitants could be counted. Just like in a developing country of the 1990s, Norway had a young population – a fact which, of course, had a heavy impact on the extent and nature of the medical and social problems encountered at the time.

That a population pressure existed needs no further discussion. However, the demographers do not tell the whole story. Between 1840 and 1930 about 800 000 Norwegians emigrated – almost all of them to the United States of America. Initially, this took the form of an emigration from rural Norway to rural America for demographic reasons, but there were also other elements. Later the prospects of work in American cities became more prominent pull factors, so that Norway experienced a second and larger migration wave, which mainly manifested as an urban emigration.[1]

The emigration acted as a safety valve as the population pressure increased, but it is debatable whether it was mainly people in a strained situation who were pressed out, or whether it was the more established singles and families who went, attracted by promising information about the possibilities for a better life. The very first group of emigrants, leaving as early as 1825, were seeking religious freedom in the New World. Nevertheless the population leakage caused by emigration was quite remarkable: the numbers who left between 1866 and 1873 could be compared to 60 per cent of the birth surplus and, for some years, mortality rates and emigration rates were approximately the same.

It is important to bear these demographic data in mind when looking at health and poverty. In addition it must be noted that 19th century Norway was largely a rural society and, for a long time, a major part of the population lived in just one of the counties, in the rural county of Akershus in the south-east (in 1801, 43 per cent of the total population of 883 603). Most of the increase in population during the 19th century also took place in this south-eastern region. Although half of the Norwegian population still lives in the south-east (in 1995, 4 347 695), this is mainly due to the growth of the cities.[2]

The village structure found in many other European countries was never typical for Norway, nor were big estates run by large landowners, as in neighbouring Sweden and Denmark. Family farms scattered over the cultivable area were, and still are, the dominating pattern of settlement in rural Norway. However, the cultivable areas make up only some 3 per cent of the land surface. Only in the south-east, in the middle of the country around the old city of Trondheim, and to a certain degree in the south-west near Stavanger, are there continuous agricultural areas of any extent. This means that the rest of the farms were found in the valleys or by the coast, often where farming could be combined with forestry and fishing. Thus the settled areas could be separated by large distances, and forests, fjords and waters had to be overcome. As the individual farms were often inhabited by large families, supplemented by cotter families living in the neighbourhood, it might be rather crowded on the single settlement, but a good distance to the next.

At the outset of what can be called the period of modern Norway, in 1815, 9.8 per cent of the population lived in densely built-up areas – a percentage not basically different from the 6.8 per cent in 1664–66. But in 1875, when the number of inhabitants had reached 1 813 424, still only 24.4 per cent were city-dwellers. This distribution of the population in urban and rural areas, and the special distribution within rural Norway give quite special preconditions on the one hand for the occurrence and spread of disease and for vulnerability to factors triggering poverty and, on the other hand, also for setting up effective health services, and for providing health care for the poor.

With the steady increase in population in the 19th century the percentage increase in urban-dwellers was greater. The population pressure on the sustainability of the small communities, of course, represented a push factor for migration to towns. Pull factors were prospects of work and a better personal standard of living than what could in future be expected in the countryside. To obtain education also required moving to a city, and the education received there often led to a decision to remain there because of the availability of suitable work. Some important structural changes in the traditional trades and industries also led to internal migration and shifts in economic opportunities: traditional Norwegian shipping could be based in small communities along the coast as long as sailing ships could compete in the market, but the introduction of costly steamers required a financial and professional base which small communities could not provide. A major push factor, of course, was the population pressure on the sustainability of the small communities. For example, in the period 1875 to 1900, the capital of Christiania (now Oslo) doubled its population from around 120 000 to around 240 000. In 1900, 35.7 per cent of Norway's 2 240 032 inhabitants lived in densely populated areas – a substantial increase in the numbers of urban-dwellers, but still also a proof of the strong rural traditions in Norway. These demographic facts indicate that if one looks for urban health and poverty problems on a large scale, one has to concentrate on the last decades of the 19th century. But, compared to many other European nations, most Norwegian agglomerations were still on a small scale.

Social and cultural background

The description of the historical, demographic, economic and geographical set-up of Norwegian society in the 18th and 19th centuries indicates that it must have been rather egalitarian. Class differences in the rural population, as represented through the numbers of cotters and land workers, are most visible in the central farming districts. In the cities before the major urbanisation, the social differences were mainly between an élite, usually immigrant, families from Denmark, or people of other foreign descent, and the rest. And as a certain degree of social difference is often a prerequisite for a poverty problem (for instance) to become visible, this special trait of Norwegian society helps explain why, for a long time, both problems and solutions were different in the various parts of the country. Since the sources do not reveal how they were handled, problems may remain concealed from the historian in a rural society with rather evenly distributed living conditions and capacities to absorb failures in health and subsistence.

On the ideological side, Protestant Christianity had a strong position, setting moral standards for the duties owed towards one's fellow human beings. In the second half of the 18th century the waves of Enlightenment also broke over Norway, and a new interest in society as such was aroused. Preventive medicine was propagated, as were practical measures to support, for example, agriculture and food production. The extent of the impact exerted by the introduction of the potato into Norwegian households during this period has been somewhat disputed among historians. However, in the long run there is no doubt that the effect on the calory supply was substantial.

The Industrial Revolution in Norway took place in the 19th century. However, this delay in comparison with other countries does not preclude another important development in Norway. What has been called an 'industrious revolution'[3] took place in the 18th century. Work and workmanship became predominant virtues. And as trade and the economy allowed greater freedom for initiatives towards the end of the century, living conditions and prosperity could be enhanced by means of long and varied working days for large groups of the population. There is also a linkage to religious life which has to be noted: Hans Nilsen Hauge (1771–1824), an influential lay preacher, not only led a revivalist movement which spread throughout most of the country, he also eagerly promoted homeworking, trade, and the establishment of new industry. Considering idleness as a sin, he even knitted while walking and participated in farmwork in places he visited to preach.

But this industriousness also influenced attitudes towards its counterpart – towards those who were not inclined to work or to those who were unable to work, the sick and the poor. Thus the workhouses in the cities and the arrangements for the poor in the countryside also had an eye towards exploiting the working capacity of their clients and towards correcting the unwilling and teaching them the blessings of work.

The health of the Norwegians

We do not have too much exact information about the health situation in Norway in the first half of the 19th century. Of course, there are mortality figures available, as well as some materials which may shed a certain light also on morbidity,[4] but the data are mostly linked to a diagnostic system which is not suited for more detailed etiological studies. A reporting system for health matters on the local level gradually developed in the course of the century and, especially from 1868 onwards, quite comprehensive information is available not only about deaths and other vital statistics, but also about transient diseases, the health services and the like.

What is crucial to the understanding of the development, shape and extent of health services is how the health situation was perceived by the population. In the 1801 census, health personnel cannot be traced among the listed professions. At the end of the century, Norway had a quite modern health system for the period, however. Either a fatalistic view on life, well-being and death or, on the other hand, strong, generalised priorities linked to other values, such as religion, the economy or even the adventures of life, may leave severe health conditions rather underestimated, and a change will both take time and require the emergence of a new way of thinking.

For the period 1868–1900 we have tried to assess disease perception by means of a content analysis method, comparing the verbal parts of the medical officers' reports to the corresponding figures.[5] The results indicate, with due precautions taken, that concern about health decreases in the period of economic growth up to around 1890, when the concern index increases again. For the whole period an appalling difference between urban and rural districts can be noted: the concern for health in the capital of Christiania, the node for economic growth and modernity, is lower than for the country as a whole.

The calculation of the health concern index was based on the available figures for infectious diseases. This is unproblematic, because infectious diseases were by far the most prevalent health hazards at the time. A major concern for the health services was to stem ravaging epidemics, and possibly prevent their occurrence. One might believe that epidemics would only spread slowly, because of the local settlement pattern, but this is not quite true. Along the coast, the sea made relatively swift communication possible. In addition, when the great fisheries took place off the coast, thousands of fishermen from some distance away set out in their vessels. Temporary villages of very low housing standards were built, and these primitive agglomerations acted as nodes for the distribution of infections to large parts of Norway. Among the serious intestinal diseases, the nervous fever – an infection historically interpreted as salmonellosis – had an especially easy ride in the indescribably awful sanitary conditions.

Among the special medical problems of Norway in the 18th century was the so-called *radesyge*, a disease which, however, gradually disappeared. This was probably a non-venereal syphilis-like infection which attracted considerable contemporary attention and led to the building of several dedicated hospitals in small cities along the coast. In addition, leprosy persistently occurred, especially in western Norway. A centre for treatment and research in leprosy was established in the city of Bergen on the western coast, and it was here that the physician Gerhard Henrik Armauer Hansen (1841–1912) discovered the leprosy bacillus in 1873.

The impact of nutrition on the health of the population is difficult to assess and consequently an issue for discussion among historians. For a mainly rural population like that of Norway, calculations of food intake will always be compromised by an unknown supplement of fish and game. The introduction of the potato in the 18th century is given credit for the fact that famine, even in periods when food supplies were scarce, has never been an important health factor since the end of the Napoleonic Wars. However, the abrupt fall in mortality in 1815 indicates that the previous social conditions had caused larger parts of the population to live just on the brink of subsistence level, and that the effect on health of a rise in living standards was revealed through a fall in mortality.

The epidemics of Asiatic cholera also hit Norway – for example, in 1832–33 and in 1853. The most important impact of these epidemics on the health of the Norwegians was not the death tolls, but the interest in, and efforts to develop, preventive medicine which followed. Tuberculosis was also an ever-present scourge with important social consequences; the main efforts here, however, were set in train only after 1905, partly because the broad grassroots engagement in preparing for a possible war with Sweden shifted its focus to tuberculosis and public health.

What sort of health care?

To provide evenly distributed health care in the strict sense of the word – care for the individual in both sickness and health for all Norwegians – was an impossible public task in the 19th century due to the demographic and economic structure of the country. Care for the sick simply had to take place at home on the farm or in the cotter's hut in rural Norway.

Running a medical practice in the countryside was difficult not only because of the great distances and slow communications, but also because the population was not used to calling for services which had to be paid for, and they only had little to pay with. In addition, they had centuries of tradition of managing without physicians. Folk medicine, quacks and people with some medical knowledge gained not least from popular books published in the spirit of Enlightenment in the last decades of the 18th century obviously met part of the demand. The same reaction was seen when a public midwife system was proposed and actually introduced. Substantial difficulties arose: why pay for birth services which since time immemorial had been taken on by local women?[6]

The needs were more clearly perceived by the authorities, which had established a system of medical officers, a sort of public health service, as early as 1603 when the first public health officer was appointed. It goes without saying that serving, for example, a district in northern Norway with hundreds of kilometres between the different settlements could only offer very little to the population in cases of disease. In 1815 there were 100 medical doctors in Norway; 90 years later, there were 1200, and a modern medical profession had been established.

However, the build-up of a primary health care and also a hospital system was tightly linked to the pushing forward of a national, academic medicine. This again was part of an old conflict with the Danes – the university issue. In Norway strong local forces in the 18th century wanted to open a national university not only to meet upcoming demands in research and education, but also to strengthen national identity. And, for this latter reason, proposals for a university were repeatedly refused by the authorities in Copenhagen. Only in the turmoil of wartime did clever negotiators manage to establish a university, the Royal Frederik's University in the Norwegian capital of Christiania. When the essential document was signed by the king on 2 September 1811, this event was celebrated all over Norway in a way that seems quite out of proportion to all those who are not familiar with its background and context.

Among the branches of the university was the small, new, medical faculty, which started its teaching in the autumn of 1814 with a staff of three professors and three students, but aimed to achieve a sufficient capacity to educate doctors for the local needs – an objective which was fulfilled only a few decades later. It is a matter of discussion within the history of science to what extent a national medicine in the strict sense was developed, or if it was a mere copy of what was going on in other places. It is beyond the scope of this chapter to go into this topic; suffice it here to state that the medical curriculum was more or less taken over from the Royal Surgical Academy in Copenhagen. However, this fact must not be interpreted as only using a blueprint: the curriculum in Copenhagen was brand new in 1785 and represented the modern merger of surgery and internal medicine, offering just that combination of theory and hands-on training of skills that Norway needed.

The public health system could be taken over from the old administration, but there were also local efforts to keep up with the new ideas in the field abroad. An adapted version of the Austrian medical policy of Johann Peter Frank (1745–1821) was presented by a Norwegian medical officer, Rasmus Frankenau (1767–1814). And the first professor of hygiene from 1824, Frederik Holst (1791–1871), eagerly studied principles and practices from abroad to evaluate them and introduce at home what he found relevant for Norwegian medicine and Norwegian health care. Studies of the numerous study travels undertaken by Norwegian physicians also reveal a remarkable medical internationalism, which is in sharp contrast with the tendency to present almost all scientific papers and medical reports in the Norwegian language, and in that way cutting off a reciprocity which probably would have given mutual benefits.

The build-up of family medicine in Norway was based on a system of general practitioners. Payment was a problem. Details have to be omitted here, but a combination of a private fee for service practice with official public health services, services for the poor, military duties, arrangements with emerging industry, and – late in the 19th century – also with different types of health insurance systems made it possible for the doctors to enjoy an admittedly modest lifestyle, even in the countryside.

The establishment of a hospital system was driven by three forces. One of them was the new university which required a teaching hospital to be built in Christiania. A military hospital, which had existed in the capital since 1807, was among the temporary teaching premises which had to be used until the first buildings of the National Hospital, the teaching hospital, could be opened in 1826.

The second force was urbanisation. In the cities, caring for the sick at home was not possible to the same extent as in the countryside, and hospitals were built. In the larger cities, such as in the capital of Christiania, these hospitals were of course larger, particularly *Ullevål Sykehus* in Oslo, which opened in 1887 and developed into a mammoth institution with around 2000 beds by the first decades of the 20th century. In the more built-up rural communities, some similar hospitals were opened – for example, the one in Aker, outside the capital, in 1871. County hospitals were often small, but the patients found there were, as a rule, admitted for the same reasons as in the city: they were workers, craftsmen or widowed; in short, they typically came from categories of the population which were less likely to have access to care at home, as was the case for members of rural farming families or the more well-off bourgeoisie in the towns.

The third force was the developments within medicine itself and the changes in general attitudes towards the concept of disease. As in other countries, in Norway much of the effort in the fields of preventive medicine originated in the fears caused by the cholera epidemics. Of particular importance was the epidemic of 1832–33 and the larger one in 1853. Largely as a result of experiences with cholera, a law of sanitary commissions was passed in 1860. This law, which was in force until 1984, gave an efficient basis for preventive health services led by the local medical officer. Later on, the fight against tuberculosis implied public sanitation, and this fitted well into the prevailing visions for a modern society and for a matching form of health education setting high standards for personal hygiene.

The poverty problem

Responsibility for the poor had traditionally been linked to the family, which seems obvious to the historian in light of the population structure. After the Reformation, the commitments of the Church went hand-in-hand with public and private arrangements. In the 18th century similar attitudes and similar legislation to that in other European countries were also found in Norway. The poor who were sick, frail or disabled were entitled to support, but the attitudes against people who were able and had the capacity for work were rather harsh.

In the last part of the 18th century social conditions worsened. At the turn of the century, Norway experienced years of war and blockade, but an internal process was also beginning – the population growth. The local rural societies had to absorb the increase as the numbers of cotters rose, but as the means of subsistence could not follow suit at the same pace, increasing social inequalities were an unavoidable consequence. The efforts against poverty on the public level were intensified in 1735, as a response to an initiative taken by King Christian VI (1730–46) in Copenhagen.[7] The king, known for his Pietistic religious views, and for his concerns about public enlightenment and education, had been touring Norway in the summer of 1733 when he had observed a considerable number of beggars. In a letter of 2 September 1735 to the Norwegian governor, Count Christian Rantzau (1648–1771), he requested that the problem be taken up, which was done immediately. After collecting information on the extent and nature of the poverty problem, a policy was introduced which had three aspects: care and support for people without the means to live; restrictive regulations against people unwilling to work; and the establishment of a labour market to absorb the increasing numbers of lower-class inhabitants.

Thus, from 1741, work was a duty, with referral to the workhouse as the threatened option if this duty was violated. Such an arrangement gave a cheap and stable workforce to the benefit of the upper classes, and was a form of social security for the lower classes. Poverty legislation was enacted first in 1741, initially for the diocese of Akershus, the most densely populated area, but later extended to the rest of the country: Bergen in 1755, Christianssand in 1786 and Trondhjem in 1790. Other regulations of the labour market followed suit. Some workhouses were built, following an old arrangement, as the city of Trondheim had been allowed to build a workhouse as early as 1639, and Bergen in 1646.

The urban and rural faces of poverty were different, and so were the regions of rural Norway. Nor did the pressure of poverty even mount simultaneously. This fact required different solutions. However, after 1789 the regulations were given a more human touch. A symptom of this was a duty laid on the state that everyone who could not care for themselves was entitled to support for subsistence. But workhouses with the dual functions of providing work and of serving as ordinary jails still existed. The public costs for handling the poverty problem were mostly taken from taxes, but the taxation system was not very developed at the end of the 18th century. In the countryside, outdoor relief on the parish was the traditional method, while confinement in institutions was used in the cities. In the 1820s around 50 such institutions existed. As the chronically ill and the disabled were also entitled to support, it was quite natural that health care and care for the poor were mixed together. Doctors had to give their services free of charge to people with no means to pay, and several institutions served as hospitals and as housing for the poor at the same time.

But what was the extent of the poverty problem? It has been calculated from the 1801 census that 1.3 per cent of the inhabitants in the rural but densely populated diocese of Akershus were receiving financial support. In the nearby city of Christiania this figure fluctuated around 6–7 per cent at the end of the 18th century. In 1828 the number of poor people supported in the country as a whole has been calculated at 3.1 per cent, which is regarded as relatively normal for comparable countries. But a steady increase in the number of poor people took place, discussions about new legislation for poor relief progressed, and a new poor law was passed in 1845. Now the responsibility was laid on the municipalities. This principle, of course, linked poor relief to the local community to which the poor belonged. However, the possible advantages of handling of these matters locally was probably outweighed by the frail dependence on local resources and the local economy. The community-based principle was made even more fundamental in a revised poor law passed in 1863.

The public debate in Norway from the 1860s was profoundly influenced by the theologian and sociologist Elert Sundt (1817–74). By means of wide travelling and fieldwork, and through his extensive writings, he drew public attention to the poverty problem, as well as the problems connected with the existing poor relief system, and suggested the application of systems from abroad. In particular, he promoted voluntary systems, but these failed to achieve a strong foothold in Norway.

The skewed distribution of poverty and also of poverty relief was a constant concern in Norway. In 1872 four out of five people who received public support for poverty were women and children. And in a municipality where the funds for poverty relief were modest, this was not necessarily a positive sign, as poor communities with low tax revenues had only a little to spend on poverty. By contrast, a high poverty relief budget might indicate emerging wealthiness and better support for the indigent individuals.

After 1870 the poor relief system of Norway was even more closely linked to the build-up of a modern welfare state of the European type. Insurance arrangements were established, and new legislation covered more and more of the public responsibility for life, health and subsistence. But this belongs to the history of the 20th century and lies outside the framework of this chapter.

Diseases and poverty: parts of a totality

In Norway, as in comparable countries, the handling of health and poverty was part of the total set-up of the society and cannot be considered separately from the developments in other fields.[8] Looking at medical history, it is quite clear that the perceived importance of the preservation of health shows variation in time and place. Correspondingly, care for those who were in need, of course, was dependent on economy, demography, geography and so forth. But most important were the shifting attitudes which occurred in the prevailing policy – elements of religious charity, such as the Protestant emphasis on such virtues as modesty and diligence, but also elements of the exploitation of the available workforce, opposed by the strengthening lower classes. It should also be noted as a national peculiarity that politics in Norway, despite urbanisation, modernisation and economic growth in industry and trades was tilted towards agriculture throughout almost the entire 19th century. Poverty, and also parts of the health problems, not surprisingly were most predominant among the lower classes.

Politically, Norway experienced a similar rise in the influence of the lower classes as did other European countries. And in 1849 the revolutionary teacher Marcus Thrane (1817–1890) wrote in his newspaper: 'Wake up, workers! Unite!' Thrane succeeded in setting up a political movement, but it was curbed, and lost most of its power when the leaders were imprisoned. However, from the 1880s a new labour movement and the shaping of a political labour party put inequality in living standards and social problems for the lower classes on the agenda in a new way.

Clearly, the contemporary contacts which had been set up to learn from experiences in other countries were extensive, so that Norway, in her early efforts to build up a modern welfare state at the end of the 19th century, probably succeeded in her objective of catching up with her neighbours.

Notes

1. O.S. Lovoll, *The Promise of America: A History of the Norwegian-American People*, Minneapolis, 1984.
2. S. Dyrvik and O. Feldbæk, *Mellom Brødre 1780–1830 (Between Brothers, 1780–1830)*, Aschehougs Norgeshistorie, Vol. 7, Oslo, 1996.
3. S. Sogner, *Krig og Fred 1660–1780 (War and Peace, 1660–1780)*, Aschehougs Norgeshistorie, Vol. 6, Oslo, 1996.
4. A.E. Imhof and Ø. Larsen, *Sozialgeschichte und Medizin*, Oslo and Stuttgart, 1975.
5. Ø. Larsen, O. Berg and F. Hodne, *Legene og samfunnet (The Physicians and Society)*, Oslo, 1986; Ø. Larsen (ed.), *The Shaping of a Profession. Physicians in Norway Past and Present*, Canton, MA, 1996; Ø. Larsen, H. Haugtomt and W. Platou, *Sykdomsoppfatning og epidemiology 1860–1900 (Infectious Diseases in Norway 1860–1900, and the Attitudes of the Health Authorities towards them – a Presentation of the Data)*, Oslo, 1980.
6. K. Kjærheim, *Mellom kloke koner og kvitkledde menn: jordmorvesenet på 1800-tallet (Midwives in Norway in the Nineteenth Century)*, Oslo, 1987.
7. S. Dyrvik in K-G. Andersson, S. Dyrvik, G.A. Gunnlaugsson, U. Johanson, H. Jørgensen, J. Kowalik, S. Malmberg and P. Pulma, *Oppdaginga av Fattigdommen (Discovering Poverty. 18th Century Social Legislation in Scandinavia)*, Oslo, 1983.
8. L. Seip, *Nasjonen Bygges 1830–1870 (Building of the Nation 1830–1870)*, Aschehougs Norgeshistorie, Vol. 8, Oslo, 1997; F. Hodne, *An Economic History of Norway, 1815–1970*, Trondheim, 1975.

PART FOUR
Britain

CHAPTER TEN

Health Care and Poor Relief in Provincial England

Anne Crowther

Enlightenment, political economy and poor relief

Provincial England seems an unpromising field in which to study the influence of the Enlightenment, since the very word 'provincial' carries with it a suggestion of isolation from the mainstream of intellectual life. In fact provincial England of the 18th and early 19th centuries had important intellectual, scientific and medical centres, of which the Lunar Society in Birmingham is the best known for its association with Joseph Priestley, James Watt and Mathew Boulton.[1] There were also active societies in Liverpool, Newcastle and Manchester, and Manchester was home to the learned Thomas Percival whose views on medical ethics reached out to continental ideas of medical police via his Edinburgh contacts.[2] Yet provincial England is not conventionally associated with what might be termed the European 'High Enlightenment'. Bertrand Russell's populist *History of Western Philosophy*, for example, dismissed English thought during the period of industrialisation in a few words as 'individualistic in intellectual matters, and also in economics, but ... not emotionally or ethically self-assertive'.[3] Elie Halévy's description of intellectual England (which he contrasted firmly with Scotland) at the end of the 18th century represents another widely held view: he argued that the social exclusiveness of England's ancient universities forced intellectual life into the provinces, where its emphasis was chiefly scientific. Noting the weakness of the English educational system, Halévy argued that, as far as the higher learning was concerned, even London 'was merely a large provincial town'. European ideas were transposed into a British context by philosophers such as Jeremy Bentham whose aim was to translate the European Enlightenment into practical policy. Halévy believed that government, attracted by this eminently practical philosophy, was particularly influenced by 'Utilitarian propaganda' during the 1830s and 1840s. Although this rather mechanistic view of how philosophers may influence government has been much debated, the direct influence of the political economy on the treatment of the poor in 19th-century England is less open to dispute.[4] The reform of the Poor Law in 1834, although precipitated by economic and social problems, owed its characteristic shape to a long debate developed by the political economists.[5]

European visitors admired the ingenuity of industrialising England, but were discouraged by its apparent lack of Enlightenment virtues. They admired the celebrated rural retreats of the Romantic poets, but reacted against the sordid appearance of the industrial towns, pervaded, as they often were, by the dour culture of the Dissenting sects. Many English writers also developed a profoundly ambiguous view of their own industrial regions. Revulsion from the squalor of industrialisation could be found in the Romantic poets, in the moral fictions of Disraeli, Dickens or Mrs Gaskell, or in the influential essays of Thomas Carlyle. Carlyle, the correspondent of Goethe, saw himself specifically as the purveyor of Weimar Enlightenment to the incorrigibly practical English. He wrote in 1829:

> ... the wise men, who now appear as Political Philosophers, deal exclusively with the Mechanical province; and occupying themselves in counting-up and estimating men's motives, strive by curious checking and balancing, and other adjustments of Profit and Loss, to guide them to their true advantage ... But though Mechanism, wisely contrived, has done much for man in a social and moral point of view, we cannot be persuaded that it has ever been the chief source of his worth or happiness.[6]

The above description would, of course, have been seen by the provincial leaders as typical of the patronising and uninformed views of a metropolitan-based critic, albeit a Scottish one. The most dynamic cities of provincial England – especially Liverpool, Birmingham, Leeds, Manchester and Bristol – certainly lacked some of the peculiar social and educational advantages which made Edinburgh the centre of Enlightenment culture in Britain. None had a university like Edinburgh's, and the learned societies had to compensate for this. As in Edinburgh, medical men played a part in the general culture, as well as forming their own professional institutions.[7]

It is not surprising that, in the expanding industrial towns of England, the aspects of the Enlightenment with strongest appeal were those rooted in economics. The thinkers who prevailed in these grimy regions were Adam Smith and Jeremy Bentham, associated respectively with the ideas of commercial freedom and enlightened self-interest. Both were essentially optimistic writers, believing that society operated through powerful natural laws which government must understand in order for society to profit. Yet Adam Smith's hopeful view of economic development in *The Wealth of Nations* (1776), had been countered by the alarming theory of Thomas Malthus in his *Essay on the Principle of Population* (1798), that all human progress would be checked by the unalterable laws of population.[8] Smith envisaged a commercial society where increasing population indicated new wealth, but Malthus, who looked back to an agricultural past, believed that the unchecked growth of population would rapidly cause misery by pressing too heavily on limited supplies of food. Both Smith and Malthus were very widely read in their own time, and stimulated a large body of critics and admirers. Malthus's more pessimistic view seemed especially convincing during the lengthy period of the French wars when Britain was much affected by the dislocations of early industrialism, disruption of trade and sudden shocks to the agricultural economy.

Adam Smith's views were employed selectively by many in the industrial towns of England to justify free trade and the ending of restraints in the workplace: they were less drawn to his Scottish faith in universal education as the necessary basis for a prosperous society. Equally, Malthus could be culled for his more congenial opinions such as his attack on the English system of poor relief, for, he argued, compulsory levies given to the poor encouraged reckless early marriages and overpopulation. His ideas were further endorsed in the political economy of David Ricardo, whose work was mainly responsible for economics being branded as 'the dismal science'. Poor relief, argued Ricardo, was a form of taxation which interfered with the natural level of wages, and he endorsed Malthus's belief in the relationship of poor laws to population growth.[9] The first censuses of 1800 and 1810 confirmed that the population was indeed expanding: at the same time, the poor were apparently becoming more riotous in both town and countryside, while the rising cost of poor relief caused many critics to rethink the basis of the Poor Laws. By the late 18th century a number of English regions, particularly in the old industrial towns of Nottinghamshire, were already experimenting with ways of imposing moral restraint on the poor through making it more difficult and humiliating to apply for poor relief.[10] Neither political expediency nor ordinary humane feeling made it possible to abolish the Poor Law completely, but political economy, as it appeared in its everyday guise in newspapers or pamphlets, favoured a more stringent approach to the poor. By the 1840s those who believed themselves to be the heirs of Smith and Bentham were given a title which stressed their provincial affiliations: the Manchester School.[11] Apart from the obligatory attachment to free trade, this school of thought remained antagonistic to poor relief, viewing it as an incentive to indolence and vice amongst the ablebodied poor. Confronted with the sick poor, its response was more ambiguous.

A traditional response to the problem of supplying health care to the poor in many towns was to gather local resources, often on a generous scale, to support charity hospitals and dispensaries. Since even the most generous of charities was not sufficient to meet the demands for treatment, each parish paid for free medical treatment under the Poor Law. It was hard to sustain such a system effectively in the emerging industrial towns, which were also faced with the problem of defending the public health by expensive preventive measures such as improved water supplies, cleansing and drainage. Although the division between charitable medical care and poor relief was also apparent in London, the metropolis was exceptional in its concentration of population, wealth and charity. The strains of rapid growth were felt most severely in smaller towns where population overwhelmed traditional systems of both charity and civic government. London, whose problems were immense, was nevertheless able to build on an existing network of charity hospitals, dispensaries and poor law infirmaries, many of them developing from the mid-18th century or even earlier: provincial cities which had recently been small towns, had a much less elaborate heritage. Help from longstanding charitable endowments was more common in the older cathedral cities such as York or Canterbury, but rapidly expanding industrial towns, like Manchester or Huddersfield, had to build from scratch. Local government, imbued both by a strong desire for economy and a Ricardian suspicion of poor relief, was slow to respond. John Pickstone entitles one chapter of his history of health care in Manchester, 'Small town ways and large town problems', and this encapsulates the situation.[12]

The division between voluntary and state assistance is currently much discussed by British historians, especially in terms of the 'mixed economy of welfare'. This phrase was first used to describe the development of British social services in the 20th century, especially as governments from Attlee to Thatcher took different views on what the components of the social assistance should be.[13] The 'mixed economy' of family, state and charitable assistance, has been readily projected back into earlier centuries, since the Poor Laws in Britain meant that an official system of relief, although dominated by local rather than central government, existed alongside older forms of charitable assistance, and also aimed to support, rather than supplant, family help. This was particularly important in medical assistance from the late 18th century. On one side was the voluntary hospital or dispensary, endowed by public subscription, run by local élites, attended by the more prestigious medical practitioners (usually for free), and used only by the poor. On the other side was Poor Law medical relief, offering some basic medical attendance in the workhouse, but mainly giving medical treatment or nursing help to the poor in their own homes. Although this service, too, was intended only for the poor, the doctor was paid by the parish, and his status was correspondingly less than the doctor who offered his services free to a charitable institution. The poor took advantage of both systems when they could, and Mary Fissell has described 18th century Bristol as offering a complex set of choices to the poor, as they steered their way around several charitable institutions.[14] Yet the idea of a 'mixed economy' of welfare is rather too neat for the period of industrialisation, suggesting, as it does, some element of conscious choice or planned strategy not to be found in the chaotic and overlapping medical services of the time.

The history of health care for the poor from the 18th century onwards might be seen as a struggle between high Enlightenment and low political economy. Charitable hospitals in the towns of course stemmed from ancient Christian ideals, but increasingly aimed at the combination of civic virtue and scientific curiosity which was associated with the Enlightenment.[15] They provided free services for the public good, were a focus of medical education and scientific inquiry, were the natural home of medical innovators, particularly in surgery, and they were the testing ground for new medical techniques. In many cities during the 19th century they also developed formal links with the new civic universities. But they also struggled to provide stable and coherent health care, since their finances were frequently precarious and unpredictable. Hence they increasingly depended on emergency state assistance, and were effectively nationalised in 1948. The Poor Laws, where the motives were mainly economic, had much more modest medical ambitions, but rested on more secure finance. Without much conscious planning, and under pressure from medical reformers, the Poor Law by the end of the 19th century produced an extensive system of health care employing ever larger numbers of medical professionals. It is usually the more stable, if unattractive, state-controlled systems of Poor Law and public health, joined in 1911 by national health insurance (funded from national rather than local taxation), which are described as the foundations of the modern welfare state in Britain.[16] This view might be challenged, since after 1834 poor law medical services, like the rest of the English Poor Law, had to accommodate the notion that relief must be made as unattractive to the poor as possible. In fact, the National Health Service even after 1948 had to deal with a lingering public hostility to many of the remaining poor law institutions, however effective their medical services.

Industrialisation and poor relief

Although industrialisation ultimately made possible an extensive network of health care for the poor, and supported the large infirmaries of the 19th century, its immediate influence should not be exaggerated. Just as 'Enlightenment' is a convenient shorthand for quite diverse intellectual developments, so 'industrialisation' is a word which gives a superficial unity to a process which reached the English provinces in different ways. Britain in the mid-18th century was a wealthy commercial country by European standards; it also had a large industrial output. The widespread domestic manufacture of textiles, for example, supplemented rural incomes. Unlike most European nations, England already possessed a system of poor relief which, even though frequently abused in practice, gave some kind of legal right to assistance. The claims of the sick and 'impotent' (mainly the handicapped or those too old and infirm to work) were enshrined in the original enactment of 1601. Hence industrialisation, and the movements of population which accompanied it, affected the English provinces in different ways. The legal form of poor relief was based on a parish or borough system of administration, yet the effect of industrialisation was both to accelerate and distort the urbanisation already characteristic of pre-industrial England. Textiles, including both wool and cotton, became focused on the northern counties. Yet there had been many thriving textile areas in other parts of England, and so communities in the south, where agricultural incomes also depended on domestic manufacture, suffered a severe economic shock. By the beginning of the 19th century, the Poor Law had to deal both with cities like Manchester or Leeds, where a rapidly expanding population pressed on an ancient administrative structure, and old, formerly prosperous counties like Dorset or Gloucestershire, where domestic industries collapsed, underemployment in agriculture put pressure on the Poor Law, and the rural poor became increasingly discontented.

The effects of industrialisation were also felt in cities which were not themselves industrial in origin, such as Bristol or Liverpool. Before the Industrial Revolution these were great ports, reflecting Britain's importance in international trade and the spread of its colonial empire, but Britain's ever-expanding commerce caused these towns to grow as well, and they were also the destination of large numbers of impoverished immigrants.[17] Industrialism caused difficulties for poor relief both in the centres where it flourished, and those it had passed by. Some of the old market and trading towns in the south and home counties, or the most successful centres of agricultural improvement, such as East Anglia, had substantial poorhouses which took in both the sick and the insane, although they also offered medical services to the poor in their own homes. Depending on the size of the population, the poorhouses might range from a few dozen to 100 or more inmates. Cities such as Bristol and Liverpool already had big workhouses: by the early 1830s, Liverpool's housed over 1600 inmates, and was one of the largest institutions in the country – no charity hospital, prison or asylum could compare to it in size. An institution of this kind took in inmates of all conditions, and was both a hospital and an asylum. The parish of St Mary's in the town of Nottingham had also developed a complex system, with a hospital attached to the workhouse, a dispensary and home attendance. There seems to have been an effort to harness the voluntary principle to the old Poor Law, since consultants gave their services free if the parish doctor required assistance. The whole was managed by one full-time, resident surgeon. However, the effectiveness of the system should not be exaggerated, as one contemporary report shows:

> ... a great proportion of the patients, especially vagrants, are attended only once. ... Many cases were so slight as to cost little, not averaging more than three pence each; but this was at a time when the duty devolved upon one medical officer, whose time was so fully occupied, as to render the simplest treatment necessary, and the use of any except the most indispensable remedies, almost impracticable. and yet, with all this economy, this Institution was popular among the poor; and many who required no other kind of parochial aid, anxiously resorted to its assistance.[18]

Then there were the towns at the centre of the Industrial Revolution, where the population rose most rapidly and traditional poor law arrangements had been modest. Manchester had a sizeable workhouse by the early 1830s, holding around 600 inmates, and employing an apothecary and lunatic keeper amongst its staff, but this was small in relation to need, and its medical services were very limited. Other expanding towns, such as Rochdale or Todmorden, were making no concessions to demand and had very modest buildings with a few dozen inmates; medical assistance at home was favoured as a cheaper alternative.[19] The traditional parish governments in these towns were often inflexible in dealing with rapid expansion and new social problems.

The old Poor Law

Before 1834 the habit was already well developed of contracting with a local medical practitioner to treat paupers. He was usually paid a fixed sum for his attendance on the poor, though he was paid per case for assistance with childbirth and for vaccination. It was assumed, of course, that he would not attend at childbirth unless the case was difficult, but the parish would pay the lesser costs of a midwife. Very small parishes simply paid the doctor his fee for each case. Payment for a nurse was also common; it seemed sensible to the parish authorities to pay a widow, who would herself otherwise be on poor relief, to attend a sick person at home. Nursing payments might also be made to relatives of the invalid, so that the nurse would not have to go out to work. Hilary Marland has shown that, in the West Riding of Yorkshire, payments to medical men were often quite generous and that poor law work was attractive to local practitioners. Payments might also be made to specialists, bonesetters or unconventional practitioners, while the workhouse was hardly ever used as a centre for the sick. Many local medical men were involved with occasional treatment of paupers, while the vestry also funded the cost of special diets, including alcohol.[20] Where there was no suitable workhouse accommodation, the parish would often pay a subscription to the nearest charity hospital in order to ensure hospital treatment for its poor, and subscriptions extended also to friendly societies providing medical insurance and burial clubs.

The extensive use of home-based medical care and the close relationship with local charities can be explained in a number of ways: pauperism had not been a major problem in the smaller towns before the onset of industrialisation, and it was easier to pay intermittently for personal services rather than meet the costly and permanent overheads of a large workhouse. Decisions about the level of treatment were highly individual and personal, and it was assumed that that the applicant would be known to the overseers. There were no standard scales of relief, and parishes adopted a wide variety of approaches to the sick poor, just as they did to the healthy. Amongst the considerations which might affect the generosity of treatment might be the sick person's moral character, the attitudes of local magistrates (to whom the applicant could appeal if not given sufficient help), or even whether the applicant had influence with the vestry through personal relationships. Hilary Marland has written of the very low uptake and minimal cost of medical relief in industrialising Yorkshire: the cost in the West Riding was the lowest in the country. Even before the New Poor Law, the Yorkshire parishes were tightening up on expenditure for poor relief, given their rapidly expanding populations. In this argument, industrialisation has a negative effect on health care provided by local government, and it was the least important method of assisting the poor with medical treatment. The working class in this area was better paid than in many parts of the country, and they developed alternative methods of paying for a doctor, particularly under their own friendly societies or medical clubs. If the doctor was involved with the poor, it was more because they employed him directly through their own self-help organisations, than through the Poor Law.[21] Indeed, in Malthus's original view, one of the main benefits of abolishing the Poor Laws altogether would be to further encourage such provident associations.[22]

Marland's description of industrialising Yorkshire relates particularly to towns with no experience of providing large infirmaries: here, the earlier medical services provided from local taxation were given in the pauper's home. This contrasts with the prototype poor law hospitals in the workhouses of Bristol or Liverpool. However, it should be stressed that all this poor law assistance was intended for the settled poor. Settlement was a most complex legal issue: the settled poor were defined as those born in the parish or who had acquired a settlement by some legal form such as marriage or apprenticeship. Settlement was, in the real sense of the word, a parochial issue, for the law assumed that all paupers had a place of settlement, even if they had not lived in it for many years, and the place of settlement carried the financial responsibility for its own wandering poor. Yet the towns of the Industrial Revolution depended on a constant supply of immigrants who had no legal right to relief. An examination of census returns shows that many of the immigrants had not come very far; they moved from the Lancashire countryside or adjacent counties to the nearest large town – the main exception being the Irish, whose desperate plight drove them over longer distances to find work.[23]

The medical treatment of incomers was a sore point. Sometimes it was given quite generously, either because the applicant was a long-term resident and his treatment not expensive, or because the parish expected to recoup the cost from the immigrant's place of settlement. The parish doctor was told to make out his bill and send it to the parish of origin, frequently resulting in long and expensive legal battles between parishes. But the Irish, Scots and other foreigners had no fixed place of settlement, and the cost of treating them could not be recouped. It was still not unknown for a sick or pregnant pauper to be put on a cart or cattle boat and returned to another parish, or to Ireland, or dumped across the Scottish border. But such practices had been prohibited by law in the early 18th century, and removal was not to be carried out if the pauper were too sick to move. For the sick poor and their families without a settlement, the decision on where to seek relief was a delicate one; parish relief could not be refused, but it might be followed by ejection – in some cases, to a place of origin which had been left many years previously. Because private charity offered no such threat, it was important to this group in times of sickness.[24]

Poor law medical care, or the lack of it, was much criticised by poor law reformers. The allegations made by the Royal Commission on the Poor Law in 1834 included comments about the neglect of the sick, and the inspectors employed under the new system frequently criticised the local administrators for their dirty and overcrowded infirmaries, failure to control their grasping or inhumane medical officers, or illegally refusing relief to applicants whose backgrounds were unknown. Several historians have qualified this picture, which was indeed much influenced by the propaganda of political economy. E.G. Thomas has argued that the sick poor in Berkshire, Essex and Oxfordshire were generally well treated: sometimes specialised services were provided, good quality food was given to the sick in their own homes, and considerable sums were spent on the local doctor, midwife and nursing. However, he admits that it was in 'the closely-knit communities, where the wants of most were known' that the system was most effective.[25] Neglectful and inconsistent treatment was more likely in the large towns – especially in the industrial areas with their constant supply of incomers – and the charity hospitals and dispensaries were often more responsive to these needs. Nevertheless, charity had limitations which were not only financial. During the 18th century, and for a considerable period afterwards, charitable institutions were selective. They would probably not turn away a worthy resident of the parish who had no legal settlement there, but they were averse to infectious diseases, venereal diseases, incurable diseases and badly behaved patients. Having no legal obligation to relieve such cases, they were able to leave them to the Poor Law, which could not refuse.[26]

The New Poor Law

Notoriously, the massive report of the Royal Commission on the Poor Laws of 1834 paid remarkably little attention to the sick poor, since it was almost exclusively concerned with ways of discouraging the healthy poor from claiming relief. Comments on medical relief were almost all concerned with finance – it was a matter of political economy, not public or personal health.[27] There was a brief section on 'out-door relief of the impotent' which noted that, since it was in no-one's interest to spend too much on medical services for the sick poor, these were usually provided economically. Ironically, in view of the heavy expense of the sick to the Poor Law in future decades, the question of medical treatment was largely ignored because of its perceived cheapness. The main problem, it seemed, was in the higher cost of treatment of sick paupers who did not belong to the parish, since the doctor was tempted to charge extortionate amounts to their parish of origin. The report added that medical relief might sabotage the natural and necessary responsibility of families to provide for their sick and elderly members.[28]

Edwin Chadwick, the disciple of Bentham, was one of the main architects of the New Poor Law. He was no admirer of the medical profession, except for those whose interests lay in public health rather than individual health care. The medical men he preferred were his friends Southwood Smith and James Phillips Kay, who were more interested in preventing pauperism through sanitation and education rather than in providing personal health services.[29] Chadwick also noted with approval the effects of the laws of settlement in discouraging immigrants from applying for medical relief:

> ... the objections to the operation of a poor's rate do not apply to the unsettled labourer, as the latter knows full well that should he neglect to provide against sickness ... his only resource would be an application to the overseer who, as a matter of course, would immediately take him before the nearest magistrate for the purpose of having him removed to his place of legal settlement ....[30]

Chadwick believed that the pressure of the settlement laws forced immigrant labourers to join provident societies to give them financial support and medical care when they were ill. There is no doubt that these societies were becoming widespread, but also that they offered help mainly to skilled workers who could afford a subscription. For the mass of poor immigrants, particularly the Irish, illness, if treated at all, would have to be a matter of charity. Chadwick's relative lack of interest in personal health care actually differed from the approach of his master Bentham, since Bentham's own proposals for a reformed institutional structure had paid particular attention to medical arrangements, and he was particularly anxious that the enlarged workhouses of his imagination should have facilities for medical experiment, by which he chiefly meant that medical men would be offered the opportunity to observe all manner of health problems, to experiment in matters of diet, and to keep detailed statistics for further guidance. The workhouses, in his view, would be places of medical education.[31]

The New Poor Law of 1834 made no special arrangements for the sick poor, and it seems to have been assumed that old arrangements would continue. The original suggestion – not in fact put into practice – was that the old workhouses be turned into purely disciplinary institutions for the ablebodied, and that 'the proper objects of relief [i.e., the sick] might be accommodated temporarily in ordinary dwelling houses, and it is a fortunate district in which there are no empty tenements available for their reception'. The report was characterised by its numerous unrealistic assumptions, but in none so much as the idea that part of the discipline of the new institution might be for the medical officer to train younger pauper women to act as nurses in the infirmaries. At no stage did the framers of the new law assume that one of the most important functions of the workhouse would be as a hospital. The early structure of the law did not encourage major efforts towards a medical policy outside the workhouse. Until 1865, although each parish contributed to the cost of the workhouse and the salaries of poor law officers, the cost of maintaining an individual pauper still fell on his parish of origin, and parishes within the union engaged in frequent financial squabbles about responsibility.[32] Michael Rose has argued that this undermined policy in the provincial cities, where there was no central direction, and each of the city parishes continued to fight in its own financial interests.[33] In any case, mixing the care of the sick with the discouraging of the ablebodied made it difficult to organise the Poor Law for any major social purpose. This duty was more readily undertaken in the charity hospitals, despite their often chaotic management. Their rapid expansion, and the development of specialism within them, was a strong contrast to the all-purpose, unambitious administration of the Poor Law, which became increasingly termed a 'residual service'.

The most significant change in poor relief came in the change of scale from relatively small parishes to larger units – the poor law unions. Although the size and geography of these were often determined without any logical purpose except to suit local factions, they made possible the building of new and larger workhouses. This was done at a variable speed, since a number of unions greatly resented the expense.[34] The original intention of the Poor Law report, that the different classes of paupers – the sick, elderly, ablebodied, and children – should be housed in separate buildings, was abandoned as impractical and expensive, and so the 'general mixed workhouse' which was segregated only in terms of its internal architecture, became the norm. Despite the numerous objections to this, where buildings were large, separate sick wards with their own staff became feasible. The new system, with occasional hitches at times of economic depression, was largely successful in driving the ablebodied away, and the population of the workhouses became increasingly dominated by the sick, elderly and infirm. Many of these were elderly, incurable or chronic cases, and medical techniques could do little for them. They usually came into the workhouses because they had no-one to care for them at home. The Poor Law Commissioners preferred nursing to be done in the workhouses, and did not encourage the payment of pauper nurses to look after the sick in their own homes. It is probable, given the behaviour in London parishes which were not brought effectively under the central authority until the 1860s, that some guardians defied this instruction and continued to use pauper nurses outside the workhouses: they could defy the district auditor who examined their books by disguising such payments as outdoor poor relief to the nurse.

The changes in the Poor Law had the effect of driving a major wedge between charitable and state provision for the poor. The new workhouses – a product of Chadwick's views rather than Bentham's – did not meet Bentham's ideal of institutions which would attract high-status staff and become the focus of medical education. In fact, they were explicitly prevented from doing so, as the Poor Law Commissioners forbade any medical education to take place in them. The new law had been met with grave disquiet amongst the poor, and was greeted by riots, particularly in the industrial north. At the same time, the Anatomy Act had been passed, which gave the medical schools a legal right to dissect the bodies of poor persons whose families did not claim them. Workhouses were an obvious source of such bodies, especially as they took in so many vagrant and friendless poor people in the last stages of illness. The suggestion that their sick wards might be used for medical experiment would have made a volatile and hostile public even more danger-ous.[35] Hence medical students were banned from poor law institutions until after the First World War, even though the infirmaries could have offered valuable experience in midwifery cases, which were much more common in the workhouses than the charity hospitals. The Enlightenment heritage of scientific enquiry thus remained the province of charity, not the Poor Law. This was particularly ironic in that the New Poor Law ultimately forced the building of large hospitals in the new industrial towns where such services had previously been undeveloped.

Although the relationship of doctors to the old Poor Law is not as clear as it might be, it does seem obvious that the contemptuous attitude taken by the administrators of the new law also had the effect of lowering the status of poor law medical work. The old Poor Law did not employ élite doctors, but the close relations with medical charities suggest that several doctors could take on poor law work at a reasonable rate for the job, and that it carried no connotations of professional weakness.[36] The new Poor Law Commissioners, being very anxious that the disciplinary control of the workhouse be removed from paupers, or from people appointed through corruption, tried to 'professionalise' the roles of workhouse masters, porters and other servants. Yet, in comparison, the qualifications of the poor law medical officers and nurses received virtually no attention and, since medical relief had not been mentioned in the new law, some unions even assumed that they could stop giving it.[37] Consequently, the Poor Law Commissioners hastily passed regu-lations to confirm that the sick poor, whatever their place of origin, should be given treatment and, unlike the ablebodied poor, they did not insist that this help be given inside the workhouse. Hence the dual system of the old Poor Law, with its mixture of institutional care and home care, continued.

Poor Law medical officers, furthermore, needed an acceptable qualification from a university or one of the medical licensing bodies. Having rejected Bentham's idealistic view of a workhouse hospital, the Commissioners accepted his more pragmatic view of how doctors should be appointed and they continued the system, found in many areas before 1834, of contracting the care of the poor to the lowest bidder – a system which caused such problems that it was abandoned in 1842. Since the doctor was expected to supply all his own drugs, bandages, and so forth, and the guardians paid only for extra dietary requirements, difficult midwifery cases and surgical operations, this had the effect of lowering the rate of pay, especially in a time of rapid population expansion. The guardians were able to maintain the low pay because the doctors were, at first, hired only on an annual basis, and a new competition would be held each year. It is therefore possible that the effect of the new system was to reduce the fees of poor law doctors in many areas, but particularly in the new industrial towns of the north where the unions were particularly economical in their habits. This provoked a climate of hostility and distrust between the poor law administrators and the medical profession: the British Medical Association, itself originating in the 1830s, was the loudest voice in the medical officers' defence. The profession's chief mouthpieces, the *British Medical Journal* and the *Lancet*, ran articles on the abuses of the profession by poor law administrators, and such articles were a feature of the medical press until the Poor Law was abolished in 1948. Although the doctors did in fact gain security of employment, they continued to feel that their professional judgement could be challenged at any time by uninformed guardians or their officers. In particular, guardians might refuse to pay for surgical operations, regarding them as unnecessary or too expensive. In the charity hospitals the medical men fought a similar battle to exert their authority over lay patrons and managers and to gain the right to admit and treat patients according to their own judgement, but they won this battle more quickly and effectively than the poor law doctors. From 1867 new regulations began to dictate that the workhouse infirmaries be separated from the workhouse, and put under medical management, but this took some time to achieve. Meanwhile, the authorities tended to counter the medical attack by reporting numerous cases of indolence or callousness by poor law doctors, especially when summoned to emergency cases. The net effect was that while the medical staff in the charity hospitals associated with popular heroes such as James Simpson, Florence Nightingale and Joseph Lister continually enhanced their reputation, the poor law service was regarded as second-rate, and it was assumed that only the poorest and most desperate practitioners would engage in it.

Similar considerations applied to nursing, although poor law nursing was even slower to improve its reputation. At first, no qualification for poor law nurses was required, except for literacy and good behaviour (usually defined as keeping away from strong drink). Initially the Commissioners were prepared to allow paupers to do this work, although they objected to their employment in other workhouse positions. Nursing was regarded as an activity suitable for any well-disposed female, but also as work that was hard enough to deter women of bad character who might wish to take advantage of poor relief. This indifference to professionalism was perhaps understandable in 1834 when nursing was not recognised as a skilled occupation requiring training, but the low pay and poor working conditions of resident nurses under the Poor Law meant that low standards persisted well into the 20th century. From the 1860s onwards the central authorities tried to discourage the use of pauper nurses, and to employ more credible staff, but the low status of workhouse nursing led to a vicious circle: trained nurses would not apply for posts in workhouse infirmaries because of the low status, and the authorities could not raise the status by employing only trained nurses, since nurses refused the posts. Since the workhouses also took in fewer ablebodied women as the century progressed, the more lowly nursing tasks became the province of unmarried mothers and elderly widows who could not avoid the workhouse. In some provincial unions the guardians even insisted that younger widows with families undertake workhouse nursing as a condition of receiving relief.

The effect of the intrusion of political economy into the English Poor Law was to widen the division between charity and state medical care. Historians such as John Pickstone have charted this divided system over time: his study of the Manchester region shows a rare effort by local authorities to try to integrate the system in the 1930s before they were forcibly integrated in the 1940s. Since charities offered a much wider range of specialised treatments than did the Poor Law, guardians continued to subscribe to organisations (for the blind, for example), which would take on small groups of paupers with special problems. However, the growth of a large institutional framework in the industrial cities led, in time, to efforts to emulate the charities, especially by providing more surgical operations. This was done without the investment or back-up services provided by the charities – the ratio of professionals to patients was always lower in the poor law hospitals. Nevertheless, when the National Health Service was formed, it was usually on the basis of whether a poor law hospital provided x-ray facilities and an operating theatre that it was designated as an NHS hospital, or left under the local authority as a home for the elderly infirm. At that point, the problem was still to bring the poor law inheritance up to the standards of the voluntary system and to break down the persistent suspicion with which many professional staff viewed it. It was the voluntary system, not the state service, which the Ministry of Health wished to set as the standard for the NHS. As it was, only the largest cities were providing institutions good enough for incorporation into the new scheme.

Similarly, the experience of the Poor Law soured the attitudes of doctors towards personal services under state schemes. The only aspect of state service which achieved a high reputation was the group originally favoured by Chadwick – the public health professionals. These had many difficulties, but the medical officers of health in the cities were relatively well paid, and the law gave them considerable independence from their employers. The ill-regarded general practice work of the Poor Law led many doctors to be deeply suspicious of the national insurance scheme of 1911.[38] In practice, the panel system was better than many practitioners had expected, but the legacy of the Poor Law meant that, for many general practitioners, state medicine implied subservience and exploitation. The poor, equally, had no doubt about which part of the 'mixed economy of welfare' they preferred. By the end of the 19th century they were using, in ever larger numbers, the great poor law infirmaries which the wealth of the Industrial Revolution had made possible, although there is no indication that these services were the focus of local pride which the charity hospitals had become. Trade unions levied contributions from their members to ensure them a bed in a voluntary hospital when necessary: for the poor without such insurance, a bed in the poor law infirmary was an unwished-for, but sometimes unavoidable, alternative.

Notes

1. William H. Brock, *Fontana History of Chemistry*, London, 1992, pp. 99–100.
2. M.A. Crowther, 'Forensic Medicine and Medical Ethics in Nineteenth-century Britain', in R. Baker (ed.), *The Codification of Medical Morality*, (Dordrecht, 1995), Vol. II, pp. 175–77.
3. Bertrand Russell, *History of Western Philosophy*, 2nd edn, London, 1961, p. 580.
4. There is a useful summary of the earlier debate in Arthur J. Taylor, *Laissez-faire and State Intervention in Nineteenth-century Britain*, London, 1972.
5. Outlines of current thinking on the Poor Laws are given in J.R. Poynter, *Society and Pauperism: English Ideas on Poor Relief, 1795–1834*, London, 1969. For the specific role of the economist Nassau Senior on Poor Law reform, see Marian Bowley, *Nassau Senior and Classical Economics*, New York, 1967, pp. 291–98.
6. Thomas Carlyle, 'Signs of the Times', in *Scottish and Other Miscellanies*, London, 1964, p. 234.
7. Hilary Marland, *Medicine and Society in Wakefield and Huddersfield*, Cambridge, 1987, chapter 8, gives a particularly clear account of the complex networks which medical men developed in these two towns.
8. For a discussion of the philosophic conceptions of poverty in this period, see Gertrude Himmelfarb, *The Idea of Poverty: England in the Early Industrial Age*, London, 1984.

9. David Ricardo, *The Principles of Political Economy and Taxation*, London, 1912, pp. 61–63. The book was first published in 1817.
10. J.D. Marshall, 'The Nottinghamshire Reformers and their Contribution to the New Poor Law', *Economic History Review*, 2nd series, **XIII** (1961), pp. 382–96.
11. While the 'Manchester School' was a general term for many free traders, Manchester itself successfully provided social science with the necessary statistical underpinning, in the Manchester Statistical Society. See M.J. Cullen, *The Statistical Movement in Early Victorian Britain*, Brighton, 1975, pp. 105–18.
12. John V. Pickstone, *Medicine and Industrial Society: A History of Hospital Development in Manchester and its Region 1752–1946*, Manchester, 1985, p. 10.
13. For a general discussion, see Jane Lewis, 'Family Provision of Health and Welfare in the Mixed Economy of Care in the Late Nineteenth and Twentieth Centuries', *Social History of Medicine*, **8** (1) (1995), pp. 1–17; see also the essays in Martin Daunton (ed.), *Charity, Self-interest and Welfare in the English Past*, London, 1996.
14. Mary E. Fissell, *Patients, Power, and the Poor in Eighteenth-century Bristol*, Cambridge, 1991.
15. Or, alternatively, according to the famous reinterpretation of Michel Foucault in *The Birth of the Clinic*, a measure of social discipline.
16. This is indicated in the title of Ruth Hodgkinson, *The Origins of the National Health Service: The Medical Services of the New Poor Law 1834–1871*, London, 1967. See also Jeanne L. Brand, *Doctors and the State: The British Medical Profession and Government Action in Public Health, 1870–1912*, Baltimore, 1965. For an overview of public and private provision, with bibliography, see Steven Cherry, *Medical Services and the Hospitals in Britain, 1860–1939*, Cambridge, 1996.
17. In the early 1700s the largest towns outside London were Norwich, York, Bristol, Newcastle and Exeter, all with under 20 000 people; by 1801 Manchester/Salford, Liverpool, Birmingham, Bristol and Leeds had over 50 000; by the 1830s these were still the largest centres, but there had also been an exceptional growth of substantial towns, and the balance of provincial population in Britain had shifted to the north. See Edward Royle, *Modern Britain: A Social History 1750–1985*, London, 1987, pp. 20–22.
18. J.K. Walker, 'Statistical Observations on the Medical Charities of England and Ireland', *Transactions of the Provincial Medical and Surgical Association*, **IV** (1836), p. 477.
19. A. Redford and I.S. Russell, *The History of Local Government in Manchester*, London, 1940, Vol. II, p. 103; Felix Driver, *Power and Pauperism: The Workhouse System 1834–1884*, Cambridge, 1993, pp. 147–48.
20. Marland, *Medicine and Society* (n. 7), p. 60 ff.
21. Ibid., pp. 52–58.
22. T.R. Malthus, *An Essay on the Principle of Population*, Harmondsworth, 1970, p. 102.
23. Michael Anderson, *Family Structure in Nineteenth Century Lancashire*, Cambridge, 1971.
24. For details of how the settlement laws affected individuals, see James Stephen Taylor, *Poverty, Migration and Settlement in the Industrial Revolution: Sojourners' Narratives*, Palo Alto, Society for the Promotion of Science and Scholarship, 1898, esp. pp 9, 88, 133, 146.

25. E.G. Thomas, 'The Old Poor Law and Medicine', *Medical* History, **24** (1980), p. 3.

26. On the selective nature of charity hospital admissions, see John Woodward, *To Do the Sick No Harm: A Study of the British Voluntary Hospital System to 1875*, London, 1974, p. 45 ff.

27. Although Edwin Chadwick was, of course, to move shortly afterwards into the field of public health reform, since he came to regard sickness as a major cause of pauperism. Hence public health also became associated with political economy, since an unhealthy labourer was a drain on the state.

28. S.G. Checkland and E.O.A. Checkland (eds), *The Poor Law Report of 1834*, London, 1974, pp. 114–15.

29. S.E. Finer, *The Life and Times of Sir Edwin Chadwick*, London, 1963, pp. 157–160.

30. Checkland and Checkland, *Poor Law Report* (n. 28), p. 372.

31. Janet Semple, 'Bentham's Utilitarianism and the Provision of Medical Care', in Dorothy Porter and Roy Porter (eds), *Doctors, Politics and Society: Historical Essays*, Amsterdam, 1993, pp. 30–45.

32. S. Webb and B. Webb, *English Local Government*, Vol 8: *English Poor Law History, Part II*, London, 1929, Vol. 1, pp. 419–431.

33. Michael E. Rose, 'Settlement, Removal and the New Poor Law', in Derek Fraser (ed.), *The New Poor Law in the Nineteenth Century*, London, 1976, pp. 41–42.

34. A full account of workhouse building is given in Driver, *Power and Pauperism* (n. 19).

35. For the history of the connection between the Anatomy Acts and the workhouses, see Ruth Richardson, *Death, Dissection and the Destitute*, Harmondsworth, 1988, pp. 202, 221 ff.

36. This point requires more evidence. Despite excellent work by Marland, Fissell and others on medical services under the old Poor Law, there are still many unanswered questions about the status of poor law doctors before 1834.

37. The history of the early problems of the medical services of the New Poor Law are given in Hodgkinson, *The Origins of the National Health Service* (n. 16); Brand, *Doctors and the State* (n. 16), pp. 85–106; M.W. Flinn, 'Medical Services under the New Poor Law', in Derek Fraser (ed.), *The New Poor Law in the Nineteenth Century*, London, 1976, pp. 45–66; M.A. Crowther, *The Workhouse System 1834–1929*, London, 1981, pp. 156–92.

38. M.A. Crowther, 'Paupers or Patients? Obstacles to Professionalization in the Poor Law Medical Service before 1914', *Journal of the History of Medicine & Allied Sciences*, **39** (1) (1984), pp. 33–55.

CHAPTER ELEVEN

Medical Relief and the New Poor Law in London

David Green

The New Poor Law, medical relief and the city

The Poor Law Amendment Act of 1834, which established the New Poor Law, was arguably the most fundamental change in social policy in the 19th century.[1] It was designed primarily to deal with the mounting costs of poor relief and the growing problem of outdoor pauperism in southern agricultural districts. In contrast to the old Poor Law, which had developed from the 16th century and was based on the local administration of relief in individual parishes, the new system attempted to introduce a greater degree of uniformity of treatment and centralised control.[2] The New Poor Law established a central poor law authority, at first known as the Poor Law Commission, later the Poor Law Board and finally the Local Government Board, whose task it was to outline relief policy and monitor implementation. The 15 000 or so parishes in England and Wales responsible for providing relief were grouped into over 600 unions, each with their own elected board of guardians whose responsibility it was to dispense poor relief according to the instructions issued from time to time by the central authorities.

The main thrust of the new policy was to deter ablebodied male applicants from seeking relief, and this was to be achieved through the principle of 'less eligibility', whereby conditions for those who sought relief should be made less eligible than those for independent labourers. In practice this meant that ablebodied applicants were to be offered relief inside a workhouse whose conditions were intended to be sufficiently harsh and monotonous as to deter the poor from seeking relief in the first place. Commending the principle of deterrence enshrined in the New Poor Law of 1834, Charles Mott, the Assistant Commissioner for London, remarked that 'The Poor Law Amendment Act may indeed be called an Act of renovation for it causes the lame to walk, the blind to see, and the dumb to speak'.[3] In this way, it was argued, workers would make provision for their own welfare, leaving the Poor Law for those who, for other reasons such as sickness or old age, could not fare for themselves.

In such a complex and far-reaching reorganisation, objections were bound to occur. In some parts of England and Wales – notably in northern, midland

and southern districts – violent opposition to the formation of unions and the erection of workhouses took place.[4] In London, objections were more muted but no less important, focusing on middle-class opposition to the creation of an unelected central commission with extensive powers of supervision.[5] Uniformity of relief was also difficult to impose, and policies varied between unions. The extent to which the deterrent principle was applied, for instance, varied according to economic conditions in different districts. Places in which seasonal, as opposed to structural, unemployment prevailed, such as northern industrial towns, were more likely to have relatively lax policies towards ablebodied paupers and, in such cases, outdoor relief was often provided.[6] Similarly, historians have questioned the extent to which the New Poor Law was a departure from the old.[7] Many places, for example, had already begun to tighten relief practices prior to 1834 as a means of reducing the growing burdens on local ratepayers. In St Marylebone, for example, from the 1790s husbands and wives were separated in the workhouse and the ablebodied poor were set at task work. As costs rose in the early 1830s, stricter policies also began to be implemented.[8] Thus, it is possible to argue that whilst the New Poor Law marked a fundamental change in the administrative structure of relief, deterrent policies were already in place and that continuity, rather than discontinuity, characterised the provision of relief.

In terms of medical provision for the poor, the Act itself was virtually silent, mentioning medical relief only once in relation to the power of justices of the peace to order immediate medical relief for cases of sudden illness.[9] However, with urban growth in the 19th century came the spread of infectious disease and, by virtue of the relationship between pauperism and disease, medical provision under the Poor Law gained in importance. The fact that as much as three-quarters of pauperism in the mid-19th century was related to sickness meant that the Poor Law could not avoid sanctioning medical aid – including the provision of nourishment, as well as medicines – for large numbers of the urban population.[10] Under these circumstances, as Michael Flinn has noted, the one clause in the Poor Law Amendment Act relating to medical relief provided the narrowest of legislative chinks through which 'emerged one of the more remarkable social developments of the Victorian period'.[11]

The provision of medical treatment challenged the deterrent aspect of the New Poor Law by questioning the extent to which the stigma of pauperism should be borne by those who became destitute through ill-health rather than through improvidence. In relation to that group of paupers, poor law authorities faced a dilemma: by associating medical relief with pauperism, the Poor Law positively discouraged those in genuine need of treatment and, in so doing, may have added to their misery and indirectly encouraged the spread of disease. Conversely, although medical relief helped provide a public good by alleviating sickness and protecting society from the spread of disease, it could also be interpreted as encouraging improvidence by providing gratuitous assistance to those who could otherwise have afforded to pay for treatment. This was a view echoed by George Cornewall Lewis, one of the Poor Law Commissioners:

> If the pauper is always promptly attended by the skilful and well-qualified medical practitioner; if such practitioner is not only under the usual responsibilities of his profession, but is liable to reprimand or dismissal from office in case of neglect or error; if the patient be furnished with all the cordials and stimulants which may promote his recovery, it cannot be denied that his condition in these respects is better than that of the needy, but industrious ratepayer....This superiority of the condition of the pauper over that of the independent labourer as regards medical aid will, on the one hand ... thus tempt the industrious labourer into pauperism and on the other, it will discourage sick clubs and friendly societies and other similar institutions....[12]

In relation to medical relief, the Poor Law thus found itself in a dilemma that was especially acute in 19th-century cities. Resolving this issue, particularly in London, occupied the attention of the central poor law authorities for much of the century.

The issues surrounding medical treatment and poor relief were especially problematic in London. The capital provided a unique challenge to the centralising efforts of the 19th-century Poor Law. Its size, political complexity and social heterogeneity created immense difficulties for the Poor Law in general and medical relief in particular. London was by far the largest city in the country: at the start of the 19th century its population numbered nearly 1 million rising to over 4.5 million by the end. Indeed, throughout the period, it accounted for about one in eight of the English and Welsh population. Similarly, it also accounted for a significant share of poor law expenditure, particularly as the century progressed: in 1813 approximately 8 per cent of the total expenditure on poor relief occurred in London, rising to nearly a quarter by the end of the century.

Given its quantitative importance, no national policy could claim to be comprehensive unless it tackled the problems of the capital. Equally, the fragmentation and political intransigence of separate metropolitan authorities created serious difficulties for the implementation of poor law policies. Middle-class distrust of centralised authority was strongest in the capital, especially in those districts where parochial reform had most recently taken place, and for much of the century this opposition dogged the efforts of the Poor Law Commission to implement a uniform policy in the city. At the same time, however, these difficulties offered opportunities for the modernising and centralising state: if social policies could succeed in the unwieldy and overgrown capital, then they could succeed anywhere.

As the century unfolded, London became the focus for new approaches in poor law policy, notably concerning the provision of medical relief. How these approaches emerged and how the city's poor law authorities resolved the dilemma of providing medical treatment under the Poor Law is the subject of this chapter.[13] First, it considers the relationships between ill-health and poverty and examines the provision of medical treatment for the sick poor in London prior to 1867. Second, it explores how the structure of poor law administration in the city strained the capacity of local authorities to provide relief. Finally, it examines how the retreat from the deterrent principle of the New Poor Law after 1867 ushered in a new, and specifically metropolitan, approach to the treatment of the sick poor.

Ill-health, poverty and the Poor Law

For the urban working class, the risks of sinking into poverty as a result of ill-health were significant. Even relatively healthy male workers could expect to spend a significant part of their working lives off sick. In the 1830s and 1840s, for example, male steam-engine makers aged under 30 were absent from work on account of sickness on over 3 per cent of working days rising to over 10 per cent for those aged over 60.[14] Similarly, William Farr found that labourers employed in the East India Docks spent nearly 8 per cent of their lifetime in illness.[15] For women, the dangers of repeated pregnancies and childbirth added to the ravages of disease. Not surprisingly, therefore, in mid-19th century London, at least one-third of applications for private charity and an even higher proportion for poor relief may have been the result of sickness or death of the main wage-earner.[16] Dr Southwood Smith, physician at the London Fever Hospital, noted that one-fifth of all paupers in London unions in 1837–38 had suffered bouts of fever, rising in poorer districts, such as Bethnal Green, to one-third and even higher in places such as Whitechapel and St George Southwark.[17] Similarly, in St Giles between 1832 and 1862, sickness was cited as the cause of over half the applications for relief.[18] Although urban death rates fell and the situation improved in later decades, nevertheless Charles Booth's survey of the poor in the late 1880s and 1890s showed that, after casual work, the main cause of poverty for households in chronic need was illness or infirmity.[19]

Whilst ill-health and poverty were closely associated, medical attention for the working class varied depending on individual circumstances and the nature of the problem. Three main alternatives were available in mid-19th century London: self-help through membership of sick clubs, provident dispensaries and friendly societies; private philanthropy and the voluntary hospitals; and, finally, the Poor Law, including workhouse infirmaries and lying-in wards as well as domiciliary visiting by poor law medical officers.

Self-help

In terms of medical provision, self-help was problematic for many working-class Londoners. Given the multitude of small firms and the volatility of the London labour market, few employers made any provision for medical treatment of their workforce.[20] Most workers therefore had to rely on their own resources when it came to making provision for medical treatment. Whilst insurance payments to sick clubs, friendly societies or trade unions were possible for skilled male workers in regular employment, for the less skilled and women, the prevalence of seasonal unemployment, casual labour and low pay meant that it was more difficult to maintain regular contributions. Not surprisingly, Charles Booth found that, in relative terms, class B, the very poor, paid between a half and two-thirds less on insurance as classes E and F, the 'comfortable' working class.[21] As a result of these factors, membership of friendly societies, provident dispensaries and sick clubs was less common in London than elsewhere – notably in northern and midland industrial towns – and workers were more dependent on the Poor Law and charity for medical treatment.[22] For example, the rise in the number of provident dispensaries from the mid-century to which members usually subscribed 1d (one penny) a week in return for out-patient treatment, largely bypassed London. In 1867 there were at least 39 provident dispensaries in London but after that date, when free poor law dispensaries were established, the numbers remained static.[23] Advocates of self-help, including leading lights of the Charity Organisation Society, such as Octavia Hill and its secretary Charles Loch, blamed this state of affairs on gratuitous treatment provided by poor law dispensaries.[24] According to their view, the availability of free medical aid undermined thrift, fostered improvidence and encouraged lack of foresight, arguing further that ' … by the general application of the eleemosynary principle to our London hospitals and dispensaries, they have been converted into schools of pauperism'.[25]

Private philanthropy

Private philanthropy provided the other main source of medical relief for the working class outside the Poor Law, notably through voluntary hospitals and charitable dispensaries. As befitted its role as the centre of wealth and scientific endeavour, London was relatively well provided with voluntary hospitals. In 1829 there were at least 30 hospitals, rising to 77 by 1869 and 104 by 1881.[26] As well as the larger teaching hospitals, such as University College Hospital founded in 1833 and King's College Hospital founded in 1839, which provided the majority of beds, there was a growing number of specialist institutions dealing with particular conditions, such as consumption, or with particular groups, including women and children. In total, these institutions provided 5271 beds in 1861, increasing to 9656 by 1891, and although the relative increase in provision lagged behind the growth of provincial hospitals, nevertheless London still had more than double the number of beds per thousand population than the provinces.[27]

Whilst the overall significance of hospitals should not be underestimated, especially in relation to teaching and clinical research, their role in providing medical treatment for the poor is open to question. In the first place, they were unevenly distributed in relation to population. All the principal hospitals were located within three miles of the centre whilst hardly any existed in suburban districts. Lewisham, for example, with a population of over 73 000 in 1881, only had one specialist hospital and that was for women and children. By contrast, St George Hanover Square, with a population of over 89 000, had three hospitals, including St George's with 335 beds.[28] Second, London voluntary hospitals tended to admit a far higher proportion of surgical than medical cases and a far lower proportion of chronically ill patients. In the 1860s these hospitals admitted three times more surgical than medical cases whilst the opposite was true for poor law infirmaries.[29] Furthermore, only about 4 per cent of teaching hospital patients were chronically ill compared to 34 per cent of sick paupers.[30] Age was also a factor, with hospitals typically admitting fewer children and elderly patients than the poor law infirmaries.[31] Gender also influenced admissions: male patients outnumbered females in the voluntary hospitals, whilst in poor law institutions the ratio was the same. An indication of this imbalance is provided by the number of patients who died in the main London hospitals in 1841, when deaths of males outnumbered those of females by two to one.[32] In general hospitals, pregnant women were similarly ignored. Hospital provision for the poor, therefore, was highly selective and, in the larger teaching hospitals at least, women, children and the elderly – the three main groups most liable to sink into poverty – found particular difficulty in gaining admission. For these groups, the Poor Law provided the only other alternative.

The other main providers of charitable medical treatment were the public dispensaries which, in addition to the provident dispensaries discussed above, provided out-patient care for large numbers of the working class. Treatment was normally conditional on presentation of a letter of recommendation from a governor or subscriber. Several of these dispensaries, such as the General Dispensary at Aldgate and the Westminster General Dispensary, had been founded in central districts in the 19th century. As London expanded, others were opened in the new suburbs and, by 1869, at least 39 charitable dispensaries were in existence in the capital.[33] In some cases, these dispensaries provided extensive out-patient treatment. In the 1840s, for example, staff from the Aldgate dispensary attended the sick on over 43 000 occasions, nearly half of which were visits to patient's homes.[34] In turn, home visits brought insanitary living conditions to light and encouraged the formation of specialist institutions by those involved in the dispensary movement, notably the London Fever Institution founded in 1802.[35] Midwifery was also a very important aspect of out-patient work and, in some cases, the activities of dispensaries matched, if not exceeded, those of the hospitals and the Poor Law. In east London in the early 1840s, for example, the Tower Hamlets dispensary dealt with a larger number of births than did Stepney Union.[36] Until the establishment of free poor law dispensaries later in the century, charitable dispensaries therefore provided a very important source of out-patient care for the London working class – particularly for poor pregnant women.

The Poor Law

Of even greater significance than private philanthropy, however, was the Poor Law which was the main source of medical relief for large numbers of the working class. Under the old Poor Law, medical relief had been at the discretion of local vestries and, in many cases, these authorities had dealt with the sick poor sympathetically. In varying degrees, doctors employed by the Poor Law provided a range of gratuitous medical services, including the supply of food to the poor in their own homes.[37] The fact that the Poor Law Amendment Act virtually ignored medical relief meant that these practices continued, much to the annoyance of those such as Edwin Chadwick, framer of the Poor Law Amendment Act and secretary to the Poor Law Commission, who distrusted the judgement of doctors in relation to pauperism. It was not until the early 1840s, when his power at the Poor Law Commission was waning and other views were gaining prominence, that further efforts were made to organise medical relief.[38] The General Medical Order of 1842 was the first attempt to standardise procedures, including setting a maximum size for medical districts, payment by case in place of the practice of tendering for medical services, and the requirement that poor law medical officers be fully qualified. The treatment of sick paupers was discussed more fully by the 1844 Select Committee on Medical Relief and, mindful of public criticism, the rules of provision were clarified under the 1847 General Consolidated Order.

London occupied a prominent place in these discussions, although the existence of numerous parishes which had their own local acts hindered the adoption of orders issued by the Poor Law Commission.[39] Nevertheless, throughout the period, indoor and outdoor medical relief was a particularly important element of poor law policy in the capital. Table 11.1 shows that, as early as 1837, the proportion of sick and infirm paupers in metropolitan workhouses was greater than that in provincial institutions. Although the difference can partly be explained by the fact that, in London, children were sent to separate establishments thereby increasing the proportion of elderly

Table 11.1 Paupers in workhouses, 1837

	Sick %	Infirm %	Healthy %
Metropolitan workhouses (10)	14.5	50.1	35.4
Provincial workhouses (100)	10.3	31.3	58.3

Source: W. Farr in J. McCulloch, *Statistics of the British Empire* (1837), cited in Ruth Hodgkinson, *The Origins of the National Health Service: The Medical Services of the New Poor Law 1834–1871*, London: Wellcome Institute, 1967, p. 171.

and sick paupers in the workhouse, nevertheless the figures suggest that indoor medical relief in London was important from an early date. In the following decades, the difference between London and provincial workhouses was maintained. By the 1850s and 1860s the proportion of sick paupers in London had risen to between 32 and 48 per cent of the indoor poor compared to about 28 per cent in provincial workhouses, reflecting the growing practice in many metropolitan poor law authorities of providing separate accommodation for the sick poor.[40]

Although nursing provision and sanitary arrangements in the sick wards of many workhouses were inadequate and neglect undoubtedly occurred, nevertheless treatment offered a promise of at least rudimentary medical care and conditions in infirmaries were often an improvement on those experienced by the poor in their own homes.[41] Moreover, sensitive to scandals, such as that in the Andover workhouse in 1845 when starving paupers fought for rotting bones, and wary of public scrutiny on the part of anti-Poor Law campaigners – notably Dr Thomas Wakley, radical MP for Finsbury and editor of the *Lancet* – the central authorities were keen to oversee conditions of treatment. Thus, under the General Consolidated Order of 1847 the Poor Law Commission took a keener interest in workhouse medical provision, issuing guidance not only on how the sick poor should be treated in relation to other categories of paupers but also in the qualification and duties of medical officers and their powers to order additional food for the indoor sick. Although relatively few London unions were included, it marked the start of much closer attention on the part of the central authorities to the provision of medical relief inside the workhouse.[42]

Insofar as the Poor Law provided the main sources of institutional relief for the chronically ill, aged and infirm, it was inevitable that it should also act as the last place of refuge for the poor. Whilst fear of a pauper's funeral haunted the working class, nevertheless a growing proportion of the London poor ended their days in the workhouse or being cared for in other ways by

Table 11.2   Deaths in the workhouse, 1841–1901 (percentage of total deaths)

	1841	1851	1861	1871	1881	1891	1901
England and Wales	n/a	n/a	4.60	5.08	5.81	5.79	6.36
London	9.41	8.92	8.82	8.29	13.07	14.86	16.63
Deaths in London workhouses as a percentage of all workhouse deaths	n/a	n/a	33.81	30.20	44.54	45.83	43.19

Source: *Annual Reports of the Registrar General*, 5th (1843), 14th (1855), 24th (1863), 34th (1873) 44th (1883), 54th (1892), 64th (1901).

the Poor Law. William Farr's belief that, in the late 1830s, about 10 per cent of deaths in London occurred in the workhouse whilst about 20 per cent of all deaths came under the auspices of the Poor Law, confirms this view.[43] In keeping with the larger proportion of aged and sick poor in metropolitan workhouses, rates of mortality were generally higher in London workhouses than those in the provinces. In 1837 mortality rates per 100 indoor paupers in London were 32.1 for males and 26.2 for females compared to 20.9 and 15.1 respectively in provincial workhouses.[44] Moreover, death in a London workhouse became more common as the period progressed. As Table 11.2 shows, not only was the proportion of deaths that occurred in London workhouses approximately double that for the country as a whole but, over time, the capital's workhouses accounted for an increasing proportion of all deaths in the workhouse.

Care of the sick inside the workhouse, however, was dwarfed by the amount of outdoor relief provided by the Poor Law. In Whitechapel and Stepney during the early 1840s at least 70 per cent of the total medical cases were relieved in their own homes, although in wealthier districts, such as Marylebone in the 1850s, the proportion was somewhat lower.[45] In Stepney in the early 1840s, nearly 10 per cent of the population received medical aid in the course of a year.[46] Furthermore, over time there was a general relaxation of the conditions under which outdoor medical relief was granted. Accidents and midwifery had always been granted free medical relief, whilst the General Outdoor Relief Prohibition Order of 1844, which disallowed outdoor relief to the ablebodied, made an exception in cases of temporary sickness. In 1852, the Outdoor Relief Regulation Order provided outdoor relief in cases of sickness of the family, even if the head of household was also earning wages. Under these circumstances, the numbers of sick poor receiving outdoor relief rose and, by the 1860s, the majority of the outdoor ablebodied poor were relieved on account of widowhood, sickness, accident or were families dependent on sick men.[47]

Under the terms of the Poor Law Amendment Act, Guardians were allowed to provide sick relief outside the workhouse and any magistrate could sanction an order for medical attendance in cases of sudden and dangerous illness. In addition, medical officers could also recommend to relieving officers that food be provided for the sick poor and, unlike medicines, the cost of which came from the medical officer's salary, such expenditure was borne by the rates. Although expenditure on medical relief was relatively small compared to overall expenditure, averaging about 3 per cent between the 1840s and 1860s, nevertheless the amounts in kind could be substantial.[48] In one month in 1844, for example, medical officers in the East London Union ordered over 1500 lbs of meat, 736 lbs of oatmeal, 1030 quarts of milk, 7lb 9oz of tea, 29lb 12oz of sugar, 431 glasses of wine plus sago, arrowroot and other 'little comforts' for the poor.[49] Inevitably, such practices gave rise to the suspicion that medical officers were inadvertently pauperising the population through the liberal relief in aid of sickness – a view endorsed by Edwin Chadwick who believed that 'medical relief is the avenue to all pauperism', and subsequently echoed by the Poor Law Board and supporters of the Charity Organisation Society in the late 1860s.[50]

For women, medical treatment under the Poor Law had added significance in relation to childbirth. Although the proportion of births in London under the Poor Law was relatively small, nevertheless, for poor pregnant women, outdoor relief and midwifery were extremely important. In St Giles between 1832 and 1862, for example, one in five women applied for relief on account of pregnancy or childbirth.[51] During the 1860s approximately 3 per cent of births in London took place in workhouses, although this figure was probably between two and three times greater if outdoor midwifery cases were included.[52] In Stepney during the early 1840s, for example, the Poor Law accounted for approximately 6 per cent of all births in the district, three-quarters of which took place outside the workhouse.[53] Whilst the decision to provide indoor or outdoor relief to poor pregnant women rested with the relieving officer, and as such practices varied considerably between unions, childbirth under the Poor Law was nevertheless clearly of some considerable importance to large numbers of working-class women.

Childbirth in the workhouse also had an added significance when considering institutional maternal mortality. Compared to that of lying-in hospitals, maternal mortality in London workhouses was relatively low, although it was still higher than that of home deliveries.[54] In the 39 workhouses in 1865, maternal mortality was about 6 per 1000 live births, compared to an average of 29.6 between 1857 and 1874 in Queen Charlotte's hospital.[55] In part, the variations reflected differences in the type of patients treated, with the tendency for lying-in hospitals to take more emergency cases. Nevertheless, death rates from puerperal fever, the most important cause of maternal mortality, were significantly lower in workhouses than in the specialist lying-in hospitals.[56] The reasons for this were twofold. First, workhouse lying-in wards were usually separate from the infirmaries, which helped reduce infection. Second and more importantly, midwives outnumbered doctors in workhouses and were also less likely to interfere during the birth, again reducing the chances of infection. Indeed, lack of intervention was also the reason why maternal mortality was generally lower amongst the working class than the middle class, and why women who delivered at home had lower mortality rates than those who gave birth in the workhouse.[57]

In addition to medical treatment and midwifery services discussed above, the other important activity of the Poor Law at the mid-century concerned the role of medical officers in providing vaccination against smallpox. Although the impact of vaccination on smallpox mortality has been questioned, there is little doubt that it played an important role in helping reduce the spread of infection.[58] The Vaccination Act of 1848 provided free public vaccination organised through the Poor Law although it was not made compulsory until 1853. From that date, vaccination became far more common although significant regional variations in coverage existed, notably in London compared to the provinces.

The progress of vaccination in London well illustrates the specific problems arising, first, from the association of medical services with the Poor Law and, second, from the lack of coordination in the capital between the multiplicity of separate poor law authorities. Despite statements to the contrary by the Poor Law Commission and the Poor Law Board, the practice of organising vaccination through local boards of guardians meant that it was always associated with the stigma of pauperism.[59] Given the choice, parents usually took their infants to vaccinators who were not associated with the Poor Law.[60] However, since all but five of the 39 metropolitan unions appointed the poor law medical officer as the public vaccinator, parents were given little choice but to take their children to a poor law establishment. In 1844, for example, the guardians of St George Southwark resolved that all vaccinations should henceforth be provided at the workhouse. The Poor Law Commissioners objected on the grounds that this would associate vaccination with pauperism and would thereby deter the general population from vaccinating their children. Sure enough, the numbers of children vaccinated in the district fell from 1079 in 1844 to 42 in the following year.[61] Second, the fragmentation of poor law administration in the capital meant that there was no overall planning of the location of vaccination stations. In several cases, outlying stations in inconvenient locations hardly attracted anyone whilst some central stations were often so close to others, such as the three located in Dean Street in Soho, that attendance at each was low.[62] In total, 260 stations had been created by 1862, although only 19 achieved an average attendance of 500 per annum – the minimum total considered to allow efficient working of the station.[63]

Largely for these reasons, London had a relatively low rate of vaccination and a correspondingly high incidence of smallpox. Between 1845 and 1890, public infant vaccination rates in London never rose above 500 per 1000 live births and, for much of the period, vaccination rates were the lowest in the country.[64] Although private vaccinations were more common in London than elsewhere, nevertheless between 1873 and 1877 the percentage of infants not vaccinated was twice as high in the capital compared to the rest of the country.[65] In turn, smallpox mortality in London, prior to the adoption of stricter isolation policies from 1885, was generally between two and three times higher than for the rest of the country.[66] It was not until the isolation of smallpox victims and the administrative reorganisation of the machinery of prevention from the late 1880s that the disease was largely banished from the capital.

London and the New Poor Law: fragmentation and crisis

The significance of the Poor Law in relation to medical treatment of the poor, and the specific issues raised concerning vaccination rates, prompt questions about the way in which the New Poor Law itself operated in the capital. London posed a particular set of problems for the Poor Law Commissioners. Its size alone meant that it could not be omitted from the Poor Law Amendment Act of 1834 yet, at the same time, the administrative fragmentation of the city into innumerable local bodies responsible for poor relief created immense difficulties regarding the implementation of a uniform poor law system. Added to this were the strong anti-centralisation sentiments of many London vestries that influenced the nature of metropolitan government for much of the century. Indeed, so entrenched were parochial interests and so strong the distrust of central government that Lord Althorp, whose task it was to pilot the Poor Law Amendment bill through parliament, initially considered omitting metropolitan vestries from the legislation. It was only upon Edwin Chadwick's urging that he was eventually persuaded to do otherwise.[67] Anti-centralisation sentiment and administrative fragmentation, therefore, provided the context in which medical relief operated and it is important to understand these limitations if we are to make sense of the way that poor law policy subsequently developed in the capital.

Prior to 1834 a large number of local authorities were vested with the power to distribute relief in the capital, varying in size from city parishes with populations of less than a few hundred to districts such as St Marylebone and St Pancras, both of which exceeded 150 000 by the mid-century. Many parishes provided poor relief under local acts which the Poor Law Commissioners found impossible to overturn without the agreement of local ratepayers.[68] Whilst in the majority of cases agreement was forthcoming, a significant number of parishes objected, rallying around the cry of local democratic self government as opposed to the perceived tyranny of rule by unelected commissions.[69]

Whilst the rallying cry of local self-government found support in several quarters, it created immense problems over the introduction of the Poor Law Amendment Act in London. Although 28 new unions had been formed by the end of 1837, 11 vestries, accounting for about a third of London's population, and the equivalent expenditure on poor relief, continued to operate under local acts for the relief of the poor. This gap in the Commissioners' jurisdiction included some of the largest and wealthiest districts, such as St George Hanover Square, St Marylebone and St Pancras. In terms of size, wealth and poor relief, several of these districts were of national, let alone local, significance (see Figure 11.1).[70] In 1837, for example, poor relief expenditure in St Marylebone was exceeded only by Birmingham and Liverpool, whilst St Pancras spent a similar amount to Leeds.[71] Such omissions were therefore of enormous significance in relation to poor law policy and continued to frustrate the central authorities until the 1867 Metropolitan Poor Act eventually brought them under the control of the Poor Law Board. The measures ushered in after 1867 – notably the formation of the Metropolitan Asylums Board (MAB) and separate asylums for the sick poor – thereafter placed London at the centre of poor law reform for the remainder of the century.

What added to the difficulties, however, was the nature of poor relief in the capital. Expenditure on indoor relief was higher in London than elsewhere. In 1850, for example, in relative terms London unions spent twice as much on indoor relief as Lancashire and nearly four times as much as the West Riding of Yorkshire.[72] This situation was even more marked later in the century: between 1882 and 1904 an average of 60 per cent of paupers in London were relieved inside the workhouse compared to only about 23 per cent in the rest of the country.[73]

This emphasis on indoor relief created additional problems in London, which in turn influenced the provision of medical care under the Poor Law. Indoor relief entailed significantly higher costs than outdoor assistance, largely on account of the need to construct and run workhouses as well as to pay salaries of poor law officials.[74] The cost of constructing new workhouses was exceptionally high in London, especially in the more impoverished districts. Between 1835 and 1850 the average cost of new workhouses in England and Wales was £5422, but in London the cost rose from £17 131 for those built between 1835 and 1839 to £21 715 in the following decade and to £28 676 in the 1850s.[75] Because of the expense involved, London lagged behind other regions in terms of new workhouse construction. By 1847 only eight unions had sought permission to construct new workhouses, although a far larger

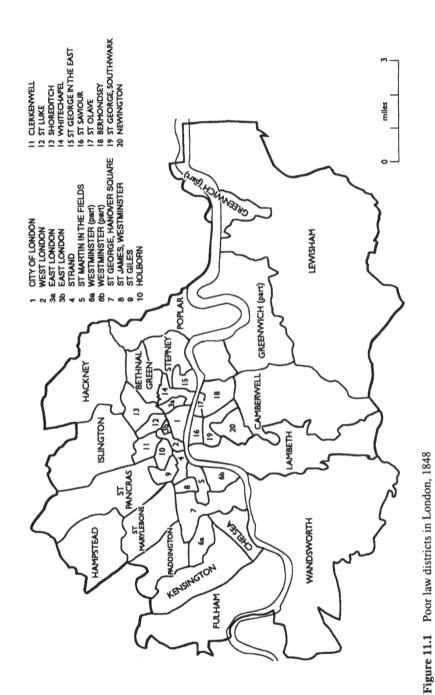

Figure 11.1 Poor law districts in London, 1848

1 CITY OF LONDON
2 WEST LONDON
3a EAST LONDON
3b EAST LONDON
4 STRAND
5 ST MARTIN IN THE FIELDS
6a WESTMINSTER (part)
6b WESTMINSTER (part)
7 ST GEORGE, HANOVER SQUARE
ST JAMES, WESTMINSTER
8 ST GILES
9 HOLBORN
10

11 CLERKENWELL
12 ST LUKE
13 SHOREDITCH
14 WHITECHAPEL
15 ST GEORGE IN THE EAST
16 ST SAVIOUR
17 ST OLAVE
18 BERMONDSEY
19 ST GEORGE, SOUTHWARK
20 NEWINGTON

number had enlarged or altered their old ones.[76] Even as late as 1868, ten of the 39 metropolitan unions steadfastly refused to construct new workhouses, despite the fact that Henry Farnall, the poor law inspector for London, had previously noted in 1861 that 16 establishments were inadequate both in terms of size and internal arrangements.[77]

From the mid-century the inadequacies of London workhouses and the inability of the Poor Law in some districts to deal with the demands for relief became increasingly evident. The problem was essentially threefold. First, the fact that workhouses were largely filled with the aged, infirm and sick meant that they could hardly function as a test of destitution for the ablebodied. Even where sufficient room existed to accommodate the ablebodied, the internal arrangements of older workhouses were inadequate to meet the Act's requirement that paupers be separated into four classes and each housed in a separate building. In turn, lack of workhouse accommodation meant that during periods of high demand poor law authorities had little choice but to dispense outdoor relief to the ablebodied – a situation that was anathema to the spirit of the New Poor Law.[78] Second, changes in the laws of removal from 1846 made it progressively more difficult for local poor law authorities to remove paupers without a settlement.[79] The outcome was that districts in which the poor resided, or into which they had moved, experienced sharp increases in the number of irremovable paupers and correspondingly large increases in expenditure. In eastern districts, such as Whitechapel and Poplar, and southern districts such as St George Southwark, a third or more of poor law expenditure from the mid-1850s was committed to the relief of the irremovable poor. It was in the context of this worsening situation that guardians set about trying to tighten relief practices and enforce stricter workhouse regimes.[80] Finally, middle-class flight undermined the fiscal basis of the Poor Law, particularly in eastern and southern riverside districts into which the poor, made irremovable by changes in the law, had been displaced. In such districts, boards of guardians were all but overwhelmed by the high costs of providing relief.

The Metropolitan Poor Act and the retreat from deterrence

These structural problems of poor law expenditure came to prominence in the 1860s, as economic downturn and outbreaks of disease forced large numbers to apply for relief. A harsh winter in 1861, during which the Poor Law in eastern districts broke down, was followed in 1866 by an even more serious crisis brought about by the collapse of the Thames shipbuilding industry and an outbreak of cholera in eastern districts. Between 1865 and 1867 the numbers of paupers and cost of relief in London rose by nearly 50 per cent, with eastern districts witnessing the steepest rises.[81] In the face of such increases it was quite evident that the poor law authorities could not operate an effective deterrent policy, far less provide relief to those in need, without significant changes in the administration and funding of poor relief. The problem was how to achieve such changes in the context of fragmentation and opposition to centralisation whilst at the same time maintaining the principle of deterrence.

From a metropolitan perspective the principal question was how to redistribute the costs of poor relief between districts without encouraging unnecessary expenditure on the part of recipient authorities. A limited measure of redistribution had taken place in 1864 when the Metropolitan Board of Works had been given powers to reimburse guardians for the cost of building casual wards, but more fundamental change came in 1867 with the Metropolitan Poor Act which laid the basis for a complete overhaul of both medical relief and the London Poor Law. This Act had two distinct purposes: first, to separate the sick poor from other workhouse inmates through the provision of sick asylums and, second, to distribute the charge for poor relief across the city as a whole. It also established the Metropolitan Asylums Board (MAB) whose responsibility it was to coordinate the working of the Act and to arrange the redistribution of money through the Metropolitan Common Poor Fund. Middle-class fears that the centralisation of relief expenditure would remove local control and thereby prove to be a bottomless pit strongly influenced the nature of reform and ensured that members were drawn largely from poor law unions and parishes, with a minority from the Poor Law Board and its successor, the Local Government Board. Of all the options advocated, the new Act represented the least centralised solution to the problem.[82] Finally, the ten remaining parishes which had continued to operate under separate local acts were instructed to dispense with other administrative arrangements for relief and to elect boards of guardians.

In terms of medical relief, the Act was immensely important and laid the basis for the treatment of the sick by the Poor Law for the remainder of the century. Its main objective was to isolate sick paupers from the rest, either, in the case of infectious cases, in separate poor law hospitals or in workhouse infirmaries. To allay fears of profligacy on the part of recipient districts, and to discourage boards of guardians merely from increasing outdoor relief, the Act stipulated that the money was to be used solely to support indoor relief and to construct separate asylums for sick paupers. However, because it was clearly impossible for poorer districts to support extra expenditure, let alone sustain their current levels, additional funds had to be provided. This was achieved by redistributing the product of a one penny rate based on the rateable value of districts, thereby allowing the MAB to channel resources from wealthy to poorer districts. As Figure 11.2 shows, the main beneficiaries of the system were eastern and southern riverside districts whilst the wealthier city and West End unions were net contributors.

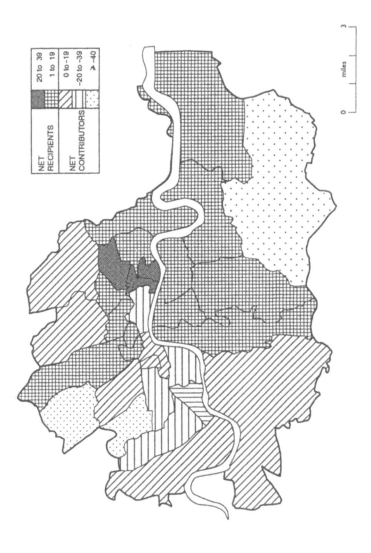

NET RECIPIENTS		NET CONTRIBUTORS		
20 to 39	1 to 19	0 to -19	-20 to -39	> -40

0 _____ 3 miles

Source: Poor Law Board, annual reports (1869–70)
Local Government Board, annual reports (1871–78)

Figure 11.2 Metropolitan Common Poor Fund receipts and contributions 1869–1878 (percentage of total poor relief expenditure)

The new funding made possible the construction of new workhouse infirmaries and also new poor law hospitals run by the MAB. By the late 1860s
London workhouses had become primarily places for the care of the sick and
elderly, with nearly 90 per cent of inmates falling into that category.[83] Rising
levels of pauperism and consequent overcrowding in workhouses had exacerbated the problems of providing indoor treatment for the sick poor and
investigations by the Poor Law Board and the *Lancet*, together with pressure
from people such as Florence Nightingale and Louisa Twining, founder of
the Workhouse Visiting Association, had brought to public attention the insanitary state and inadequate treatment in many sick wards and infirmaries.[84]
Whilst some improvements had been made, it was not until additional funding became available that widespread rebuilding could take place. In 1868,
for example, St Pancras was allowed £40 000 to construct a new infirmary at
Highgate. New infirmaries were also started in Poplar, Stepney, Kensington
and Newington and, in the following decade, the construction of new wings
and infirmaries took place throughout London.[85] By 1877 only six unions
still treated the sick within mixed workhouses, the remainder having already
designed or constructed separate infirmaries.[86]

More significantly, the Metropolitan Poor Act allowed for the construction
of separate asylums for the treatment of infectious diseases, primarily smallpox and fever. The city was divided into separate asylum districts and, by
1877, five new hospitals had been built at Fulham, Hampstead and Homerton
to the north and Stockwell and Deptford in the south. The main emphasis in
the treatment of infectious disease, particularly smallpox, had already swung
away from vaccination towards isolation and therefore the new hospitals
were built in peripheral locations, leaving workhouse infirmaries and sick
wards in more central areas to deal with the chronically sick poor.

Whilst the Metropolitan Poor Act marked a decisive shift in terms of
medical provision for the sick poor, separation of such relief from the stigma
of pauperism was not immediately achieved. Indeed, the very fact that the
new institutions were designated 'asylums' rather than 'hospitals' emphasised the fact that receipt of medical relief under the Poor Law still constituted
pauperism. This was in keeping with the prevailing ideology of the Charity
Organisation Society (COS) which opposed any attempts to extend the operation of the Poor Laws or to remove the stigma of pauperism from the receipt
of relief.[87] According to this view, profligate and indiscriminate almsgiving,
coupled with the availability of outdoor relief, weakened thrift and undermined the sense of family responsibility. Accordingly, supporters opposed
any attempts to sever the link between medical relief and the deterrent aspect
of the Poor Law on the grounds that free medical aid to those who could
afford it was the route to dependence, 'for which', noted Sir Charles Trevelyan,
a prominent member of the COS, 'our London population is unhappily distinguished beyond the rest of their countrymen'.[88]

Despite the stigma of pauperism, the new asylums attracted large numbers of patients, the majority of whom were not paupers prior to being admitted, and this in turn helped to create pressures for reform. Strictly speaking, the admission of non-pauper cases by the new asylums was illegal, but in practice anyone suffering from an infectious disease, irrespective of their social status was admitted. Thus, up to mid-1872, of the 16 459 admissions to metropolitan asylums, 71 per cent were not paupers.[89] Although the charges for such patients were to be passed on to their own unions, in practice the sheer volume overwhelmed the administrative capacity and in 1876 the charges were waived. In 1879 sanitary authorities in the capital were allowed to contract with MAB institutions to admit non-infectious patients from their districts and, following the Royal Commission of 1881 on smallpox and fever hospitals, further legislation progressively separated the treatment of infectious diseases from the Poor Law. In 1883 the Diseases Prevention (Metropolis) Act removed civil disabilities from patients admitted to MAB hospitals, thereby finally ridding receipt of medical relief in such institutions from the stigma of pauperism.

These changes, together with the compulsory notification of infectious disease to medical officers of health and the MAB in 1889 and the opening of new hospitals, resulted in large increases in admissions. Fever admissions rose from 1207 in 1877 to 21 654 by 1900 whilst the proportion of infectious cases admitted to MAB hospitals rose from 33.6 per cent of the total in 1890 to 84.6 per cent by 1905.[90] Better notification of infectious disease and stricter isolation of patients, notably those suffering from smallpox in three hospital ships moored 18 miles downstream on the Thames, helped to reduce significantly outbreaks of disease and infectious mortality, bringing London's rate into line with the rest of the country.[91] Indeed, by reducing the incidence of smallpox in London, the new hospitals also helped limit the spread of the disease into the surrounding hinterland and this, in turn, was likely to have had a wider impact on regional and national mortality rates.

Whilst the MAB hospitals catered for ever-increasing numbers of patients, their efforts were still dwarfed by the number of chronically sick and aged poor who received treatment in workhouse infirmaries or as outdoor medical relief. The construction of new workhouse sick wards and infirmaries had gathered pace during the 1870s, and by 1881 there were 10 000 beds in workhouse infirmaries compared to 1500 in MAB institutions and about 8000 in voluntary hospitals.[92] The number of workhouse infirmary places continued to rise, and by 1906 there were about 16 300 beds compared to 10 224 in voluntary hospitals. In terms of national significance, this was more than double the number of infirmary beds available in Liverpool, Manchester and Birmingham combined.[93] Furthermore, in contrast to the voluntary hospitals, most of which were concentrated in the inner districts, many of these new infirmaries were located in suburban locations, mirroring the outward expansion of the city's population and more closely reflecting the changing geographical pattern of need. For the chronically sick, therefore, poor law infirmaries remained the major institutional source of treatment.

Finally, we should not forget the impact of the Metropolitan Poor Act on the provision of outdoor medical relief. In addition to the changes noted above, the Act allowed poor law authorities to open free dispensaries and, by 1877, at least 57 were operating in London.[94] Opponents of free dispensaries, notably the Charity Organisation Society, argued that by undermining habits of thrift and foresight by those who could otherwise have afforded to pay for treatment at provident dispensaries, free medical assistance was the first step towards pauperism.[95] Only by thoroughly investigating all requests for medical relief by relieving officers, it was argued, could imposture be prevented and such habits be preserved. However, by the 1880s the tide had finally turned, such views were losing support and the separation of medical relief from pauperism had become an accepted part of the Poor Law. Under these circumstances free dispensaries, similar to the MAB hospitals, became a major source of medical services to the London working class.

Conclusion: resolving the dilemma of medical relief

Overcoming the ravages of disease in 19th-century cities was as much a function of developing suitable administrative structures as it was of gaining better medical knowledge or improving the urban infrastructure. This was especially true in relation to the sick poor who relied heavily on the Poor Law for much of their medical needs. However, providing such treatment raised some difficult questions about the nature of poor relief. For the urban middle class the critical issue was how to maintain the balance between the deterrent principle of the Poor Law whilst providing adequate care for the sick poor. Too harsh an application of deterrence might have meant that the sick failed to receive treatment, resulting in additional suffering and the further spread of disease. Over-generous relief, on the other hand, might discourage thrift and encourage pauperism. The critical question facing urban poor law authorities during this period was how to resolve this dilemma.

This question was both particularly acute and especially difficult to resolve in London. The threat posed by infectious disease could not be ignored by sanitary authorities, nor could the close relationship between pauperism and ill-health be ignored by the Poor Law. At the same time, however, the administrative structures to deal with disease and poor relief were wholly inadequate, largely because of the fragmented nature of metropolitan government. Improvements in infrastructure from the mid-century – notably the construction of an integrated sewer network by the Metropolitan Board of Works – helped considerably to cleanse the urban environment. However, in view of the moral issues surrounding poor relief, both in terms of middle-class concerns over encouraging pauperism and working-class hostility towards the Poor Law itself, providing medical treatment for the sick poor was more problematic. Separating medical relief from the stigma of pauperism involved recognising that comprehensive treatment for the sick poor was a public good. From the 1860s such a view became more common and the state provision of medical services for the population as a whole, irrespective of the ability to pay, was seen as increasingly acceptable. The new administrative structures established after 1867 provided an entirely new metropolitan approach to paying for medical treatment. In this way London can justifiably claim to have been at the centre of reforms that subsequently laid the basis for the state's responsibility for the health care of its citizens.

Acknowledgements

I am very grateful to Anne Crowther and Graham Mooney for their helpful comments on an earlier draft of this chapter. Any errors that remain are, of course, my own.

Notes

1. *An Act for the Amendment and better Administration of the Laws relating to the Poor in England and Wales* (4 & 5 Will IV. Cap. 76).
2. Recent studies of the New Poor Law include G. Boyer, *An Economic History of the English Poor Law 1750–1850*, Cambridge, 1990; F. Driver, *Power and Pauperism*, Cambridge, 1993; D. Fraser (ed.), *The New Poor Law in the Nineteenth Century*, London, 1976; L. Lees, *The Solidarities of Strangers*, Cambridge, 1998; M. Rose (ed.), *The Poor and the City: The English Poor Law in its Urban Context 1834–1914*, Leicester, 1985; K. Williams, *From Pauperism to Poverty*, London, 1981. The classic account remains S. Webb and B. Webb, *English Poor Law Policy: Part II, The Last Hundred Years*, Vols 1 and 2, London, 1963, (1st edn 1929).
3. Quoted in R. Hodgkinson, *The Origins of the National Health Service; The Medical Services of the New Poor Law 1834–1871*, London, 1967, p. 8.
4. The anti-Poor Law movement is discussed in N. Edsall, *The Anti-Poor Law Movement 1834–44*, Manchester, 1971; John Knott, *Popular Opposition to the 1834 Poor Law*, London, 1986; M. Rose, 'The Anti-Poor Law Movement in the North of England', *Northern History*, I (1966), pp. 70–91; idem, 'The Anti-Poor Law Movement', in J.T. Ward (ed.), *Popular Movements 1830–1851*, London, 1970, pp. 78–84.
5. A. Brundage, *The Making of the New Poor Law*, London, 1978, pp. 145–80 has drawn attention to the importance of different forms of protest, including those in London.
6. See Boyer, *An Economic History* (n. 2), pp. 237–39.
7. See P. Mandler, 'The Making of the New Poor Law Redivivus', *Past and*

Present, **117** (1987), pp. 131–57 and the subsequent debate that this article generated in *Past and Present*.

8. See A.R. Neate, *The St Marylebone Workhouse and Institution 1730–1865*, London, 1967, pp. 8–9. The weekly number of poor relieved in St Marylebone fell from a peak of 8108 in February 1833 to 2846 in October 1834. See St Marylebone, vestry minutes, 1833, 1834.

9. See M. Flinn, 'Medical Services under the New Poor Law', in D. Fraser (ed.), *The New Poor Law in the Nineteenth Century*, London, 1976, p. 48.

10. A. Digby, *Making a Medical Living*, Cambridge, 1994, pp. 44–45. According to Digby, between half and two-third of patients in the nineteenth century received medical treatment from the Poor Law or charity. Poor law records tend to conflate the sick with the infirm, and it is therefore extremely difficult to separate out the effects of sickness from old age.

11. Flinn 'Medical Services' (n. 9), p. 48.

12. Parliamentary Paper (PP), 1844, IX *Select Committee on Medical Poor Relief*, third report, q. 5

13. Attention here is confined to medical relief of disease rather than the treatment of lunacy under the Poor Law.

14. H. Southall, D. Gilbert and C. Bryce, *Nineteenth Century Trade Union Records*, Historical Geography Research Series, **27**, (1994), p. 30.

15. William Farr in J. McCulloch, *Statistics of the British Empire*, Vol. II (1837), cited in Hodgkinson, *The Origins of the National Health Service* (n. 3), p. 53.

16. In 1844, for example, of the 204 persons relieved by the St Andrew's district visiting society in Holborn, 63 (30.9 per cent) received help on account of sickness, accident or lameness. See *Association for Promoting the Relief of Destitution in the Metropolis, First Report*, 1844, p. 23.

17. Poor Law Commission, *Fourth Annual Report*, 1838, Appendix A, Number 1, Supplement 2, pp. 129–38; idem, *Fifth Annual Report*, 1839, Appendix c, Number 2, p. 164; H. Gavin, *Sanitary Ramblings*, London, 1848, pp. 94–95.

18. D. Green and A. Parton, 'Slums and Slum Life in Victorian England: London and Birmingham at Mid-century', in M. Gaskell (ed.), *Slums*, Leicester, 1990, p. 75.

19. C. Booth, *Life and Labour of the People of London*, Poverty Series, Vol. 1, London, 1902, p. 147. Based on friendly society claims statistics drawn from the Ancient Order of Foresters, James Riley has recently argued that the late 19th-century decline in mortality was accompanied by an increase in sickness. See J. Riley, *Sick not Dead*, Baltimore, 1997.

20. There were exceptions to this, notably amongst the dock companies. See Hodgkinson, *The Origins of the National Health Service* (n. 3), p. 53.

21. Class B paid 2.6 per cent of their weekly household income on insurance compared to 3.5 per cent for class E and 4.4 per cent for class F. See Booth, *Life and Labour* (n. 19), p. 138.

22. PP 1844 IX *S. C. Medical Poor Relief, Third Report*, q. 13, 17, 22, 31, 35. Despite having a larger population, for example, friendly society membership in London and Middlesex in 1818 was lower than in Lancashire. See P. Gosden, *The Friendly Societies in England 1815–1875*, Manchester, 1961.

23. K. Waddington, 'Unsuitable Cases: The Debate over Outpatient Admissions, The Medical Profession and Late Victorian London Hospitals', *Medical History*, **42** (1998), p. 41.

24. PP 1888 XV *Select Committee of the House of Lords on Poor Law Relief, Report*, p. viii.

25. C. Trevelyan, *Metropolitan Medical Relief*, London, 1879, pp. 4–5.

26. The figure for 1829 is taken from S. Low, *The Charities of London*, London, 1861; for 1869 see S. Low, *A Handbook to the Charities of London*, London, 1870 and for 1881 see F. Mouat, 'On Hospitals – Their Management, Construction and Arrangement', *Lancet*, 16 July 1881, pp. 79–80.

27. In 1891 there were 1.71 beds per 1000 population in London compared to 0.85 elsewhere. See R. Pinker, *English Hospital Statistics 1861–1938*, London, 1966, pp. 81, 84.

28. Mouat, 'On Hospitals' (n. 26), p. 79.

29. London was unusual in this respect since in provincial and Scottish hospitals medical cases outnumbered surgical until the mid-1860s. Greater specialisation in London hospitals and their refusal to admit patients suffering from contagious disease may also have reinforced the significance of surgery. I am grateful to Anne Crowther for drawing my attention to this point.

30. Pinker, *English Hospital Statistics* (n. 27), p. 93.

31. Ibid., pp. 93–94.

32. Registrar General, *Fifth Annual Report*, 1843, p. 460.

33. See Low, *The Charities of London* and Low, *A Handbook* (n. 26).

34. Hodgkinson, *The Origins of the National Health Service* (n. 3), p. 210.

35. Digby, *Making a Medical Living* (n. 10), p. 242.

36. In 1842 the Tower Hamlets Dispensary dealt with 246 midwifery cases compared to 172 in the Stepney Union. See PP 1844 IX *S. C. Medical Poor Relief, Third Report*, p. 173; Hodgkinson, *The Origins of the National Health Service* (n. 3), p. 210. By way of comparison, between 1856 and 1863 the outdoor midwifery department of St George's Hospital in west London dealt with 2800 cases of childbirth, averaging 350 a year. See G. Gathorne-Hardy, 'Workhouse Death-rate in Childbirth', *Journal of the Royal Statistical Society*, **30** (1867), p. 172.

37. See, for example, E. G. Thomas, 'The Old Poor Law and Medicine', *Medical History*, **24** (1980), pp. 1–19.

38. For this episode in Chadwick's life see S. Finer, *The Life and Times of Sir Edwin Chadwick*, London, 1952, pp. 243–91; A. Brundage, *England's 'Prussian Minister'*, London, 1988, pp. 113–20.

39. The 1842 General Medical Order, for example, was only issued to 13 of the 39 local poor law authorities in London.

40. In 1867 there were only 15 counties in which sickness accounted for over 30 per cent of workhouse inmates. See Poor Law Board, *Twenty Second Annual Report*, 1870, p. xxvi

41. See M.A. Crowther, *The Workhouse System 1834–1929*, London, 1981, pp. 160–62. For a description of conditions in a London workhouse see J. Rogers, *Reminiscences of a Workhouse Medical Officer*, London, 1889.

42. The unions to which it was issued in London included Greenwich, Lewisham, City of London, East London, West London, St Olave's, Poplar, St Saviour's, Stepney, Strand and Wandsworth.

43. Hodgkinson, *The Origins of the National Health Service* (n. 3), p. 62.

44. Ibid., p. 171.

45. PP 1844 IX S. C. *Medical Poor Relief, Third Report*, q. 838; PP 1854 XII *Select Committee to inquire into the mode in which medical relief is now administered*, minutes of evidence, q. 618; Hodgkinson, *The Origins of the National Health Service* (n. 3), p. 86; E. Chadwick, *The Sanitary Condition of the Labouring Population of Great Britain*, ed. M. Flinn, Edinburgh, 1965 (1st edn 1842), p. 213.

46. In 1842–43, medical officers in Stepney attended 9025 patients in a district with a population of 91 078 in 1841. PP 1844 IX *S. C. Medical Poor Relief, Third Report*, q. 838.

47. By 1860, 24 500 adult ablebodied male paupers out of a total of 26 290 in London were in receipt of outdoor relief on account of sickness or accident. See Hodgkinson, *The Origins of the National Health Service* (n. 3), p. 270.

48. This figure is calculated by averaging the amounts spent on medical relief compared to the total relief expenditure in London unions in 1842, 1849, 1855 and 1867, as provided in the annual reports of the Poor Law Commission and Poor Law Board.

49. PP 1844 IX, *S. C. Medical Poor Relief, Third Report*, q. 600.

50. Quoted in S.E. Finer, *The Life and Times of Edwin Chadwick*, London, 1952, p. 245. The phrase is attributed to Edward Tufnell, one of the assistant inspectors. See also Poor Law Board, *Twenty Second Annual Report*, 1870, p. xxviii.

51. Green and Parton, 'Slums and Slum Life' (n. 18), p. 75.

52. L. Marks, 'Medical Care for Pauper Mothers and their Infants: Poor Law Provision and Local Demand in East London 1870–1929', *Economic History Review*, second series, **XLVI** (1993), p. 537.

53. PP 1844 IX *S. C. Medical Poor Relief, Third Report*, q. 838.

54. Maternal mortality rates remained at between 4 and 5 deaths per 1000 births throughout the 19th century, although rates in most London districts were lower. See R. Woods and N. Shelton, *An Atlas of Victorian Mortality*, Liverpool, 1997, p. 117.

55. G. Gathorne-Hardy, 'Workhouse Death-rate in Childbirth', *Journal of the Royal Statistical Society*, **30** (1867), p. 172 ; I. Loudon, 'Deaths in Childbed from the Eighteenth Century to 1935', *Medical History*, **30** (1986), p. 21.

56. Marks, 'Medical Care for Pauper Mothers' (n. 52), p. 526.

57. During the 1830s and 1840s, maternal mortality for women aided by the Royal Maternal Charity, which operated within a three mile radius of St Pauls, varied between 1.96 and 4.6 per 1000 births. Mortality rates for outdoor deliveries in general in London between 1867 and 1891 varied between 1.5 and 3.6. See Loudon, 'Deaths in Childbed' (n. 55), p. 16.

58. For a fuller discussion see A. Hardy, 'Smallpox in London: Factors in the Decline of the Disease in the Nineteenth Century', *Medical History*, **27** (1983), pp. 111–38.

59. In 1849 the Poor Law Board pointed out that the 4 & 5 Vict. c. 29 expressly stated that vaccination was not to be deemed poor relief. Poor Law Board, *Official Circular*, 30, (October 1849).

60. A. Hardy, *The Epidemic Streets*, Oxford, 1993, p. 118.

61. Poor Law Commission, *Thirteenth Annual Report*, 1847, p. 15.

62. G. Mooney, '"A Tissue of the most Flagrant Anomalies": Smallpox Vaccination and the Centralization of Sanitary Administration in Nineteenth-century London', *Medical History*, **41** (1997), p. 274.

63. The effectiveness of vaccination depended on the length of time that the vaccine lymph had been kept. The fewer patients, the longer the period the lymph was kept and the less effective was the vaccine. A high level of attendance was also required to facilitate arm-to-arm vaccination.

64. Mooney, 'A Tissue' (n. 62), p. 268.

65. Between 1873 and 1877, 8.1 per cent of infants in London were not vaccinated compared to 4.1 per cent for the rest of England and Wales. See, PP 1881 XLV Local Government Board, *Tenth Annual Report*, 1880–81, p. 416.

66. Hardy, *The Epidemic Streets*, (1983), p. 120.
67. See A. Brundage, *The Making of the New Poor Law 1832–39*, London, 1978, pp. 54–57.
68. The Poor Law Amendment Act was permissive rather than mandatory. In 1837 an objection by the Directors of the Poor in St Pancras against forcible adoption of the Act was upheld, thereby limiting the Poor Law Commissioners from imposing their authority on unwilling parishes.
69. The most vociferous anti-centralisation advocate was Joshua Toulmin Smith. See, for example, J.T. Smith, *Government by Commissions: Illegal and Pernicious*, London, 1849; idem, *Local Self-government and Centralization*, London, 1851; idem, *The People and the Parish: The Common Law and its Breakers*, London, 1853.
70. The 11 districts were St George Hanover Square, St Giles and St George Bloomsbury, St Luke Middlesex, St James Clerkenwell, St James Westminster, St Leonard Shoreditch, St Margaret and St John Westminster, St Marylebone, St Mary Islington, St Mary Newington and St Pancras.
71. The figure for Birmingham was £32 837; Liverpool was £32 020 and Leeds was £18 640 compared to £27 907 for St Marylebone and £18 296 for St Pancras. See Poor Law Commission, *Thirteenth Annual Report*, 1847.
72. D.R. Green, *From Artisans to Paupers*, Aldershot, 1995, p. 215.
73. See PP 1904 LXXXII *Pauperism (England and Wales)*, half-yearly statement.
74. In 1861, for example, the average per capita cost of indoor relief in London was 4s 5d a week compared to 1s 4d for outdoor relief. See Green, *From Artisans to Paupers* (n. 72), p. 224.
75. The figures for England and Wales are calculated from F. Driver, *Power and Pauperism*, Cambridge, 1993, pp. 78, 88; the information for London is taken from the Poor Law Commission, *Annual Reports*, 1834–47; Poor Law Board, *Annual Reports*, 1848–59. The cost is based on the amount authorised by the Poor Law Commission and Poor Law Board for the construction of new workhouses. See also Green, *From Artisans to Paupers* (n. 72), pp. 215–23.
76. The eight were St Saviour's (1837) Wandsworth, Greenwich (1838), Bethnal Green, Lambeth, St Olave's (1841), Kensington, Paddington (1845). See Poor Law Commission, *Annual Reports*, 1838–47.
77. PP 1861 IX *Select Committee on Poor Relief* (England), q. 3015–17, 3029.
78. Poor Law Board, *Twentieth Annual Report*, 1868, pp. 14, 126.
79. Paupers, other than the casual poor, were entitled to receive relief only if they had a settlement in a parish. The grounds for settlement varied but included birth or apprenticeship in a district. Wives took the settlement of their husbands. Non-settled paupers were always liable to be removed to their place of settlement. In 1846 a new category of 'irremovable' poor was created whereby paupers without a settlement in a parish but resident there for five continuous years gained entitlement to receive relief without the threat of removal. In 1861 the period of continuous residence was reduced to three years and in 1865 to one year. See M.E. Rose, 'Settlement, Removal and the New Poor Law', in D. Fraser (ed.), *The New Poor Law in the Nineteenth Century*, London, 1976, pp. 25–44.
80. Green, *From Artisans to Paupers* (n. 72), p. 226.
81. Ibid., p. 235.
82. P. Ashbridge, 'Paying for the Poor: A Middle Class Metropolitan Movement for Rate Equalisation 1857–1867', *London Journal*, **22** (1997), p. 118.
83. G. Ayers, *England's First State Hospitals and the Metropolitan Asylums Board 1867–1930*, London, 1971, p. 18.

84. See PP 1866 LXI *Report of Dr E. Smith on metropolitan workhouse infirmaries and sick wards*; PP 1866 LXI *Report of H. B. Farnall on infirmary wards of metropolitan workhouses*; PP 1867 LXI *Report of U. Corbett and W. O. Markham relative to metropolitan workhouses*; Poor Law Board, *Nineteenth Annual Report*, 1867, p. 17; 'Commission to inquire into the state of workhouse hospitals', *Lancet*, (15 April, 3 June, 1, 15, 29 July, 12, 26 August, 9, 23 September, 4, 18, 25 November, 23 December 1865, 20, 27 January, 17 February, 3, 10 March, 15 April 1866); E. Hart, *An Account of the Condition of the Infirmaries of the London Workhouses*, London, 1866); Hodgkinson, *The Origins of the National Health Service* (n. 3), pp. 468–99; Driver, *Power and Pauperism* (n. 75), pp. 69–70.

85. Poor Law Board, *Twenty First Annual Report*, 1869; Hodgkinson, *The Origins of the National Health Service* (n. 3), p. 505. National expenditure on sick wards was disproportionately concentrated in London from the 1860s. See Driver, *Power and Pauperism* (n. 75), pp. 88–90.

86. Trevelyan, *Metropolitan Medical Relief* (n. 25), p. 105.

87. For a discussion of the role of the Charity Organisation Society in London see G.S. Jones, *Outcast London*, Oxford, 1971, pp. 256–80.

88. Ibid., p. 3

89. Ayers, *England's First State Hospitals* (n. 83), p. 63.

90. PP 1909 XL *Royal Commission on the Poor Laws*, Appendix II, 336; Ayers, *England's First State Hospitals* (n. 83), p. 286. The proportion of patients who died from smallpox in their own home rather than in an MAB institution fell from nearly 67 per cent in 1871–72 to less than 34 per cent ten years later. See G. Rivett, *The Development of the London Hospital System 1823–1982*, London, 1986, p. 91.

91. See Hardy, 'Smallpox in London' (n. 58) for further discussion of smallpox mortality and the effects of isolation.

92. F. Mouat, 'On Hospitals' (n. 26), p. 80.

93. PP 1909 XXXVII *Royal Commission on the Poor Laws, Part V: Medical Relief*, p. 255.

94. Trevelyan, *Metropolitan Medical Relief* (n. 29), p. 16.

95. Ibid., pp. 3–5.

CHAPTER TWELVE

Poor Relief and Health Care in 19th Century Scotland

Rosalind Mitchison

Scotland's 19th century system of poor relief, like England's, had a major discontinuity, the passing from the 'Old' Poor Law and the hesitant start of the 'New' in 1845. The particular importance of the change is that the 'New' embodied concepts which had not been part of the Scottish way of life in the 16th century when the 'Old' was set up. Such concepts included the idea that statutes should be obeyed, that workers should carry out the instructions of their employers and approach work in a professional way, that the law should be taken to mean what it said, and that new legal principles should not be invented by those supposed to be carrying it out.

The Scottish break with the Old Poor Law took place 11 years later than the English one and was a much more drastic change. It was based on a thorough investigation, and was less doctrinaire than the English. The investigation showed the deplorably inadequate support system in many places, so, whereas the intention of the English New Poor Law was to reduce the amount of aid given to the labouring classes, that of the Scottish was to increase it. Both new laws were influenced by Benthamite principles.

The Scotland of the early 19th century was not accustomed to legislative change. There had been almost no legislation which touched Scotland since the Union of 1707. True, there had been a small outbreak of parliamentary interventions after the rising of 1745 and, in the late 18th century, Henry Dundas had made some desirable changes. But law had been altered by other means than statute – mainly by legal cases decided in the interests of landowners and subsequently adhered to. The judges had all been landowners and had accepted the legal interpretations put up by advocates, nearly all of whom were also landowners. Except in the larger cities it was the Church which administered the Poor Law and so the Law reflected the fashions in religious thought. During the famine of the 1690s the kirk session of one small parish had set out its policy in strictly religious terms:

> Whereas the Word of the Lord requires our Collection to be for the saints, and what is given to such in Extremitie helps them to praise and glorifie God, and may have its owne influence on the rest of the poor of the parish (who ordinarily are the Scumm and Refuse of the people) to set upon a Course of Reformation and may be more also for the Honour

of religion and peace of our Consciences Therefor the Session unani-
mouslie appoints that the Collection, for hereafter, be for the supplie
first of all, of such as truelie fear the Lord, when reduced to straits and
necessities, and next of such as have endeavoured honestlie to gain a
livelihood to themselves, but have been blasted upon by providence; and
failing these, of the Poor of the parish that beg from Door to Door, but
with these provisions, that they get none of it but in time of great
extremities and Dearth, to preserve their lives.[1]

It is rare for the executive organ of any system to state so clearly the principles of their actions. This statement shows that the Enlightenment, with its
emphasis on humanitarianism and civic, rather than religious, principles, was
still a long way off.

The climate of opinion, at least among the upper classes, was to change in
the 18th century. By the date of this statement, with landowners indulging in
a considerable amount of foot-dragging, the old Scottish Poor Law was
already keeping some of the old and infirm and other handicapped people
alive, paying for the schooling of poor children and joining with other parishes to provide bursaries for poor students at the universities. Even before
the adoption of Enlightenment ideals, landowners, though unwilling to pay a
regular poor rate, as demanded by statute, would intervene to support their
peasantry in hard times – as, for instance, during the harsh climate of the
years 1739–41 – provided that their generosity was well-publicised. Such
action was part of civic duty. The Enlightenment emphasised the obligations
on the citizen's role in society. A citizen was a man of independence – in
other words, a gentleman in secure possession of an income, usually from a
landed estate.

Examples of generosity to tenants are numerous through the whole period
of Enlightenment dominance, but that does not mean that landowning bore its
proper share of relief. By the mid-18th century many landed families had
acquired, through marriage with heiresses, estates in other areas. Such families would usually confine their generosity to the area where their principal
residence lay. Non-resident landowners had little interest in the needs of
outlying communities and gave little aid to such places when they were in
need. Nevertheless, there was a slow increase in the number of parishes
which had managed to raise an assessment for the poor, whereby they placed
half of the financial burden of relief on the landed gentry. Most of the
parishes of the Border area and many of those round the Forth estuary were
supporting their poor by assessment by the end of the eighteenth century.

The economic change known as the Agricultural Revolution which began
in the 1770s had drastic social effects. Landowners reorganised their estates
in the expectation of enhanced incomes. Larger farm units reduced the need
for labour, but also altered the type of labour most required. Improved agricultural techniques demanded a selective labour force and there was no
concern for the less useful, who were left to find what niche they could. As a

result, the large class of cotters – subtenants with small plots of land who also worked for others – disappeared. Some became full-time agricultural labourers; others moved away to work on the roads or in industry. The availability of this labour force, living in small towns or in farm cottages, made the Industrial Revolution possible.

The economic changes which made up the Industrial Revolution had even more marked social effects. There was a drastic acceleration of change. The first cotton mill, based on water power, in Scotland began work in 1777. It and its successors gave work to the displaced cotters. Then, in the early 19th century, steam power came to supplement and eventually supplant water power. The factories could now move to town, and their owners no longer had to provide housing for the workers. Scotland had been the least urbanised country in western Europe; now she lay second only to England. The vast industrial town, characteristic of the 19th century, had arrived.[2]

It is well known that rapid urban growth produced social problems and a high risk of infectious disease. Also, as the swings of the business cycle drew closer together and became sharper, the risk of unemployment rose. In Scotland these changes were accompanied by a change in the interpretation of Christian duty. The old hard line of 17th century Calvinism was modified by a stronger emphasis on personal religion, and less on community. Evangelical Christianity stressed the obligations of individuals. The working man was held to have the same obligation as his social superior; he was responsible for the survival, care and behaviour of his family. He was expected to stand up to outside forces. Those who managed to do this came to be termed as 'independent'. It was assumed that economic stresses should be foreseen. Indeed the particular line of thought promoted by Thomas Malthus held that parents should not marry and have children unless they could be sure of supporting them through the stresses of economic change.

The new emphasis on independence has already been investigated by Professor Mary Lindemann for Hamburg.[3] The practical result of such a belief was to leave the relief of poverty wherever possible to voluntary funding, and to discourage any claim against government-based funds. Scotland seems to have held by this theory even more strongly than did Hamburg. The country was able to reduce the funds available to support the poor because, early in the 1820s, a group of young Whig lawyers had managed to obtain lawsuits on useful themes and, through these, had established that the Scottish Poor Law did not support any one who was not disabled. The word 'disabled' covered the old, women with large families and no husband, orphans and foundlings, the blind and the insane. For adult men it covered only those with some serious and permanent physical disability. The statute phrase 'poor, aged and infirm' as a definition of those who should be supported by relief was interpreted to mean 'poor and aged' and 'poor and infirm', and not simply poor.[4]

The new definition took over. Landowning sympathy for the workforce in years of bad harvest did not extend to regarding an economic slump as the equivalent. Some longstanding Scottish beliefs about Scotland's position in the world remained unmodified by the Enlightenment. One was that Scotland had the purest form of Reformed religion and thus must have the most moral basic institutions, including the Poor Law. The country also possessed the most influential preacher of the age, the minister Thomas Chalmers, installed in the influential University of St Andrews, where he had had much to do with the training of future parish ministers. Chalmers had set up what he called an experiment in a large working-class parish in Glasgow. Here middle-class businessmen and others were specially imported from other parishes to control, and for the most part reduce, the number of those dependent on relief. In some cases, this was done by the offer of work. Two deacons had to agree before any money was passed over.[5]

Very little came to be passed as relief in that parish, and Chalmers claimed that the whole system proved that rate-based relief was largely unnecessary: what little remained could instead be handed over to the Church to manage. The great majority of ministers, as their evidence to the Royal Commission of 1844–45 shows, accepted Chalmer's ideas and statements. However, the ministers' verbal enthusiasm for the system did not count for much because their evidence revealed that they had very little idea of the scale of destitution in their own parishes. In the event, only one parish out of Scotland's 900 or so followed the line proposed. (There are three other parishes whose records do not survive, which may also have come into the system. The two we know about, and any others that may have tried it, gave it up after a few years.)

In the early 1840s a devastating recession highlighted the inadequacy of the Scottish system of relief. Large numbers of the unemployed tramped the roads looking for work and begging, alarming rural society. A substantial amount of money was voluntarily supplied, but proved insufficient. The town of Paisley, which specialised in producing elaborate and expensive cottons, was in danger of starvation because funds for relief had run out. It was saved only by covert aid from members of the government.[6] A pressure group of professional men, mostly Edinburgh doctors, and including a distinguished professor of medicine, was set up to lobby the government for a Royal Commission to inquire into the workings of the Poor Law. In response to this, a large group of landowners from all parts of Scotland met and initiated inquiries, published reports based on these and declared that all was well and that giving relief to the unemployed would be unscriptural (although no specific biblical text to this effect was quoted).[7] The government set up a small Royal Commission of inquiry, made up of very conscientious men who made a thorough investigation. The Commission, or its individual members, visited all parts of Scotland and interviewed the minister or parish clerk in all parishes. The published record of its work shows answers to a lengthy questionnaire and interviews with 872 ministers of religion, about 100 medical men, eight skilled workers and one woman. Over 4000 paupers were visited in their own homes, but landowners with special information or opinions were interviewed. Information about the level of relief was sought from all available sources.[8]

The main conclusions of the evidence were inescapable – that in most Scottish parishes the level of relief was too low to cover even basic food and shelter. In the big cities the diet and shelter provided in the 'hospitals' (poorhouses) was adequate, but these hospitals could not cope with all of the destitute, and, for those left on outdoor relief, allowances fell below what was needed for survival. The local authorities, however, were determined not to raise the general cost of relief. There is little evidence of influence by the principles of the English New Poor Law, but in a few places it was acknowledged that it gave a more generous standard of living than did the Scottish.

Although it had become generally accepted that relief for adults depended on their being permanently disabled, very little of the relief money was spent on medical or surgical aid. Some aristocrats, such as the Duke of Sutherland, paid a salary to surgeons to provide some care in remote areas, and some large collieries supported doctors on a compulsory contribution from their workforce, but generally a doctor available to treat the poor was the exception rather than the rule. Parishes might use a local voluntary dispensary: for instance many Border parishes sent their sick to the Kelso dispensary, to the funds of which most of them did not contribute. A common pattern of action was for a kirk session to let a doctor know that somebody was ill, but not formally to call him out. On this basis the parish could then fail to pay him or, alternatively, pay for any medicaments or drugs that he used but not for his time. A doctor in Wick remarked to the Royal Commission that attendance on the poor was a 'heavy assessment on the medical profession'.[9]

The Church might give aid more directly. A Shetland minister claimed that the poor did not need any treatment that could not be supplied from his own medical chest. Indeed, several ministers had undertaken part of a medical training. The minister of Dores in Moray had had vaccinia sent to him from London and had vaccinated over 100 children. (In the early years of the century the Church had circulated instructions to ministers on how to vaccinate if there was no other organisation ready to take on giving the protection.) In Torosay an elder bled the sick and a local landowner had a medicine chest. Some urban parishes had agreements with the local infirmary to which they might subscribe, which would enable them to place a few sick paupers in care. No parish gave any help in childbirth. Overall, the availability of medical aid was only occasional.

More serious was the fact that the sick had to subsist on inadequate allowances, and that these might be reduced by a bout of economy. Extreme examples of this had occurred in Oban in the west Highlands where, following on a decision to stop raising assessment, allowances had been drastically cut. Consequently, in the next few months three-quarters of the bedridden poor had died. There were other examples of neglect and squalor. Scone parish used the house of one known locally as 'Dirty Meg' for its sick; one man had been found dead in bed along with 'the Excrements and other Evacuations of his body'; another pauper placed there had killed himself.

It was the inadequate level of basic allowances that was the most serious shortcoming of the old Poor Law, for medicine had relatively few useful treatments available. Opium was a powerful drug, and there was enough malaria around for quinine to have its uses. There was also, of course, the incalculable aid of what we would today consider placebos and which recent opinion has suggested might be of real use. Surgery had more claims to be effective, but it had no part to play in treating the infections that proliferated in urban areas.

The general impression of the level of medical aid is surprising. At this time, the early 19th century, Scottish medicine was considered to be at the forefront of development: Scottish medical writings and Scottish practitioners were considered to be leading elements in medical development. Yet very little of this prestige helped those under the Poor Law.

The Report of the Royal Commission was very hesitant about change. Basically it held that the creation of a central Board of Supervision which would receive annual reports from all parishes, and from them compile its own report, would remove the shortcomings and evils of the parish system: these reports would create a public opinion powerful enough to demand improvement. Yet public opinion cannot have been entirely unaware of aspects of the existing provision, and had done very little. The Commission published over 2000 folio pages of evidence, reporting interviews and home visits, besides the two volumes of replies to the questionnaire. One or two particular scandals caught the attention of the London newspapers, and the cumulative evidence stimulated MPs to demand a more drastic and effective reform to be effected by rapid legislation. In this, the duty of the parish to pay for medical and surgical aid was expressly stated.

One particular area of ill-health with a temporary influence on the old Poor Law was lunacy. This is not an aspect of ill-health which is evenly distributed and, as a local burden, could be very heavy. The movement towards gentleness in treatment was marked in Scotland and, as a result, asylums were set up in the early 19th century. However, the difficulty, from the point of view of poor law authorities, was the cost of keeping a lunatic clean, clothed and safe; it worked out at between six and seven times the cost of supporting an ordinary pauper. There was also considerable concern in the upper reaches of society that the care of upper-class lunatics might be misused to enable unscrupulous people to gain their property. Under this influence an act was passed by parliament in

1840 insisting that all lunatics had to be supported in suitable institutions. This forced some parish landowners to accept assessment solely for this section of the poor. Meanwhile the larger cities in the west of Scotland had found a cheap solution for pauper lunatics – shipping them out to farms on the island of Arran. Unmodernised farms were thus kept going through the work of lunatics living in primitive conditions; this was an easier way for the landlord to make a holding pay than agrarian modernisation.

The New Poor Law in the first place put pressure on parishes and towns to be more generous with allowances. There was, however, little pressure on them to do much about the health of their clients. But other events conspired to reduce the influence of the evangelical movements. The presence and power of the Church of Scotland was drastically reduced by the great split of 1843, the 'Disruption' after which the established Church became merely the Church of approximately a third of the population. It was impossible to accept the claim that poor relief could be restored to its management and control.

At the same time, middle-class Scots proved more susceptible than they had been before to the tenet of less eligibility. It was thought that the recipients of poor relief should be discouraged by making the reception of aid unpleasant and demeaning. Ablebodied men were still considered as ineligible for relief, so the main group of people now affected were unmarried mothers. As poorhouses became more common under the encouragement of the central Board of Supervision, the policy of insisting on indoor relief for this group was generally accepted. As members of parochial boards stated to a Select Committee on the Poor Law in 1869, insistence on indoor relief was 'helpful' in such cases.[10] It is not clear who they thought had been helped, but, in any case, those with several illegitimate children and no male support could not hope to maintain their family by means of their own labour.

An interesting confusion over the correct application of the Benthamite principle is shown in the report of an inspector of the Edinburgh suburban parish's hospital in 1861. Besides some comments on the level of cleanliness, the hospital was criticised for allowing paupers to have private possessions and spare clothes with them in the wards, letting them go out and meet friends on 'liberty days', allowing them to bring in food, cook it in the dormitories and wear clothes that were not uniform.[11] The hospital was the residence of the old and infirm. To those not infected by Benthamism it sounds rather comfortable.

Simple meanness allied with 'less eligibility'. An issue which persisted until the 1880s was the refusal of poor law hospitals to employ professional nurses, rather than inmates. These were untrained and not particularly clean, so that hygiene in the wards was low.

Another aspect of parsimony was on the diet for children in poorhouses. Most children were farmed out to rural areas – Arran in particular had replaced its lunatics with children – but for those remaining in the institution, food was restricted. It was discovered in 1884 that children in English work-houses had almost twice the food allowance of those in Scottish poorhouses, and were more healthy. The Scottish diets were some 40 years out of date, and it was time to abolish cornmeal and buttermilk.[12]

One area of development which seems to have been underappreciated by historians of the 19th century, is the growth of professionalism. Some employments in earlier centuries demonstrated this feature – the navy, for instance, and the Church of Scotland's ministry. It also becomes noticeable very early on in the administration of the New Poor Law: early on in Scotland the parish inspectors set up their own society and soon began to publish a journal, *The Poor Law Magazine*. Its papers are not very sprightly but they contain a great deal of information and were clearly an important element in the creation of formulas for dealing with particular types of case.[13]

The relationship between the Board of Supervision and the development of public health in Scotland did not spring from the recognition that communic-able disease was a likely source of poverty, but rather from the limitations of the structure of government. The organisation of civil registration in England was placed under poor law authorities – there being no other area of government with complete local coverage – so in response to a threat of a cholera epidemic in 1859 the government turned to the Board of Supervision, and the Board of Supervision turned to Henry Littlejohn for a short and localised study. Littlejohn was then known as a bright young doctor of some academic achievement, and his personality and thoroughness were to be the main force behind the public health movement. His particular skills were in his ability to see the practical implications of the slowly developing knowledge about the communication of disease and his talent for writing vigorous reports on which even the most unwilling local authority felt that something had to be done.[14]

Eventually the Board was to take on more staff and carry out further health investigations. Then, in 1867, public health was given its own Board, but until the reorganisation of local government in 1889 the Board of Supervision dominated the new Board and instructed its servants to put matters of poor relief before those of public health.[15] By the end of the century, Littlejohn had achieved what he had long demanded, the compulsory notification of infectious diseases so that authorities could be alerted to epidemics in their early stages. By then, also, the Board had gained more inspectors and had become skilled in coercing parishes to accept a level of interference. It had not, however, managed to overcome the major weakness of the Scottish definition of entitlement to relief – its exclusion of the ablebodied. In the 1860s the Board had pressed parishes to ignore this: one famous letter of instruction had pointed out that if a man was truly destitute though ablebodied 'no long time' would elapse before he was disabled by want of food. But aid to such people had to come under special and partly disguised headings.[16]

Such a penal attitude to the unemployed was ceasing to be applicable by the end of the century because of new political developments. Some parts of the working class obtained the vote in 1884, and this led to pressure for a more democratic approach to relief. The Boer War caused concern over the physical quality of the working class, on account of the number that had been rejected as recruits for the army.[17]

There was an increased knowledge about disease, although this did not prevent the Dundee poorhouse suffering an outbreak of scurvy in 1898.[18] It was no longer acceptable for prison diets to be more generous than poor law ones. National fitness as a cause was incompatible with less eligibility. An Inter-departmental Committee on Physical Deterioration was investigating national fitness, handicapped to some degree by Lamarckian theories about the hereditary effects of urbanisation. There were new ideas about insurance and state pensions. And the start of the discovery of new drugs and treatments was to make personal medicine, rather than public health, the new growth area.

Notes

1. Scottish Record Office, CH2/569/1. Kiltearn Kirk Session Register, Vol. 1, August 1697.
2. Ian D. Whyte, *Scotland before the Industrial Revolution*, London, 1995, chapter 10.
3. Mary Lindemann, 'Urban Growth and Medical Charity: Hamburg 1788–1815', in Jonathan Barry and Colin Jones (eds), *Medicine and Charity before the Welfare State*, London, 1991, pp. 113–32.
4. John Guthrie Smith, *Digest on the Law of Scotland relating to the Poor*, Edinburgh, 1859, p. 39.
5. R.A. Cage and E.O.A. Checkland, 'Thomas Chalmers and Urban Poverty: The St John's Experiment in Glasgow, 1818–1837', *Philosophical Journal*, 22 (1976), pp. 37–56.
6. T.C. Smout, 'The Strange Intervention of Edward Twistelton: Paisley in Depression, 1843', in T.C. Smout (ed.). *The Search for Wealth and Stability*, London, 1979, pp. 218–42.
7. *Report of a Committee appointed on the 20th April 1846 at a general meeting in Edinburgh of landed proprietors connected with the different parts of Scotland called in consequence of an association for obtaining an official inquiry into pauperism in Scotland*, nd.
8. The material evidence of the Royal Commission's work is contained in *PP 1844*, Vols. XX–XXV. The report and verbal evidence occupy the first three of these volumes, and the replies to the questionnaire the second three.
9. *PP* 1844 Vol. XXI, p. 352, evidence of Mr Henderson, surgeon.
10. *PP* 1868–9. Vol. XI, *PP* 1870, Vol. XI, *PP* 1871, Vol. XI
11. Ian Levitt (ed.), *Government and Social Conditions in Scotland, 1845–1919*, Edinburgh: Scottish History Society, 1988, pp. 43–44. This chapter is much indebted to Dr Levitt's work.

12. Ian Levitt, *Poverty and Welfare in Scotland 1890–1919*, Edinburgh, 1988, pp. 37–38.
13. *The Poor Law Magazine* was started in 1858.
14. Ian Levitt, 'Henry Littlejohn and Scottish Health Policy, 1859–1908', *Scottish Archives*, **2** (1996), pp. 63–77.
15. T. Ferguson, *Scottish Social Welfare*, Edinburgh, 1958, p. 11.
16. Levitt, *Poverty and Welfare* (n. 12), pp. 14–16.
17. *Report of the Interdepartmental Committee on Physical Deterioration*, *PP* 1904, Vol. XXX, p. 11.
18. Levitt, *Poverty and Welfare* (n. 12), p. 84.

PART FIVE

The Netherlands

CHAPTER THIRTEEN

Dutch Approaches to Problems of Illness and Poverty between the Golden Age and the *Fin de Siècle*

Marijke Gijswijt-Hofstra

'Charity seems to be very national among them.' These were Sir William Temple's words in 1673.[1] He had served as English ambassador at the Hague, and 'them' were the Dutch. Temple was not the only foreign observer who was impressed by the Dutch charitable diligence.[2] Nor were the Dutch over-modest. With evident self-satisfaction it was stated around 1800 that Dutch poor relief in general, and Amsterdam poor relief in particular, enjoyed an excellent reputation.[3] Moreover, this reputation was thought to be well-deserved. As one of the Dutch authors remarked in 1792: 'It is undeniably true that our *Nederland*, if it does not deserve priority over all other nations in the exercise of the duty of charity, it may at least be put on a par with the most charitable nation.'[4]

This rosy picture makes one suspicious. For what did Dutch poor relief actually amount to? And, for that matter, to what extent was health care provided for? Was the provision of health care just one aspect of poor relief, or were health care and poor relief distinct, although partly overlapping, fields? Unfortunately, Dutch historical research has tended to focus either on health care or on poor relief. Insufficient light has been shed on connections between the two. The history of poor relief has been the domain of social historians who have paid relatively little attention to problems of health care, while health care has been the domain of medical historians who have mainly concentrated on the medical professions and the public organisation of health care, and much less on medical poor relief.[5] Another problem may as well be pointed out at this stage: the available research on Dutch health care and poor relief is fairly unevenly spread over time and places.

This chapter will discuss Dutch approaches to problems of illness and poverty in the course of the 18th and 19th centuries – the period between the Dutch 'golden age' and the *fin de siècle*. What were the problems considered to be in both these fields? How were these problems defined in the first place? Which solutions were proposed, which measures were actually taken, and with what results? As in the rest of this volume, the focus will be urban, which in the Dutch case means that a substantial part of the population will be covered anyway. In 1675, 45 per cent of the Dutch population lived in towns of more than 2500 residents, although this percentage slightly decreased to about 40 per cent in 1800.[6] The Dutch population in the 18th century amounted to about 2 million, then grew to 2.6 million in 1830, to over 3 million in 1850, and to over 5 million in 1900.

The following discussion of Dutch health care and poor relief arrangements is chronologically structured. The periodisation is mainly based on political and, to a lesser extent, economic developments. The first period to be discussed comprises the 18th century until the end of the Dutch Republic in 1795, by which time demands for reforms of the existing system of poor relief had become numerous. The second period covers the so-called Batavian and French time, starting in 1795 and ending with Napoleon's defeat in 1813, during which attempts to reform and centralise health care and poor relief proved to be largely futile. In fact, the same applies to the third period which begins with the (United) Kingdom of the Netherlands, which initially also comprised the present Belgium (the Belgian revolt in 1830 marked the actual dissolution of the union), and ends roughly halfway through the 19th century. At that time – to be precise in 1848 – the Constitution was thoroughly revised, which meant less power for the king, the establishment of a parliamentary system and a victory for liberalism. From then on, the Netherlands very gradually began to develop into a state which held itself responsible for the welfare of its subjects. Undoubtedly this process received an important impetus from the belated take-off of Dutch industrialisation during the last decades of the 19th century. Even so, both health care and poor relief would, to a large extent, remain local responsibilities.

Health care and poor relief in the Dutch Republic, 1700–1795

The Dutch Republic would never become a unified state. It always remained a federation of united, but sovereign provinces – seven in all. The mainly Catholic provinces of northern Brabant and Limburg, the *Generaliteitslanden* or Generality Lands, which had been incorporated after the formation of the Dutch Republic, had a special, subordinate status and were directly ruled by the Estates-General. Especially in the western provinces of Holland and Zeeland the towns had an important say, with Amsterdam being by far the most influential. Local privileges were cherished all through the Dutch Republic. Indeed, this local orientation would very much continue to direct the way in which public matters were settled during much of the 19th century.

The Dutch Republic was a professedly Calvinist country, although its Reformed Church did not obtain the status of a state Church, and a considerable percentage of the Dutch population remained Catholic or belonged either to one of the smaller Protestant denominations or to one of the Jewish communities.[7] Although freedom of religion was not formally granted, non-Calvinists met few obstacles in this respect, at any rate by the 18th century.[8] The actual practice of religious tolerance implied that non-Calvinist denominations could also be forced to look after their own ill and poor members. And this is exactly what happened from around 1700 onwards.[9] Apart from its strongly local orientation Dutch political culture was therefore also characterised by the organisation of (semi-)public activities along religious lines. Thus it appears that the Dutch process of 'pillarisation' in the 19th and 20th centuries has its roots way back in the 18th century, or even earlier as S. Groenveld has suggested.[10] Pillarisation refers to the formation of 'pillars' – that is, population groups whose members perform a significant proportion of their social, cultural and political activities within their own religious or ideological circle. These pillars also include the organisations (from political parties to schools, hospitals or sporting clubs) which have been established to facilitate this kind of behaviour.

The Dutch 'golden age' of the 17th century was followed by a still fairly prosperous 18th century. Trade and shipping remained the principal economic activities, but, with the deterioration of the economic situation from the 1770s onwards, the Dutch Republic lost its leading status. Prices rose and the number of unemployed increased. The ensuing strain on poor relief resulted in a stream of publications on how poor relief should be reformed and how the problem of poverty should be tackled. As a result, a number of 'enlightened' solutions were proposed particularly by the anti-Orangist camp of the *Patriotten* – the movement which wanted to democratise and revitalise the Dutch Republic – and the numerous learned societies which had by then sprung up.[11] Poor relief, which only resulted in laziness, was rejected in favour of setting people to work. Work should therefore be provided for, as well as education and moral edification.

But what did poor relief in the towns actually amount to during the 18th century? The regions or towns which have been best covered by historical research are the northern province of Friesland, the South-Brabant town of Den Bosch or 's-Hertogenbosch (Bois-le-Duc), and both Amsterdam and Leiden in the province of Holland, the province where about half the population – some 1 million people – lived.[12] The general image which can be distilled from this research is that poor relief was primarily meant to be for fellow townspeople rather than strangers, for fellow believers, and for the 'deserving' or 'traditional' poor – that is, ill people, invalids, the elderly and widows with children.[13]

Except for Amsterdam, which depended on a steady stream of immigrants for shipping and related activities, the towns (as well as the countryside) tended to do their utmost to avoid having to provide poor relief for people coming from elsewhere, nor were they inclined to allow begging.[14] From the late 17th century onwards, immigrants were required, by acts of indemnity, to show so-called letters of surety or indemnity from their former place of residence. These letters contained a guarantee that the costs of poor relief for the immigrant would be refunded up to a certain period after his or her departure. However, in practice, these arrangements proved fairly difficult to enforce.

An exclusionist policy also became common practice as far as poor relief on the part of the various Churches was concerned. Poor relief was only provided to members of one's own Church, and recipients could also be subjected to restrictive measures such as a minimum period of membership. On the other hand, poor relief provided by the Church could even include assistance to the less poor – the so-called genteel or shamefaced poor who could no longer afford to live a decent life and risked social degradation. In Friesland, for example, where the Churches' obligation to provide poor relief for their own members was regulated by provincial law in the 1750s, the Reformed and the Mennonites are known especially to have assisted their members relatively generously, while at the same time exercising an increasingly restrictive admission policy for new members.[15]

The organisation of poor relief differed regionally, both from town to town and over time. Responsibility could be either concentrated or more or less spread over Churches and public authorities. In Friesland the various Churches became primarily responsible for rendering poor relief to their own members, while public poor relief was reserved for the remaining poor. In Amsterdam similar arrangements evolved. In Den Bosch, on the other hand, public poor relief was offered to all the local poor, irrespective of their religious affiliation. Indeed, in the mainly Catholic southern parts of the country, poor relief was to a large extent financed from public funds, whereas church funds played a much bigger role in the rest of the country.[16]

On the whole, poor relief was far from generous; in fact, it was fairly minimal and by no means sufficient to live on.[17] People were expected to earn at least some money themselves, and to call on relatives or neighbours for assistance. Already long before the late 18th century, when warnings were aired that poor relief resulted in laziness, it was commonly understood that those who could work should do so, whether in urban workhouses or elsewhere. The great majority of those receiving poor relief lived somehow on their own. Poor relief consisted mainly of food and money, but fuel and free medical care and education were usually provided as well.

Thus health care, or rather medical care, was one of the forms of poor relief. In the case of public poor relief, medical care was usually provided by specially appointed town doctors, surgeons or midwives. Orphanages and the charitable agencies of particular denominations (*diaconieën*) could also appoint their own medical personnel, or they paid for medical services on an incidental basis. If things developed badly, the sick poor could eventually be sent to the town hospital.

However, health care comprised more than just the provision of medical care to the poor. Increasing attention would be paid to the prevention of disease. By the beginning of the 18th century the plague belonged to the past, and cholera would only make its appearance much later, in the early 1830s. But diseases such as smallpox could still develop into real epidemics. Although the introduction of variolation in the second half of the 18th century was supported by enlightened intellectuals and Huguenots, it would not become common practice. In Groningen, to give but one example, it was introduced in both orphanages in 1770, but in many other towns variolation was prohibited by the local authorities because of the medical risks.[18] The safer vaccination with cowpox would become much more widely propagated and applied from the beginning of the 19th century onwards. Moreover, towards the end of the 18th century, medical doctors became increasingly active in proposing various hygienic measures to the local authorities. Having organised themselves in the *Correspondentie-Sociëteit* in 1778, they carried out extensive studies of the environmental causes of diseases and modes of prevention.[19]

If, towards the end of the 18th century, the provision of work for the poor was being promoted with renewed vigour as the best solution for the problem of poverty, then it could have been expected that the physical condition of the poor would have received as much attention. For was it not a matter of course that poverty and illness represented two sides of the same coin? Clearly, illness kept people from working, and therefore caused poverty. But the other way round? It seems that medical doctors or other contemporaneous commentators were much less inclined to point out that poverty could easily lead to illness. Apparently solutions for the problem of poverty were only seldom sought in the provision of both work and healthy conditions for the poor.

Prospects of renewal: the Dutch and the French, 1795–1813

The demands for reforms of the existing system of poor relief, however, remained largely ineffective. Nor did suggestions to improve health care and illness prevention come to much. The ideas were there, but however enlightened, the economic and political situation had been far from favourable for their realisation. The Patriot Revolution (1780–1787) had been ended by Prussian troops and followed by an Orangist restoration. When, in early 1795, the French revolutionary army marched in, the *Patriotten* – or the *Bataven* as they called themselves by then – seized the opportunity to start another revolution, the Batavian Revolution, resulting in the foundation of the Batavian Republic which would last until 1806. In 1806 the Netherlands became a monarchy with Napoleon's brother Louis Bonaparte as its king. In 1810 the Kingdom of the Netherlands was incorporated in the French Empire. This situation would last until Napoleon's defeat in 1813.

Times were turbulent and economically difficult. Nevertheless, the foundations for a unitary state were finally being laid. In 1798 a national Constitution was proclaimed which implied, amongst other things, the unity of law, the separation between Church and state and the abolition of the guilds. What followed was a constant tussle between unitarians and federalists. As it turned out, it was by no means easy to enforce centralist measures on a traditionally non-centralised country. Provincial, local and Church autonomy continued to be cherished.

What difference did the Batavian and the French periods make to the fields of health care and poor relief? Research into the actual practice of health care and poor relief is relatively scarce for this period. Somewhat more is known about the successive attempts at legislation.[20] With respect to health care, special attention has been paid to smallpox epidemics and attempts to control this disease throughout the 18th and 19th centuries.[21] As regards poor relief the most information is available on Maastricht in the south-eastern province of Limburg, as well as on Den Bosch, Amsterdam and Leiden.[22]

It is particularly interesting to see what happened to legislation. In Article 62 of the unitarian Constitution of 1798, which was specially dedicated to health care, it was stated that the representative body should by means of 'wholesome legislation' extend its care to anything that could generally contribute to the health of the citizens, while removing, as far as possible, all barriers. Between 1801 and 1804 departmental (provincial) and local medical committees were installed which were to take over the supervisory and training tasks of the former corporative bodies – namely, the medical or medico-pharmaceutical colleges and the surgeon's guilds. After a brief interlude (1811–1813) during which French public health laws were in force, the departmental and local medical committees were restored in 1814. Although it had been the intention of the Batavian reformers to introduce uniform regulations for medical training and practice, these intentions had not come to pass. Nor would they materialise within the foreseeable future, for the medical state settlement of 1818 would more or less replicate the Batavian regulations. The unintended effect of all this was that Dutch medical training and practice were in fact in a worse state than before 1795. Before long, new generations of physicians would sound the alarm.[23]

However disappointing the results of medical legislation may have been, more progress was made with regard to smallpox. In 1801 smallpox was decreed to be public enemy number one. Variolation was outlawed in 1808, and vaccination was strongly promoted. At least half of the children born during the French period were vaccinated – about half of them free of charge.[24] King Willem I would continue this policy.

A similar story can be related about the legislation on poor relief. In Article 47 of the unitarian Constitution of 1798 it was stated that society supplies work to the industrious and assistance to the needy. But, it continued, those who are wilfully idle have no right to assistance and begging is to be banned completely. These were familiar words, except for the role allotted to 'society' and the implied right to work or poor relief. However, it proved to be difficult to reach consensus about the contents of the law which was to be elaborated along these lines within six months. What should be the tasks of the state, the municipalities and the Churches? And how was poor relief going to be financed? In 1800 the Poor Law was finally passed. Only those poor people who did not receive poor relief from other institutions would be considered as 'children of the state'. This meant that there was still a role for the Churches, albeit that they were going to be subjected to a mild form of government control. Furthermore, the acts of indemnity were abolished, which resulted in many problems.[25]

The new Constitution of 1801 partially restored the autonomy of the towns and the provinces. By 1802 it was decided that the acts of indemnity were to be preserved. For the time being, this meant that attempts to centralise poor relief and make it uniform had come to nothing. In 1811, after the Netherlands had become part of the French Empire, the system of the acts of indemnity was substituted by the Law on the Domicile of Relief which prescribed that poor relief had to be provided by the municipality where one was born. However, if the person in question had moved to another municipality and had lived there for one year, then such provision would become the responsibility of this other municipality. In 1818 another Law on the Domicile of Relief was passed, extending the term of residence to four years.

In the meantime several inquiries had been held into the organisation, financing and actual provision of poor relief in different parts of the country. Not surprisingly, they showed that the differences between both regions and charitable institutions were considerable. Uniformity and centralisation were still far away. In every case the financing of poor relief, resistance on the part of the Churches and the tradition of local autonomy proved to be the main obstacles.

From royal rule to constitutional monarchy, 1813–1848

Disregarding the Belgian part of the United Kingdom of the Netherlands, which lasted from 1815 to 1830, the main developments to be noted are the fairly authoritarian rule by King Willem I (until 1840), aimed at state- and nation-building, and gradual but overall uneven economic growth during most of the 19th century. Although the Belgian revolt and the agrarian crisis due to potato disease in the 1840s gave rise to financial and social problems, the Netherlands was still one of the richest countries in Europe and, for that matter, the world. The exploitation of the Dutch East Indian colonies proved to be a true goldmine, providing up to 30 per cent of the public money.

International trade and finance, as well as the agrarian sector and small-scale industry, were still important. Only towards the end of the 19th century would industrialisation really get going.

During the reign of the 'merchant king' Willem I, only limited progress was made in the field of health care. The medical state settlement of 1818 proved to be highly unsatisfactory, but it would be 1865 before new medical laws would be passed. Also in 1818 a Royal Decree was issued containing exhortations for improving care of the insane in institutions.[26] This decree is known as the 'humane decree'. For the first time it was officially established that mental institutions had as their aim healing 'these unfortunates' – the insane. Although enquiries into the situation of the insane and proposals for drastic reforms were made, the Belgian revolt paralysed further action on the part of the Dutch government for the time being. Only after the passing of a law in 1841, containing provisions about the institutions for the insane and procedures for their admission and discharge, would conditions gradually improve. A number of institutions were closed down, some others were modernised and, in 1849, a new mental institution, Meerenberg, was opened in the dunes of North-Holland.

While three decades earlier the alarming publications of the Amsterdam physician C.J. Nieuwenhuys[27] on the health conditions in Amsterdam had been to no avail, and the first, fairly small, cholera epidemic of 1832 had only resulted in minor government measures, the time had now become ripe for action on the part of the physicians. In 1849 they organised themselves into the Dutch Society for the Advancement of Medicine. Their aim was to achieve a radical renewal of medical legislation in order to improve the material position and expertise of the medical profession. The so-called hygienists amongst them were also intent on reforming public health care. It was from their circles that the initiative had come to found Meerenberg and to do so according to modern insights into psychiatric treatment and care. However, the hygienists' concerns reached much further.[28] They wanted to improve material living conditions, especially of the poor, in order to improve the physical condition of the people and thus to combat poverty. Simple poor relief and the moral education of the poor were deemed to be insufficient. Initially, the hygienic movement attempted to improve living conditions by publishing hygienic recommendations. However, it would soon become clear that much more was needed – namely, public measures to improve housing, sewerage, conditions at work and the like.

With respect to poor relief, the Constitution of 1815 contained a provision which obliged the king to report yearly to the Estates-General on poor relief and the education of poor children. Poor relief remained locally and segmentedly organised. A general Poor Law would be passed only much later, in 1854. It soon became clear that the 1818 Law on the Domicile of Relief gave rise to many problems, one being the question whether the law should also be applied to poor relief by the Churches. By 1822 this was indeed decreed to be the case.[29] But actual practice proved to be different. The *diaconie* of the Reformed Church in Rotterdam, for example, would until 1853 continue refusing poor relief to members who had been born elsewhere.[30]

The only new initiative which should be mentioned was the foundation of the *Maatschappij van weldadigheid* (Benevolent Society) in 1818 by Johannes van den Bosch, with the support of the King's son, Prince Frederik.[31] This society started a number of agricultural colonies in the north of the country. Initially its aim was to provide the urban poor with a means of existence. However, because it was not sufficiently successful, the emphasis was soon shifted to forced employment of marginal groups such as beggars, abandoned children and also orphans. The central government guaranteed the yearly supply of a group of these people. Already in the early 1830s it became clear that this new formula did not function as well as had been hoped.[32] Except for the *Maatschappij*, work was provided for the destitute in charitable workhouses. Between 1832 and 1850 the number of charitable, mostly urban, workhouses increased from 27 to 50.[33]

Research on urban poor relief in the first half of the 19th century has again been concentrated on Amsterdam, Leiden, Den Bosch and Maastricht, but this time Rotterdam and Haarlem have been included as well.[34] From Marco van Leeuwen's substantial research on Amsterdam it can be learned that in the period 1829–54 one-quarter of the Amsterdam population received poor relief on a more or less regular basis, which amounts to some 55 000 men, women and children.[35] The majority of the destitute were sick or infirm, aged, widows with children or workers with large families. Most poor relief, some 90 per cent, was outdoor relief. As in the 18th century, poor relief was by no means sufficient to live on; the poor had to rely on other 'survival strategies' as well.[36] The Churches distributed charity to about three times as many persons as the municipal authorities. The share of the Reformed Church was by far the largest, offering relief to over one-third of the destitute.[37]

In Rotterdam about 17 per cent of the population received poor relief both in 1796 and in 1859, which is a somewhat lower percentage than in Amsterdam. About one-third of them received charity from public institutions, while the rest were cared for by Church or, to a much lesser extent, private institutions. The share of the Reformed Church appears to have been somewhat bigger than in Amsterdam.[38]

In Maastricht, on the other hand, it was primarily the civil poor administration (*Burgerlijk Armbestuur*) which provided assistance. The *Burgerlijk Armbestuur* assisted, irrespective of Church membership, about 40 to 50 per cent of the destitute.[39] Charitable institutions of the churches, the large majority of them being Catholic, could provide additional relief for their own parishioners. Religious charity had an even smaller share in poor relief in

Den Bosch than in Maastricht. However, in Maastricht the share of public poor relief was still much larger than in most Dutch towns.[40] This division of labour would be reversed by the introduction of the Poor Law of 1854 which gave priority to poor relief by the Churches. The share of public poor relief in Maastricht then decreased to some 10 to 15 per cent. Medical poor relief would, however, primarily remain the responsibility of the *Burgerlijk Armbestuur*. It also spent much money on schools for children of the poor, and on assistance to the elderly.[41]

Haarlem, west of Amsterdam in the province of North-Holland, employed yet another system. While the Churches provided poor relief to their own members, the care for the so-called *stadsarmen* – those poor who were not members of a Church – was contracted out to the *diaconie* of the Reformed Church. In fact, all poor administrations were to a large extent subsidised, and also financially and otherwise controlled, by the municipal authorities.[42]

In whatever way poor relief was organised, it is certainly clear that poverty remained a serious problem in Dutch society. Health conditions were problematic as well, with, for example, a quite serious cholera epidemic occurring in 1848–49. We shall now turn to the various solutions which were suggested by contemporaries.

Poverty, the most serious of diseases: changing views on old problems, 1848–c.1900

The Constitution of 1848 marked the establishment of a parliamentary system and the victory of liberalism at central level. Already during the preceding years there had been much discussion over the problems of both health care and poverty. Hygienists would continue to discuss these problems, shocked by their own observations of the living conditions of the poor, while they also compiled health statistics to provide a factual basis. S. Sr. Coronel, for example, until 1860 town physician at Middelburg in the province of Zeeland and from 1860 to 1866 at Amsterdam, published in 1859 a pamphlet on poor relief in this town. He wrote that poverty was actually the most serious disease at that time.[43] In 1860 the Dutch Society for the Advancement of Medicine asked him to make an inquiry into the state of medical poor relief in the Netherlands. Within a year, however, Coronel had to conclude that his task had failed because of a total lack of cooperation on the part of municipalities, charity boards and even physicians.[44] In a pamphlet on hygiene applied to the manufacturing industry, published one year later, Coronel advocated prevention with respect to both health and social problems.

> Just as medical science has recently aimed at finding the means to prevent diseases rather than curing them, and just as medical science, following this way, has produced more wholesome effects for the life of

the citizen and society than the old medical science had done during the centuries of her reign, so it should also be the task of political science to prevent social diseases.[45]

In fact, the lawyer and political scientist J. de Bosch Kemper, professor at the Athenaeum Illustre at Amsterdam from 1852 to 1862, had already set an example in this direction with his historical research on poverty in 'our fatherland', published in 1851. Having partially attributed the poor state of health of many members of 'the lower orders' to 'immorality' (alcohol abuse scored highly) and previous poverty, he counted health care for 'the lower orders' – that is, health care in a broad sense, including better housing, hygiene and food – as one of the most powerful means of preventing poverty. He concluded that 'much as ill health may be a result of poverty, it is also a continuous cause of poverty. Improve the health of the people, and you will have removed a major, a very great cause of poverty.'[46]

Old ideas also kept cropping up, such as De Bosch Kemper's view that poor relief caused laziness and that the problem of poverty could only be solved by setting the poor to work, and by indeed providing work and seeing to their moral edification.[47] Especially on the part of the Reformed Church it was increasingly stressed that poverty was caused by sin. This meant that the poor should be taught and stimulated to lead a morally irreproachable life. Indeed, to an increasing extent this became a precondition for qualifying for poor relief, irrespective of who provided it.

Moreover, the Constitution of 1848 ordained that the administration of poor relief had to be regulated by law. Royal Decrees were to belong to the past. After much discussion the Poor Law was finally passed in 1854. It was both a compromise between advocates and opponents of state interference, and a victory for the Churches and those liberals who were against increasing state interference. It was determined that poor relief was primarily the responsibility (although not the obligation) of the Churches and that only in the last instance, if the means of the Churches proved insufficient or the poor did not qualify for charity from the Churches, it was the responsibility of the state or, rather, the municipal poor administration, the *Burgerlijk Armbestuur*. It was also decided that the destitute person's place of birth had to pay for the costs of public poor relief. This was changed in the next Poor Law of 1870: acccording to that law the present domicile of the destitute had to pay. Moreover, from 1854 onwards medical poor relief became the responsibility of the municipal authorities.

Neither of these Poor Laws included the right to relief: poor relief was considered to be a moral, not a public duty.[48] Thus poor relief remained a primarily local and private or, rather, a Church responsibility, and uniformity was a long way off. Moreover, while religious charity had been invested with the primary responsibility for poor relief, the actual costs were increasingly financed from public funds. In 1855 the Churches were paying about 50 per cent of the total costs of poor relief, versus 40 per cent by public authorities. By 1900 the public share had increased to 47 per cent, and it would further grow to 57 per cent in 1913. The share of private organisations was also growing, from 10 to 15 per cent between 1850 and 1900.[49]

Research on urban poor relief in the second half of the 19th century has again been focused on Amsterdam, Rotterdam, Den Bosch, and Maastricht and also on Alkmaar, while separate studies have been devoted to the care for the elderly.[50] Moreover, a fair amount of attention has been paid to contemporary debates on poverty and poor relief, and to legislation with respect to poor relief and related subjects.[51] In the field of health care, special mention should be made of research into the control of cholera and smallpox, the hygienist movement, health conditions in Amsterdam, hospitals, nursing, mental health care and financial and legal arrangements with respect to illness and health care.[52] In fact, only a very limited selection of this broad range of topics and studies will be discussed here. The accent will lie on changing ideas about, and ways of dealing with, the problem of poverty and poor relief towards the end of the 19th century. Much less attention will be paid to developments in the field of health care and preventive, hygienic measures, however impressive they may have been.

Already, from the late 1840s onwards, local departments of the St Vincentius Society had been founded, mainly in the southern parts of the Netherlands. The society first of all aimed at the salvation of its own members. In the second instance it aimed at other people's virtuousness and salvation, while the provision of material assistance was considered to be a means of access to the hearts of the poor. Frequent and fairly intensive personal contacts between the poor and members of the society were thought to be the best way to achieve these aims. Similar approaches could be found in other private charitable organisations, whether or not religiously based, although their aims could be different.[53] In fact, insofar as their personal approach or patronage are concerned, these organisations may be seen as precursors of the 'modern', individualised poor relief.

Private charitable societies, founded later on a non-religious basis, such as *Liefdadigheid naar Vermogen* at Amsterdam (1871), also made a point of intensively visiting and supervising the poor. Their aim was not salvation or even virtuousness *per se*, but stimulating and helping the poor to (get) work and thus become independent of relief.[54] It was primarily the Elberfeld system of poor relief that inspired the work of these later private charitable societies. As it happens, it also inspired attempts at reforming public poor relief along these lines. Educating the poor to live an industrious life was, of course, a much older idea, but the intensive way in which this was now being done was fairly new. Moreover, the coordination or centralisation of poor relief at local level scored high on the agenda of these reformers of poor relief.

Changing the habits of the poor and reorganising poor relief was one thing, but creating more favourable circumstances for the poor was another. While liberals had formerly been promoting a free market system as the best solution to the problem of poverty, socially-oriented liberals were now no longer averse to state interference. The economic depressions between the late 1870s and the early 1890s, the take-off of industrialisation and the population increase, especially in the towns, stimulated people to think of solutions to the problem of poverty and what was from then on called the 'social question'. Around 1870 the first trade unions were founded, while the Labour Law of 1889 marked the beginning of social legislation. But the problem of poverty required more than that. In the 1890s several reports were published which stressed the dire situation of the poor and the need for public measures. However, a new Poor Law, which accorded the poor the right to relief and which laid the primary responsibility for poor relief with the public authorities, failed to be passed in 1901. The liberals had lost power to confessional parties, who wanted to continue the primacy of religious charity. Not until 1912 would another attempt to have a new Poor Law passed be successful. This law, however, still affirmed the principle that the public sector should only provide subsidiary relief.[55]

The living conditions of the poor were still very bad indeed. Their poor housing, the almost entire lack of waterworks and sewerage before 1880 and their poor diet, not to mention their poor personal hygiene or frequent drunkenness, all added up to a tendency towards ill-health and disease. This had already been noticed earlier on, but, with the advance of medical knowledge, there could no longer be any doubt whatsoever about the connection between poverty, poor living conditions and illness. The problem of poverty was that it caused illness, and the problem of illness was that it caused poverty. This two-way connection between problems of poverty and illness was fully acknowledged by the end of the 19th century. Its political translation into legislation may have been tardy as far as poor relief was concerned, but this was partly compensated for by the passing, in 1901, of a Public Health Act, a Housing Act and an Industrial Injuries Act.

In fact, by that time, the economic modernisation of the Netherlands was well on its way, although it would still take a long time before poverty and the poor, illness and the ill would more fully become subject to state care. Parochialism and Church opposition would finally be overcome. Eventually, the Netherlands would even develop into 'the world's most extensive welfare state'.[56]

Acknowledgements

I am grateful to Peter Jansen, Marco van Leeuwen, Maarten Prak and Frans Smits for their generous advice on the subject of Dutch poor relief.

Notes

1. Sir William Temple, *Observations upon the United Provinces of the Nether-lands*, Cambridge, 1932 (1st edn 1673), p. 104. Cited in Jonathan I. Israel, *The Dutch Republic. Its Rise, Greatness, and Fall 1477–1806*, Oxford, 1995, p. 355.

2. See Marco H.D. van Leeuwen, *Bijstand in Amsterdam ca. 1800–1850. Armenzorg als beheersings- en overlevingsstrategie*, Zwolle and Amsterdam, 1992, p. 349 n. 5.

3. Ibid., p. 12.

4. Cited by ibid., pp. 12, 349 n.3.

5. Exceptions are two studies on poor relief: see P.A.C. Douwes, *Armenkerk. De Hervormde diaconie te Rotterdam in de negentiende eeuw*, Rotterdam, 1977; B.P.A. Gales, L.H.M. Kreukels, J.J.G. Luijten and F.H.M. Roebroeks, *Het Burgerlijk Armbestuur. Twee eeuwen zorg voor armen, zieken en ouderen te Maastricht 1796–1996*, 2 vols, Maastricht, 1997, and an article on medical care by the Rotterdam reformed (Calvinist) Church in the 17th century, M.J. van Lieburg, 'Geneeskundige zorg als kerkelijke taak. De situatie in de gereformeerde kerk van Rotterdam in de zeventiende eeuw', *De zeventiende eeuw*, 5 (1989), pp. 162–771. See also the studies on financial arrangements with respect to illness and health care: Henk van der Velden, *Financiële toegankelijkheid tot gezondheidszorg in Nederland, 1850–1941*, Amsterdam, 1993; Klasien Horstman, *Verzekerd leven. Artsen en levensverzekeringsmaatschappijen 1880–1920*, Amsterdam, 1996; K.P. Companje, *Over artsen en verzekeraars. Een historische studie naar de factoren, die de relatie ziekenfondsen – artsen vanaf 1827 op landelijk en regionaal niveau hebben beïnvloed*, Twello, 1997. See also the collection of essays on risks, risk management, and insurances: Jacques van Gerwen and Marco H.D. van Leeuwen, *Studies over zekerheidsarrangementen. Risico's, risicobestrijding en verzekeringen in Nederland vanaf de Middeleeuwen*, Amsterdam and The Hague, 1998.

6. A.M. van der Woude, *Nederland over de schouder gekeken*, Utrecht, 1986, p. 26.

7. In 1809 55.4 per cent of the population of the Kingdom of the Netherlands was Reformed, 38.1 per cent Catholic, 2.8 per cent Lutheran, 1.4 per cent Mennonite, 0.18 per cent Remonstrant, while 1.8 per cent were Jews. If the former General-ity Lands with their mainly Catholic population, are excluded, the percentages are: 68 per cent Reformed, 23 per cent Catholic, 3.5 per cent Lutheran, 1.8 per cent Mennonite, 0.24 per cent Remonstrant, 2.2 per cent Jews. J.A. de Kok, *Nederland op de breuklijn Rome-Reformatie*, Assen, 1964, p. 288. Cited in Israel, *The Dutch Republic*, (n.1), p. 1029.

8. Marijke Gijswijt-Hofstra (ed.), *Een schijn van verdraagzaamheid. Afwijking en tolerantie in Nederland van de zestiende eeuw tot heden*, Hilversum, 1989. See also Israel, *The Dutch Republic* (n.1).

9. See on Friesland Joke Spaans, *Armenzorg in Friesland 1500–1800. Publieke zorg en particuliere liefdadigheid in zes Friese steden: Leeuwarden, Bolsward, Franeker, Sneek, Dokkum en Harlingen*, Hilversum en Leeuwarden, 1998. See on Haarlem A.P.A.M. Spijkers, 'Van aalmoes to sociale bijstand. Een overzicht van de stedelijke armenzorg in Haarlem', *Haerlem jaarboek 1979*, pp. 66–98. See on Leiden G.P.M. Pot, *Arm Leiden. Levensstandaard, bedeling en bedeelden, 1750–1854*, Hilversum, 1994. See on Rotterdam C.W. van Voorst van Beest, *De katholieke armenzorg te Rotterdam in de 17e en 18e eeuw*, 's-Gravenhage, 1955.

10. S. Groenveld, *Huisgenoten des geloofs. Was de samenleving in de Republiek der Verenigde Nederlanden verzuild?*, Hilversum, 1995. See, on pillarisation, A. Lijphart, *The Politics of Accommodation. Pluralism and Democracy in the Netherlands*, Berkeley, 1968; J.C.H. Blom and C.J. Misset (eds), '*Broeders sluit U aan'. Aspecten van verzuiling in zeven Hollandse gemeenten*, 's-Gravenhage, 1985.

11. For example, the *Oeconomische Tak* (1777) of the *Hollandsche Maatschappij van Wetenschappen and the Maatschappij tot Nut van 't Algemeen* (1784). See, for contemporary publications on poverty, H.F.J.M. van den Eerenbeemt, 'Armoede in de 'gedrukte' optiek van de sociale bovenlaag in Nederland, 1750–1850', *Tijdschrift voor geschiedenis*, **88** (1975), pp. 468–500; H.F.J.M. van den Eerenbeemt, *Armoede en arbeidsdwang. Werkinrichtingen voor 'onnutte' Nederlanders in de Republiek 1760–1795. Een mentaliteitsgeschiedenis*, 's-Gravenhage, 1977.

12. On Friesland see Spaans, *Armenzorg in Friesland* (n.9). On Den Bosch see H.F.J.M. van den Eerenbeemt, *In het spanningsveld der armoede. Agressief pauperisme en reactie in Staats-Brabant*, Tilburg, 1968; idem *Armoede en arbeidsdwang* (n.11); Ton Kappelhof, *Armenzorg in Den Bosch. De Negen Blokken 1350–1810*, Utrecht, 1983; M. Prak, 'Overvloed of onbehagen? Armen, armoede en armenzorg in 's-Hertogenbosch, 1770–1850', in J. van Oudheusden and G.M.T. Trienekens (eds), *Een pront wijf, een mager paard en een zoon op het seminarie*, Den Bosch, 1993, pp. 7–44; M. Prak, 'Goede buren en verre vrienden. De ontwikkeling van onderstand bij armoede in Den Bosch sedert de Middeleeuwen', in H. Flap and M.H.D. van Leeuwen (eds), *Op lange termijn. Verklaringen van trends in de geschiedenis van samenlevingen*, Hilversum, 1994, pp. 147–69. On Amsterdam see Anne E.C. McCants, *Civic Charity in a Golden Age. Orphan Care in Early Modern Amsterdam*, Urbana and Chicago, 1997; Marco H.D. van Leeuwen, 'Amsterdam en de armenzorg tijdens de Republiek', *NEHA-Jaarboek voor economische, bedrijfs- en techniekgeschiedenis*, **59** (1996), pp. 132–61. On Leiden see Pot, *Arm Leiden* (n.9); S. Groenveld, 'Geef van uw haaf Een milde gaaf Ons arme Weesen'. De zorg voor wezen, tot 1800, als onderdeel van de armenzorg', in S. Groenveld (ed.), *Daar de orangie-appel in de gevel staat. In en om het weeshuis der doopsgezinde collegianten 1675–1975*, Amsterdam, 1975, pp. 9–51. See, for a general overview of Dutch poor relief, Maarten Prak, 'Armenzorg 1500–1800', in Van Gerwen and Van Leeuwen, *Studies over zekerheidsarrangementen* (n.5), pp. 49–90.

13. M.H.D. van Leeuwen, *Sociale zorg*, Zutphen, 1994, pp. 10–11.

14. Van Leeuwen, 'Amsterdam en de armenzorg' (n.12).

15. Spaans, *Armenzorg in Friesland* (n.9), pp. 305–14.

16. Prak, 'Goede buren en verre vrienden' (n.12), p. 160.

17. Van Leeuwen, 'Amsterdam en de armenzorg' (n.12).

18. Willibord Rutten, *De vreselijkste aller harpijen. Pokkenepidemieën en pokkenbestrijding in Nederland in de 18e en 19e eeuw*, 't Goy-Houten, 1997, p. 193; Frank Huisman, 'Genezers, magistraat en samenleving. Groninger gezondheidszorg in de tijd van de Republiek', in Frank Huisman (ed.), *Gezond weer op in Groningen. Gezondheidszorg en medisch beroep 1500–1900* Groningen, 1993, pp. 33–66 at p. 61.

19. Frank Huisman, 'De correspondenten. Medici, staat en samenleving tijdens de Nederlandse Verlichting', in Frank Huisman and Catrien Santing (eds), *Medische geschiedenis in regionaal perspectief. Groningen 1500–1900*, Rotterdam, 1997,

pp. 69–99; H.F.J.M. van den Eerenbeemt, *Arts en sociaal besef in Nederland in historisch perspectief*, Tilburg, 1969.

20. P.B.A. Melief, *De strijd om de armenzorg in Nederland 1795–1854*, Groningen and Djakarta, 1955; J.K. van der Korst, *Om lijf & leven. Gezondheidszorg en geneeskunst in Nederland circa 1200–1960*, Utrecht, 1988.

21. Rutten, *De vreselijkste aller harpijen* (n.18).

22. Gales et al., *Het Burgerlijk Armbestuur* (n.5); see note 12 for literature on Den Bosch, Amsterdam and Leiden.

23. Van der Korst, *Om lijf & leven* (n.20).

24. Rutten, *De vreselijkste aller harpijen* (n.18), ch. 8.

25. Melief, *De strijd om de armenzorg* (n.20), p. 65

26. Joost Vijselaar (ed.), *Gesticht in de duinen. De geschiedenis van de provinciale psychiatrische ziekenhuizen van Noord-Holland van 1849 tot 1994*, Hilversum, 1997, ch. 1.

27. C.J. Nieuwenhuys, *Proeve eener geneeskundige plaatsbeschrijving der stad Amsterdam*, 4 vols, Amsterdam, 1816–1820.

28. See E.S. Houwaart, *De hygiënisten. Artsen, staat & volksgezondheid in Nederland 1840–1890*, Groningen, 1991.

29. Melief, *De strijd om de armenzorg* (n.20), pp. 119–20.

30. Douwes, *Armenkerk* (n.5), pp. 45–47.

31. R. Berends et al., *Arbeid ter disciplinering en bestraffing. Veenhuizen als onvrije kolonie van de Maatschappij van Weldadigheid, 1823–1859*, Zutphen, 1984; J.D. Dorgelo, *De Koloniën van de Maatschappij van Weldadigheid (1818–1859). Een landbouwkundig en sociaal-economisch experiment*, Assen, 1964; C.A. Kloosterhuis, *De bevolking van de vrije Koloniën der Maatschappij van Weldadigheid*, Zutphen, 1981; Frances Gouda, *Poverty and Political Culture. The Rhetoric of Social Welfare in the Netherlands and France, 1815–1854*, Amsterdam, 1995, pp. 235–41.

32. Van Leeuwen, *Sociale zorg* (n.13), p. 11.

33. Gouda, *Poverty and Political Culture* (n.31), p. 234. See on charitable work-houses in the late 18th century Van den Eerenbeemt, *Armoede en arbeidsdwang* (n.11).

34. On Amsterdam see Van Leeuwen, *Bijstand in Amsterdam* (n.2); Marco H.D. van Leeuwen, 'Surviving with a Little Help: The Importance of Charity to the Poor of Amsterdam 1800–50, in a Comparative Perspective', *Social History*, **18** (1993), pp. 319–38. On Leiden see Pot, *Arm Leiden* (n.9). On Den Bosch: Prak, 'Overvloed of onbehagen?' (n.12); Prak, 'Goede buren en verre vrienden' (n.12). On Maastricht: Gales et al., *Het Burgerlijk Armbestuur* (n.5). On Rotterdam see Douwes, *Armenkerk* (n.5). On Haarlem see Nico Siffels and Willem van Spijker, 'Haarlemse paupers. Arbeidsmarkt, armoede en armenzorg in Haarlem in de eerste helft van de negentiende eeuw', *Tijdschrift voor sociale geschiedenis*, **13** (1987), pp. 458–93. See also Gouda, *Poverty and Political Culture* (n.31). See, for a general overview of Dutch poor relief in the 19th and early 20th century, Marco H.D. van Leeuwen, 'Armenzorg 1800–1912: erfenis van de republiek', in Van Gerwen and Van Leeuwen, *Studies over zekerheidsarrangementen* (n.5), pp. 276–316.

35. Van Leeuwen, 'Surviving with a little help' (n.34), p. 320.

36. Van Leeuwen, *Bijstand in Amsterdam* (n.2); Marco H. D. van Leeuwen, 'Logic of Charity: Poor Relief in Preindustrial Europe', *Journal of Interdisciplinary History*, **24** (1994), pp. 589–613. See also Catharina Lis, *Social change and the labouring poor. Antwerp 1770–1860*, New Haven and London, 1986; L.F. van Loo, *Arm in Nederland 1815–1990*, Meppel and Amsterdam, 1992.

37. Van Leeuwen, *Bijstand in Amsterdam* (n.2), pp. 170–72.
38. Douwes, *Armenkerk* (n. 5), ch. 3.
39. Gales et al., *Het Burgerlijk Armbestuur* (n.5), p. 153.
40. Ibid., p. 223.
41. Ibid., chs 5 and 7.
42. Siffels and Van Spijker, 'Haarlemse paupers' (n.34), p. 460.
43. S. Sr. Coronel, *Middelburg, voorheen en thans. Bijdrage tot de kennis van den voormaligen en tegenwoordigen toestand van het armwezen aldaar*, Middelburg, 1859.
44. Van der Korst, *Om lijf & leven* (n.20), pp. 211–12.
45. S. Sr. Coronel, *De gezondheidsleer toegepast op de fabrieksnijverheid*, Haarlem, 1861, p. 266. Cited in A.C.J. de Vrankrijker, *Een groeiende gedachte. De ontwikkeling der meningen over de sociale kwestie in de 19e eeuw in Nederland*, Assen, 1959, pp. 64–65.
46. J. de Bosch Kemper, *Geschiedkundig onderzoek naar de armoede in ons vaderland, hare oorzaken en de middelen, die tot hare vermindering zouden kunnen worden aangewend*, Haarlem, 1851 (2nd edn 1860), pp. 181, 251–55.
47. See, for a comparative analysis of the discussions in the Netherlands and France, Gouda, *Poverty and Political Culture* (n.31). See for analyses of liberal standpoints T.J. Boschloo, *De productiemaatschappij. Liberalisme, economische wetenschap en het vraagstuk der armoede in Nederland 1800–1875*, Hilversum, 1989; Stefan Dudink, *Deugdzaam liberalisme. Sociaal-liberalisme in Nederland 1870–1901*, Amsterdam, 1997.
48. Melief, *De strijd om de armenzorg* (n.20), ch. VII.
49. Ali de Regt, *Arbeidersgezinnen en beschavingsarbeid. Ontwikkelingen in Nederland 1870–1940*, Meppel and Amsterdam, 1984, p. 145; Douwes, *Armenkerk* (n.5), p. 64.
50. On Amsterdam see Frans Smits, '"Van de wind kan men niet leven". De gemeentelijke armenzorg te Amsterdam in het laatste kwart van de negentiende eeuw', *Tijdschrift voor sociale geschiedenis*, **19** (1993), pp. 94–114; Th. van Tijn, *Twintig jaren Amsterdam. De maatschappelijke ontwikkeling van de hoofdstad van de jaren '50 der vorige eeuw tot 1876*, Amsterdam, 1965. On Rotterdam see Douwes, *Armenkerk* (n.5). On Den Bosch see P.G.J. Huismans, 'Tussen armenzorg en gezondheidszorg. Het groot ziekengasthuis te 's-Hertogenbosch 1850–1920', *Noordbrabants historisch jaarboek 1987*, pp. 121–47; Prak, 'Goede buren en verre vrienden' (n.12); Th. A. Wouters, *Van bedeling naar verheffing. Evolutie in houding tegenover de behoeftige mens te 's-Hertogenbosch 1854–1912*, Tilburg, 1968. On Maastricht see Gales et al., *Het Burgerlijk Armbestuur* (n. 5). On Alkmaar see L. Frank van Loo, *Armelui. Armoede en bedeling te Alkmaar 1850–1914*, Bergen, 1986. Research on care for the elderly: M.M.J. Stavenuiter, *Verzorgd of zelfstandig. Ouderen en de levensloop in Amsterdam in de tweede helft van de negentiende eeuw*, n.p., 1993. Willem Jan van der Veen and Frans van Poppel, 'Institutional Care for the Elderly in the 19th Century: Old People in The Hague and their Institutions', *Ageing and Society*, **12** (1992), pp. 185–212.
51. Boschloo, *De productiemaatschappij* (n.12); J.C. van Dam et al., *Maatschappelijke zorg in historisch perspectief. Honderd jaren Armenwet, 1854–1954*, Alphen aan den Rijn, 1955; Dudink, *Deugdzaam liberalisme* (n.47); Melief, *De strijd om de armenzorg* (n.20); De Regt, *Arbeidersgezinnen en beschavingsarbeid* (n.49); P. de Rooy, *Werklozenzorg en werkloosheidsbestrijding 1917–1940. Landelijk en Amsterdams beleid*, Amsterdam, 1979; Siep Stuurman, *Wacht op onze daden. Het*

liberalisme en de vernieuwing van de Nederlandse staat, Amsterdam, 1992; De Vrankrijker, *Een groeiende gedachte* (n.45); Dirk Jan Wolffram, 'Vliegen in de zalf. Orthodox-protestantse principes en compromissen inzake armenzorg en schoolstrijd, 1850–1900', in Dirk Jan Wolffram (ed.), *Om het christelijk karakter der natie. Confessionelen en de modernisering van de maatschappij*, Amsterdam 1994, pp. 41–58.

52. See respectively H.F.J.M. van den Eerenbeemt, 'De "blauwe dood" als impuls tot maatschappelijke vernieuwing', *Economisch- en sociaalhistorisch jaarboek*, 47 (1984), pp. 91–104; P.D.'t Hart, *Utrecht en de cholera 1832–1910*, Zutphen, 1990; Rutten, *De vreselijkste aller harpijen* (n.18); Houwaart, *De hygiënisten* (n.28); H. van Zon, 'Nederlandse hygiënisten tussen droom en werkelijkheid, 1850–1875', *Groniek*, **131**, special issue *Medische praktijken* (1995), pp. 176–86; J.A. Verdoorn, *Het gezondheidswezen te Amsterdam in de 19e eeuw*, Nijmegen, 1981; M.J. van Lieburg, *Het Coolsingelziekenhuis te Rotterdam (1839–1900)*, Amsterdam, 1986; José Eijt, *Religieuze vrouwen: bruid, moeder, zuster. Geschiedenis van twee Nederlandse zustercongregaties, 1820–1940*, Hilversum, 1995; Nanny Wiegman, 'The Origins of Modern Nursing in the Netherlands', *Nursing History Review*, **4** (1996), pp. 83–97; Vijselaar (ed.), *Gesticht in de duinen* (n.26); Van der Velden, *Financiële toegankelijkheid* (n.5); Caren Japenga and Henk van der Velden, 'Access to Curative Health Care: Sickness Funds versus Medical Relief in the Netherlands (1850–1941)', in Hans Binneveld and Rudolf Dekker (eds), *Curing and Insuring. Essays on Illness in Past Times: the Netherlands, Belgium, England and Italy, 16th–20th Centuries*, Rotterdam, 1992, pp. 169–88; Horstman, *Verzekerd leven* (n.5); Companje, *Over artsen en verzekeraars* (n.5); D. Cannegieter, *Honderdvijftig jaar gezondheidswet*, Assen, 1954.

53. Gales et al., *Het Burgerlijk Armbestuur* (n.5), pp. 228–38; De Rooy, *Werklozenzorg en werkloosheidsbestrijding* (n.51), ch. 1.

54. De Regt, *Arbeidersgezinnen en beschavingsarbeid* (n.49), ch. VI; Smits, '"Van de wind kan men niet leven"' (n.50); De Rooy, *Werklozenzorg en werkloosheidsbestrijding* (n.51).

55. Gouda, *Poverty and Political Culture* (n.31), p. 257.

56. Ibid., pp. 256–257. Gouda cites Goran Therborn, 'Pillarization and Popular Movements. Two Variants of Welfare State Capitalism: The Netherlands and Sweden', in Francis G. Casles (ed.), *The Comparative History of Public Policy*, New York, 1989, p. 193.

PART SIX
France

CHAPTER FOURTEEN

Poor Relief and Medical Assistance in 18th and 19th Century Paris

Matthew Ramsey

Our journey to France starts in the capital, which is how the itinerary of many a hurried tourist begins and often ends, and with the sort of caveat to be found in any Baedeker. Not the usual one, which is that Paris is not France, but the more complicated observation that Paris both is, and is not, the centre. We typically think of modern France as the land of centralisation and the strong state, and yet this image is in many ways misleading. In the period before 1945, the state is better characterised as strong in the abstract but in practice only cautiously interventionist in the social and economic realms. Certain government services, including public health, poor relief and the provision of health care, were not only less well-developed than in several neighbouring European countries, but surprisingly decentralised. Here the revolutionary and Napoleonic legacy was not a powerful machine controlled from the centre, although the state did provide regulation and oversight, but rather a system that relied first of all on local institutions, private philanthropy and mutual aid. The government would second voluntary efforts, with higher levels intervening only when lower ones had proved inadequate.

Paris, capital of public assistance

Yet Paris was, in another sense, very clearly the centre, first of all as France's great metropolis and an extraordinary locus of social and cultural ferment, well before it became, in Walter Benjamin's celebrated phrase, the 'capital of the nineteenth century'. Throughout our period it was also a great commercial and manufacturing centre, though not one of the key sites for the development of large-scale industry. Paris harboured extraordinary concentrations of both wealth and poverty.[1]

Paris was also, of course, the historic political capital of France; Louis XIV's Versailles had been merely a 'royal city'. Although some alarmed conservatives talked about 'decapitalising' Paris following the revolutionary Commune of 1871, the threat was never carried out. As the experience of the Commune suggests, the political capital was also the centre of political radicalism; it was only at the very end of our period that the present more conservative pattern began to take hold. Here Tocqueville's analysis applies: Paris was periodically able to force the national agenda to the left, although actually implementing radical change throughout the country proved far more difficult. The idea of public assistance as a form of social self-defence resonated with a particular force in the capital.

Seen from a certain perspective, Paris was the capital city one would expect to find in a France shaped by centralising forces, from the Bourbon monarchy to Napoleon – although it is possible to argue that the city owed its special position in part to local autonomy and the absence of an integrated system for redistributing resources to the hinterland. It was the site of most major national institutions and, when the state did intervene, it tended to act in Paris first and to expend the most resources there. Paris absorbed the lion's share of French funds devoted to public assistance: about a quarter in 1789, and 23 per cent of total expenditures by all levels of government a century later in 1885, when the inhabitants of the capital made up 5 per cent of the total population. The per capita outlay in Paris at that time was 13.54 francs, far greater than the national average of 1.60.[2] The capital was a magnet for poor people seeking work, but also welfare, drawing 'from everywhere in France and even abroad ... the sick, the infirm, abandoned children, the unfit, indigent idiots ... ' in the acerbic words of a handbook on public assistance published in 1876.[3] Paris was also by far France's greatest medical centre; it was the leader in the public hygiene movement and the site of the most influential investigations of the working classes, poverty and differential mortality.[4] Some of the most important agencies for public health, social welfare, and medical assistance were located there – for the most part not national, but Parisian, institutions. Historians owe a particular debt to the Assistance Publique à Paris, established in 1849 to administer the hospitals, hospices, and outdoor relief systems. It maintains an extraordinary library and archive (the latter with some gaps created when the Communards burned down the Hôtel de Ville in 1871) and even operates a public assistance museum.[5]

This chapter, then, will have much to say about the centre, but less about centralisation. The city of Paris will be the principal, but not the exclusive, concern; it is not possible to write about Paris without writing to some extent about France. (For a fuller account of national developments, especially for the 19th century, see the chapter in this volume by Olivier Faure.) Paris, moreover, was not a fixed geographical entity, since it expanded several times into what had once been its suburbs. In our own time, the city exactly coincides with the *commune* of Paris – the lowest French administrative level, dating from the Revolution; there are far smaller *communes* whose population numbers in the hundreds. It also exactly coincides with the *département* of Paris – another revolutionary innovation, which for most purposes is the first administrative unit below the national level.

Throughout our period, however, Paris was the centre of various circumscriptions larger than the city and smaller than the country. During the ancien régime, it was the seat of a welter of unequal, overlapping and sometimes conflicting jurisdictions – an archdiocese, for example, and a généralité, a royal fiscal and administrative unit headed by an intendant. Paris was also the seat of the most important of the parlements, so-called sovereign courts with important administrative and political, as well as judicial, powers. The parlement of Paris was both the highest court of appeal in the land and a body empowered to issue decrees affecting many aspects of social and economic life in its own vast jurisdiction. Officials of the parlement sat on the boards that ran the major hospitals and administered outdoor relief in Paris; by our period they had ceased, in effect, to be purely municipal institutions.

In the 19th century, Paris formed part of the département of the Seine, whose territory was several times larger than the city proper, and which was itself entirely surrounded by the département of the Seine-et-Oise, which has been called the 'Parisian countryside'.[6] The Seine was administered by a prefect whose powers, together with those of his occasional rival, the prefect of police, generally outweighed those of the municipal council in the areas of public health, medical assistance and social welfare.

The ancien régime

In ancien régime France, as elsewhere in early modern Europe, poor relief and medical assistance were conflated, and the hospital had an ambiguous role – primarily as a shelter for the needy, but with some limited therapeutic functions.[7] The more medically-oriented establishments were usually known as hôtels-Dieu, as opposed to hospices or hospitals, but the terminology was loose and virtually no institution was exclusively devoted to acute care.[8] What is perhaps more distinctive about the French case is the disparity between the relatively modest public resources devoted to assistance, especially outdoor relief, and those devoted to repressing the deviant poor – although we should not allow Foucault's familiar discussion of the 'Great Confinement' to mislead us into thinking of the French hospital network as primarily a system of social control.[9] Here both the state and Paris played a prominent role. The model institution, established by royal edict in 1656, was the Hôpital-Général de Paris, which was both a shelter for the needy poor – the disabled, sick and infirm, and children – and a place of detention for beggars and other deviants. Many of the inmates came from the provinces; most provincial institutions, in contrast, took in only local residents and expelled the rest. Begging was criminalised, and the généralité of Paris had the highest arrest rates in the country.

The 18th century brought new repressive legislation on begging.[10] An act of 1724, for example, called for the poor to be interned in municipal hospitals partly at royal expense, and for the Hôpital-Général in Paris to maintain a central registry of beggars. A special commission appointed in 1764 tried to draw sharper boundaries between sturdy beggars and more deserving categories. Legislation of 1767 condemned the former to royal workhouses, called *dépôts de mendicité*. Paris was particularly well equipped to conduct a repressive campaign, with a small but active regular police force headed by a lieutenant-general of police.

The Paris hospital system

Paris was remarkably rich in hospitals, even in a kingdom notable for the number of such institutions in relation to the size of its population. (In the 16th and 17th centuries, the Crown had closed many provincial establishments considered corrupt, inefficient or superfluous, and confiscated their holdings, but France still possessed more than 2000 hospitals in the 18th century.)[11] A single council oversaw the establishments placed under the umbrella of the Hôpital-Général and the Hôtel-Dieu and its satellites, although each group had its own administrative bureau.

The largest institutions in the Hôpital-Général complex were La Salpêtrière for women and Saint-Jean de Bicêtre for men.[12] The foundling hospital, established in 1670, grew out of the charitable work of Saint Vincent de Paul. Here the state played a critical role. Perhaps a third of the foundlings were from the provinces – a practice ultimately prohibited in 1779 by a royal declaration. Many were farmed out to wet nurses in the surrounding regions, following the same routes as the children of Paris's working poor. The government took an active interest in wet nursing and closely regulated the business.[13]

By the end of the ancien régime, the capital counted about 50 hospitals of all kinds. They included the Invalides, for crippled soldiers; the Hôpital du Nom de Jésus for the aged; the Hôpital des Incurables, privately founded and endowed, which also had non-resident 'members' in the provinces; the Hôpital de la Pitié, which housed boys from the foundling hospitals and poor families; La Trinité, which accommodated Parisian boys and girls; the Hospice de Vaugirard, founded in 1780 for pregnant women with venereal disease; the Hôpital du Saint-Esprit, for orphans of master craftsmen, born in Paris and Versailles, who were taught to read and write before being sent out as apprentices; and the Hôpital des Quinze-Vingts for the blind. This last institution, founded by Saint Louis in the 13th century, was limited to about 300 members – hence the name of fifteen-score. To these must be added a range of separate and often privately endowed institutions, among them charity workshops that employed the indigent in tasks such as spinning.

When we analyse this hospital system, we find that many of our familiar dichotomies break down – not just therapeutic and custodial, but public and private, state and municipal, religious and secular. Some institutions were clearly public (the various parts of the Hôpital-Général, for example), and many at least partly private, such as the Incurables, where donors and their descendants played a role in choosing who would be admitted. But the state provided general oversight – throughout the kingdom – through the *Contrôle Général des Finances*, created under Louis XIV's minister Colbert, which had responsibility for health and poor relief and became increasingly involved in hospital administration when voluntary institutions encountered administrative or financial difficulties. Hospital boards similarly illustrate the difficulty of drawing a boundary between secular and religious establishments. Almost all consisted primarily of laymen. But the chaplain of the royal household, the Grand Aumônier, whose title literally means Great Almoner, was the director of the Quinze-Vingts and helped supervise most other Paris hospitals. Institutional finances show analogous intersections. The hospitals generally had endowments, often from the Church, but they were sometimes supplemented by state grants, including, for example, property confiscated from the Huguenots. The state also contributed to annual budgets and accepted primary financial responsibility for the care of foundlings. The municipality contributed as well, drawing mainly on the *octroi*, the duty paid on goods entering the city. Private charity – legacies, donations, and the proceeds of fund-raising events, such as charity balls and entertainments – was another important source. On the eve of the Revolution, the Hôtel-Dieu received an extraordinary bequest of 1.2 million livres, although the donor's heirs contested the will, and the hospital was ultimately left with only a quarter of that amount.[14] Another important mixing of categories was the staffing of even government hospitals by religious persons and members of the great nursing orders founded in the 17th century, notably the Sisters of Charity who also played a prominent role in home care. In some institutions, especially the Hôtel-Dieu, they increasingly struggled with the medical staff for control of the day-to-day running of the hospital.

Outdoor relief

Outdoor relief in Paris was supervised by an institution dating from 1544 known as the Grand Bureau des Pauvres, which by the end of the ancien régime had lost its ties to the municipality and come under the jurisdiction of the *parlement* of Paris. The Bureau could draw on a remarkable range of financial resources to aid the needy, particularly the elderly, children and workers who had fallen on hard times. Those who enjoyed its largesse had to be legal residents and Roman Catholics. The Bureau raised a poor tax from which only the poor – but not nobles or clergy – were exempted, and collected other funds from royal lotteries, from certain special taxes – on street maintenance, for example – and increasingly, at the end of the ancien régime, from a portion of the principal direct taxes. There was also, of course, a great deal of private almsgiving, much of it channelled through the Church; guilds and confraternities often assisted the poor as well as their own members in distress; and the government disbursed other funds in the form of pensions to reward meritorious service, to assist large families and in other special cases. In keeping with the ancien régime system of privilege and particularism, there were no fixed rights, and benefits were far from uniform. One should add to all of this the state's role in provisioning Paris; although it did not feed people directly, except on a limited basis in times of extraordinary need, it took a strong interest, for political reasons, in the price of bread. Thus, except for a few periods during the 1760s and 1770s, the government carefully regulated the trade in grain and flour.[15]

The Parisian welfare system was remarkably well coordinated by the standards of the day, although it did not depend directly on the state, the Church, or the municipality. Magistrates, ecclesiastics and certain public officials sat on its boards *ex officio*, but they enjoyed considerable autonomy from their hierarchical superiors, and elected members were typically chosen by cooptation. The resources they administered made for a rather generous allowance for the poor of Paris, even though France as a whole lacked a poor rate system like England's, and in many parts of the kingdom the least advantaged found themselves destitute during hard times.

Medical assistance

As for the provision of health care to the needy, we are brought back once again to the world of the hospitals; district and town physicians were rare in France, although the medical faculties and surgical guilds were required by their statutes to give public consultations on certain fixed days. The capital relied in particular on the Hôtel-Dieu[16] and the Charité hospital, run by the Brothers of Charity of Saint John of God, which accepted no incurables and was famed for its surgery. Starting late in the reign of Louis XIV, boxes of remedies and medical personnel, known as epidemic physicians and surgeons, were dispatched during outbreaks of disease into the countryside, including the *généralité* of Paris.[17]

Enlightenment projects

The last decades of the ancien régime saw a critical re-examination of hospitals, poor relief and medical assistance, strongly influenced by Enlightenment ideology.[18] In 1777, for example, the Academy of Châlons sponsored a celebrated competition on eliminating mendicancy. In Paris the debates reflected an awareness of the swelling numbers of the labouring poor, as described, for example, by Louis-Sébastien Mercier, in his *Tableau de Paris*.[19] Most reformers – Dupont de Nemours[20] was among the best known – hoped to move away from the hospital, which they saw as costly, inefficient and demoralising, to some form of home relief. They also reiterated the call for the ablebodied to work. But they rarely showed the harshness of some later political economists: in their view, the worthy poor deserved *bienfaisance*. What they repudiated, rather, was an older conception of charity, which they deemed indiscriminate, and the model of class providence in which the rich serve the poor but the poor also serve the rich by allowing them to save their souls through almsgiving.[21] Some reformers also expressed an interest in extending medical services to the rural poor.

Enlightened administrators put a few reforms into practice, with mixed results. At the national level, the most prominent were the physiocrat Turgot, controller-general of finance from 1774 to 1776, and Necker, who served as director-general of finance from 1777 to 1781. Turgot's many objectives included the reform of poor relief; he abolished the *dépôts de mendicité,* a move that met the same fate as his failed effort to establish free trade in grain. His economic liberalism led him to hope that prosperity would ultimately create jobs for the unemployed, but in the short run his humanity led him to accept charity workshops and other forms of relief, including local alms bureaux, though with a limited role for the state. Turgot was also godfather to the Société Royale de Médecine, which received its charter in 1778; primarily concerned with epidemics and the regulation of the remedy trade, it also served as a forum for debating health care reform. The less optimistic Necker saw a larger role for the government in providing welfare and guaranteeing bread for the people. He and his wife, Suzanne, also participated actively in hospital reform.

The debates over the design and function of the hospital, particularly after the Paris Hôtel-Dieu was severely damaged by fire in 1772, form a familiar chapter in the history of medical institutions.[22] Before Tenon's celebrated report of 1788 on the Paris hospitals, there were government commissions, several reports from the Academy of Sciences, and much more besides. Some reformers envisaged a great new Hôtel-Dieu constructed on scientific principles, but many others considered a huge hospital in the centre city unhealthy and proposed dispersing the inmates to smaller and more scattered institutions. The grand schemes for a new Hôtel-Dieu were not realised, but several new smaller hospitals emerged, including the charity hospital of the parish of Saint-Sulpice, sponsored by Mme Necker, now known as the Hôpital Necker,[23] and the hospital of the parish of Saint-Jacques-du-Haut-Pas, started by the *curé* Cochin in 1780, and now the Hôpital Cochin.

Several new institutions provided outdoor relief, among them the government-sponsored pawnbroking establishment, or Mont-de-piété, founded in

1777 as an alternative source of loans for the poor; the Société Philanthropique de Paris, established in 1780; and the Société de Charité Maternelle, for poor pregnant women, founded in 1788. The Société Philanthropique won an enthusiastic following among the highly placed. Its benefactors included the king, great nobles, Necker and the Compagnie des Indes, and prominent physicians participated in its medical programme.[24] The Société de Charité Maternelle had an even more aristocratic membership.

In the French context, the societies represented an innovative approach to the provision of poor relief and medical assistance. As voluntary philan-thropic associations, they had no direct link to either Church or government; they could freely choose what type of assistance to provide, and to whom. They imposed no religious test on recipients but, in accordance with the teachings of the liberal reformers, restricted benefits to the deserving poor. Discriminating between the worthy and the unworthy implied investigation and surveillance by the philanthropists themselves. The societies lacked the legal standing for any of these activities, which technically required authori-sation through royal letters patent. There can be no doubt, however, that they enjoyed considerable informal recognition. For several generations, commen-tators repeatedly invoked them as models for private philanthropy in the public interest.

The Revolution

The Enlightenment reform project gained new momentum at the outset of the Revolution, transposed to a wider scale and recast in terms of national re-newal: it was not just Crown and town but also the nation that had an obligation to the poor and the sick.[25] The Sociéte Royale de Médecine sub-mitted a 'New Plan' for medicine in France, which included district physicians to provide home treatment for the needy.[26] Other proposals called for a national system of poor relief. Though united in their call for change, the various projects were marked by disagreement and even internal contradic-tions. The conflicts over poor relief reflected the perennial tension between individual and communal rights and responsibilities. In the medical domain, the concept of a 'right to health', as Dora Weiner has labelled it,[27] covered competing visions, of making treatment available to all, or of developing a salubrious society and way of life that – à la Rousseau – would make doctors unnecessary. This latter theme sometimes took a more general form: in a regenerated and virtuous society, both poverty and sickness would disappear. One common denominator in many of the proposals, drawing on an Enlight-enment commonplace, was a distrust of hospitals and a preference for outdoor relief and home care.

The Constituent and Legislative Assemblies, 1789–1792

These tensions came to the fore – and found only partial resolution – in the work of two key committees of the Constituent Assembly of 1789–91. The better known was the Committee on Poverty, or more precisely on the elimination of mendicancy, headed by the aristocratic physiocrat La Rochefoucauld, duc de Liancourt, assisted by the physician Thouret, later dean of the Paris medical school. The Health Committee (*Comité de Salubrité*), chaired by Dr Guillotin, had close ties with the Société Royale de Médecine. Both committees had great aspirations.

The Committee on Poverty hoped to return poor relief to the home; even foundlings would be placed with families. Medical assistance outside the hospital, assured by a national network of physicians and pharmacists, would be an integral part of the project. In its original formulations, the programme implied a universal entitlement to public assistance. Increasingly, however, the committee focused on particular groups such as the indigent and incapacitated, diminished the government's role and emphasised the contributions of voluntary philanthropy. It studied the work of the Charité Maternelle as a possible model.

Guillotin's committee concentrated on the teaching and organisation of medicine; here its plan was close to that of the Société Royale. It also envisaged a system of district physicians to aid the poor, although it wished to avoid placing this work in the hands of a national administration that might begin to centralise the oversight of medical practice. From their different perspectives, then, both bodies expressed a distrust of a state apparatus exercising uniform control over poor relief and the provision of health care.

Neither committee saw its plans reach fruition at the national level, nor was the Committee on Poverty's detailed plan for the reorganisation of assistance in Paris fully carried out, although the capital did receive a five-member commission, essentially for the hospital system, in 1791. Although it was hardly the legislators' intent, the Constituent Assembly and then the Legislative Assembly, elected under the new Constitution of 1791, produced mainly negative results. A series of enactments weakened, or even abolished, institutions that had provided poor relief and medical assistance under the ancien régime. Local taxes, such as the *octroi,* were eliminated at the outset; Church property was nationalised, in theory so that the state could salary the clergy and take over the Church's former roles in education and assistance. Religious congregations were abolished early in 1790. None of these measures was aimed at hospitals or poor relief directly, but all took their toll.

The radical revolution, 1792–1794

The National Convention, which met after the fall of the monarchy in 1792, produced a mixed and complex record, which the Left summed up as failed hopes and the Right characterised as vandalism. The Convention intensified the commitment to assistance at the national level – the right to subsistence was written into the declaration of rights of the Jacobin Constitution – although it also cracked down on begging and almsgiving with exceptional ferocity. In theory, the deserving poor would receive aid from the state, distributed to the *départements* and from there to the *communes* according to need. The rich would be taxed to help support the less fortunate. Foundlings were declared 'natural children of the Patrie'. In the spring of 1794 the Convention called for drawing up a Grand Livre de la Bienfaisance, a roll of the deserving poor, essentially in rural districts. The government would supply money, food, medicine and the services of salaried health officers. If fully realised, this radical vision of *la bienfaisance nationale*, later derided by its Malthusian critics as 'legal charity', would have dwarfed even the English poor law system.

   In practice, the Great Book was barely opened. In the end, the Convention renounced its ambitious social projects, overcome by the financial exigencies of war at home and abroad and by real divisions within French society over the relationship between the individual and the collectivity. The radical revolution, however, had continued the negative work of dismantling old institutions to clear the ground for projected new ones. Most crucially, hospital endowments were alienated. Private charitable societies, which had flourished under the constitutional monarchy, though not formally suppressed, collapsed for lack of financial support. The poor suffered greatly, although those of Paris probably less than most, since a municipal commission and then a *comité de bienfaisance* oversaw the distribution of money, food, and medicine.

The conservative republic, 1794–1799

Following the fall of Robespierre in the summer of 1794, as the Convention steered the Republic in a more moderate direction, it turned away from the principle of *la bienfaisance nationale* toward a less statist model of assistance. In August 1795 the unsold property of the hospitals was returned. The Paris hospitals later received the proceeds of a tax on amusements in the capital and the main share of a revived *octroi*; the Hôtel-Dieu was indemnified with 'national lands' that had earlier been taken from the Church. The Directory regime, which assumed power at the end of 1795, embarked on a more far-reaching programme of reconstruction, which has sometimes been misleadingly characterised as a restoration of the traditional institutions and practices of the ancien régime. As Catherine Duprat has shown, it is better seen as a new model of *la bienfaisance **publique*** – as opposed to ***nationale*** – based on the unrealised projects of the Constituent Assembly.[28]

For the Directory, unlike the radical Convention, public assistance would not be a blanket entitlement; such a commitment would drain the government coffers, harm industry and stifle private philanthropy. Poor relief would have to stay within a budget and rely on private contributions as its primary resource – a free gift rather than a tax. Apart from supporting foundlings, whose helplessness justified special consideration, and funding a few national institutions that served the entire country, the state would provide only limited subsidies. Its main function in succouring the poor would be to set an example for the rich.

The administration of poor relief was entrusted to boards of prominent private citizens, rather than state functionaries or elected officials – an exceptional model in the context of 19th century France, as well as a radical departure from the ancien régime, in which the Church played a prominent role in poor relief. Two key pieces of legislation, adopted in October and November 1796, called for these local notables to staff municipal hospital councils and municipal or district *bureaux de bienfaisance* to collect and disburse funds for outdoor relief. Many towns subsequently assigned physicians to the *bureaux* to provide medical assistance to the poor. The entire system came under the jurisdiction of the municipal council.

At the same time, it is important to recognise the ways in which this model increased the role of the state and of government in general, compared with the ancien régime and its many autonomous institutions. The state imposed and required the localities to fund a uniform system of public assistance. The state oversaw the local budgets and had to approve appointments to the councils. Moreover, all levels of government increasingly helped sponsor and subsidise private philanthropic organisations. This mixture of private and public, central and local, was to become a characteristic feature of public assistance in 19th century France.

Assistance in the post-revolutionary world

No major new legislation on poor relief appeared between the Directory and the Second Republic (1848–1852); subsequent regimes built on the foundations laid in 1796.

From the Consulate to the July Monarchy

Bonaparte's Consulate (1799–1804) continued the work of reconstruction begun under the Directory: the government reconstituted the hospitals' domains and allowed the nursing orders to return. Under the Empire (1804–1814), a decree on foundlings (1811) affirmed the principle of state responsibility and established guidelines for institutions throughout the Empire. It is best remembered for mandating the use of the *tour*, a revolving contraption placed in the wall of a foundling hospital that allowed an adult to deposit an infant without being seen by those inside. In Paris, this work was continued by the Hospice des Enfants Trouvés – rebaptised the Hospice des Enfants Assistés in 1860, and now the Hôpital de Saint-Vincent-de-Paul.[29]

The Consulate also produced several key innovations, both at the national level and in the capital. More clearly than the Directory, the First Consul actively encouraged the voluntary philanthropic associations and made them a central part of *la bienfaisance publique*, while tightening state control; starting under the Empire, they were in principle required to secure the authorisation of the Council of State. Bonaparte, members of his family and the leading figures in what became the imperial court figured prominently on the boards of philanthropic institutions. The Société Philanthropique de Paris greatly expanded its activities, which ranged from soup kitchens to a network of five medical dispensaries and doctors who made house calls. Some of the luminaries of Paris medicine, such as Corvisart, gave their time and lent their prestige to the Society's health care programme. In 1810 the various local *charités maternelles* were organised into an imperial society under the patronage of the empress, although it was not to survive the Empire. Catholics formed their own charitable associations, since under the Concordat of 1801 the parishes could not directly collect alms for charity.

In Paris, two local institutions created under the Consulate were to play a major role in public health, poor relief and medical assistance. The Conseil de Salubrité de Paris et du Département de la Seine, established in 1802 by the prefect of police Dubois, became a model for sanitary institutions throughout France. It was not, however, directly concerned with welfare or the provision of health care, although it documented the health problems of the poor.[30] More critical for our purposes was the new hospital administration of 1801, the Conseil Général des Hospices de la Seine, proposed by the prefect of the Seine, Frochot.[31] Only the prefect and the prefect of police sat on the Council in their official capacities. In theory, the rest of its membership was made up of prominent private citizens, but in practice it included current and former government officials and the director of the Paris medical school. The capital now had a special administrative regime for poor relief and medical assistance, largely unaffected by subsequent national legislation; the only real equivalent elsewhere was the system adopted in Lyons the following year. Frochot explicitly took as his model the centralised administration of the Grand Bureau des Pauvres under the ancien régime. The Council ran the entire hospital system; its departments included a central admissions office, effectively eliminating the traditional role of charitable patrons, or staff, in handpicking beneficiaries. It also ran the *bureau de bienfaisance* in each of the 12 *arrondissements* and coordinated certain other welfare functions, such as contracting with manufacturers to employ young boys in its charge. The *bureaux*, using Council funding, distributed assistance in kind – food, clothing, fuel and medicines.

The Bourbon Restoration (1814–1830) and the July Monarchy (1830–1848), which produced few notable innovations in public assistance and the provision of health care, have not attracted the sort of attention accorded to the revolutionary and Napoleonic periods. Both regimes expanded the system of *monts-de-piété* and the network of charity workshops, and both encouraged self-help, although the legal status of mutual aid societies remained uncertain. The Restoration was more sympathetic to the Church and local notables and placed somewhat more reliance on charitable giving encouraged by the example of the king, but the changes were less dramatic than one might expect. The government did reorganise the administrative system for hospices and the *bureaux de bienfaisance* (renamed *bureaux de charité*) outside Paris, and somewhat attenuated the state's responsibility for foundlings. It also placed some Parisian institutions under the protection of members of the royal family, independent of the central hospital administration. The liberal July Monarchy kept the same basic structure, while reaffirming the principle of secular social welfare. One of its few noteworthy contributions was a law of 1838 on the confinement of the mentally ill, which separated and medicalised a function of the old hospital by requiring each *département* to establish an insane asylum headed by a doctor, though without providing funding. The asylum superintendents were state functionaries, – a rarity in the French hospital system. Until 1867 the Department of the Seine had no specialised facility for the insane within its hospital system, but it subsidised patients sent to the national psychiatric hospital at Charenton.

Although neither regime radically reshaped the welfare system to fit its ideological principles, politics was never far below the surface. Catholic charitable associations had links to ultraroyalism, which aroused the suspicion of liberals. In one notorious episode, during the cholera epidemic of 1832, the prefect of the Seine refused a charitable donation offered by the writer and politician Chateaubriand, who as a loyal supporter of the house of Bourbon wished to give it in the name of the duchess de Berry, widowed daughter-in-law of the exiled former king, Charles X. The duchess was working to topple Louis-Philippe and give the throne to her son, whom Bourbon supporters recognised as Henri V.[32]

The key providers of medical assistance outside the hospital remained the doctors attached to the *bureaux de bienfaisance*, a system formally recognised by a decree of 28 October 1813. In the Paris area, a Société Générale de Prévoyance, created in 1830 by the prefect of police, supported home medical care or office visits for the poorest members of mutual aid societies. A different model – the small neighbourhood clinic or dispensary – was foreshadowed in the emergency medical stations set up during the cholera epidemic of 1832, but they did not become permanent. The idea of a national network of district physicians was revived but rejected at a great national medical congress that met in Paris in 1845; it reappeared in a major bill on medical education and practice proposed by the minister of public instruction in 1847, but it had not yet won passage when the Revolution of 1848 intervened.

The hospital system

Under the post-revolutionary settlement, France possessed five national hospitals, which accepted patients from throughout the country. Four were located in the Paris region: the Quinze-Vingts, the institutions for the deaf and for blind children, and Charenton. (The fifth was an institution for the deaf in Bordeaux.) Throughout France, but above all in Paris, hospitals were more clearly distinguished from hospices, and both became increasingly specialised. In 1802, for example, the former Maison de l'Enfant Jésus became the first pediatric hospital anywhere; the Pitié, for acute diseases, was founded in 1809. By 1819 one commentator boasted that 'each type of infirmity and each stage of life now has its own special establishments, for each of the two sexes'.[33]

A list of Paris hospitals published in the *Almanach national et royal* for 1840[34] included, in addition to the four national hospitals, the Hôtel-Dieu (with a branch located in another part of Paris) and a series of other institutions operating under similar rules – among them, the children's hospital; the Hôpital du Midi for male venereal inpatients and outpatients; La Lourcine for women venereal patients; a Maison Royale de Santé, for paying patients; and the lying-in hospital, or Maison d'Accouchement. These examples point to the emergence of the modern hospital as the *machine à guérir*, but the single administrative apparatus at the top also makes clear the ways in which poor relief and medical care continued to intertwine.

The hospices included: the Foundlings; the Salpêtrière and Bicêtre (the first still for women and the second for men, but now primarily for the elderly); separate male and female hospices for the incurable; the Hospice de La Rochefoucauld, for former hospital employees and also paying patients; the Institution de Sainte-Périne, Consacrée à la Vieillesse, which had been founded in 1801 by a businessman as a retreat for old or infirm but not indigent men and women; the Hospice des Ménages, for indigent elderly married couples; the tiny Hospice de Saint-Michel, founded by a Paris merchant, which housed 12 old men; the Hospice de la Reconnaissance, founded by Michel Brézin, a former smelter, for elderly workers from related occupations; and the Hospice Devillas, for elderly men and women, four-fifths from lists of the *bureaux de bienfaisance*, and one-fifth Protestants.

If we were to follow the development of the Parisian system of hospitals and hospices to the end of our period, we would see an extraordinary proliferation of specialised institutions. A growing number were situated outside the city, in the Seine, Seine-et-Oise, and even further afield, to take advantage of cheaper land or local conditions. Paris acquired sanatoria on the coast and in the mountains and even an agricultural colony at Esternay (Marne), where former peasants who had failed to realise their dream of a better life in the capital could become reaccustomed to working the land.[35]

The whole system was supported by a striking mixture of public and private financing from a great variety of sources. The state played a limited role. In the Year XI of the Revolutionary calendar (1802–03), a direct government subsidy accounted for only 60 000 francs in a budget of 4 703 107.37 for the hospitals and hospices. The budget shows that rents and dividends from the hospitals' properties and investments provided the great bulk of their income, together with various special local levies such as the *octroi*, the entertainment tax, the proceeds of pawnbroking establishments and a portion of the revenue generated by fines and the sale of goods confiscated by the municipal police. Miscellaneous sources of income included the sale of articles manufactured by inmates and books published by the hospitals' official printer, including the annual budget itself.[36] Public officials sponsored fund-raising events; a charity ball held at the Opera in January 1831, organised by the mayors of the city's 12 *arrondissements* and the colonels of the Paris National Guard, netted 110 617.64 francs.[37] In addition, some establishments, such as the Hospice des Ménages and the Institution de Sainte-Périne, required either the inmate or a benevolent third party to pay for residency. The fortunes of each establishment depended to a large extent on the generosity of its benefactors and the wisdom of its administrators. The Institution de Sainte-Périne, whose overconfident founder had originally dubbed it the Retraite Assurée à l'Infortune et à la Vieillesse, was badly mismanaged and went bankrupt in 1807. The minister of the interior intervened and 'nationalised' it, entrusting its administration to the Paris Hospital Council; however, the ensuing conflicts were not resolved until 1836.[38]

One can see here the growing role of endowments and private donations, which militated against institutional uniformity. Even though the founders and benefactors of hospitals and hospices did not individually select inmates, they designated categories of beneficiaries, which could be highly specialised. A decree of July 1806 even allowed them to join the local councils in administering the institutions they had endowed. In the case of philanthropic associations that provided outdoor relief, members could still personally choose the recipients of their generosity; thus for each donation of a certain amount, the subscribers of the Société Philanthropique received a set of tickets for Rumford's economical soups and a card entitling one poor person at a time to be treated at the dispensary.

This is not to say that private income freed charitable institutions from government oversight. In addition to the decree of the Council of State that required approval for philanthropic institutions that housed inmates, a law of 3 May 1813 required government authorisation for gifts and bequests to benefit hospices or the poor.[39] According to a collection of regulations on outdoor relief published at the end of the Restoration:

> ... it is necessary for the Government's influence to be continually felt throughout the network for distributing the aid that it grants; for it to be sure that the aid is distributed in its interest and in accordance with its intentions; and, in order to reach this goal, for private establishments for outdoor relief to have a common centre to direct and oversee all the details'.[40]

Ideology and social change

This distinctively French mixture of public and private reflected a widely shared theory of *la bienfaisance publique* elaborated in the generation following the revolutionary settlement. French theorists frequently began by looking across the Channel. On the one hand, they rejected the English poor rates. On the other hand, they greatly admired and often envied the extensive use of voluntary fund-raising campaigns. As the century wore on, the widely presumed inferiority of private charitable institutions in France and Paris to those in Britain and London and the notion that the French relied almost entirely on the government were a source of hurt pride and patriotic indignation. One writer in the mid-1870s insisted that the French capital could withstand the comparison to its rival across the channel without appearing 'excessively inferior'.[41] The French also found consolation in the thought that, whatever the profusion of English philanthropies, they ordered these things better in France – a point conceded even by some British commentators, such as David Johnston, MD, fellow of the Royal College of Surgeons of Edinburgh and author of a volume on French charitable institutions (1829). In England, he wrote:

> ... every charitable establishment has an administration of its own, differing in every respect from that of any other. It is subject to no superior jurisdiction, but liable to all the abuse likely at times to arise from the disputes and jarrings that will often take place between private individuals differing in their opinions, and guided by no regularly-organized system of management.

He greatly preferred the French system.[42]

La bienfaisance publique enjoyed wide support because, whatever their other differences, most liberals and Catholic conservatives could agree on several crucial points: assistance was a social necessity; however, there should be no state guarantee, although the state could play a useful role by coordinating various governmental and voluntary efforts; assistance was a moral obligation for the donor but not a right enjoyed by the individual recipient.

The concept of social necessity – the theme of poor relief as a form of social self-defence, a bulwark against crime, class conflict and revolution – runs like a *leitmotiv* throughout the debates on public assistance in the late 18th and 19th centuries. 'In its asylums', wrote Frochot, 'society pays its debt to misfortune, old age, and infirmity; by relieving extreme need, a prudent policy prevents dereliction and despair, which can lead to crime....'[43] In 1826 the author of a volume of verse defending the hospitals and hospices of Paris against their critics argued for public assistance on political, as well as humanitarian, grounds. Any society that wished to survive had to mitigate the inequalities that were the inevitable product of 'an excessive level of civilisation'.[44]

There could be no state guarantee: theorists of *la bienfaisance publique* rejected a dominant role for the state and the principle of welfare as an individual entitlement. A Malthusian streak ran through early 19th century French liberalism and, with it, a tendency to deride government welfare programs as 'legal charity'.[45] Adam Smith's French disciple, Jean-Baptiste Say, notoriously maintained that the poor had no claim on the state or on private individuals. The liberal politician and writer, Adolphe Thiers, later voiced concern about the plight of the indigent but defended property and refused to recognise a right to work.

Yet a moral obligation remained; one could reject state programmes and legal compulsion and still leave much room for voluntary action. Even among the industrial bourgeoisie – champions of *laissez-faire* in most domains – a certain paternalism prevailed, and many provided medical assistance as well as other benefits to their employees.[46] Some shared the rival vision of a Christian moral economy, along the lines suggested by Vicomte Alban de Villeneuve-Bargemont,[47] and were in some ways closer to Sismondi, the critic of political economy and the new industrialism, than to Say.[48]

The pre-eminent theorist of *la bienfaisance publique* under the Restoration and July Monarchy was the Baron de Gérando, member of the Paris Hospital Council and author of two classic texts defending *la bienfaisance publique* as a collective, but voluntary, enterprise. The first, a short book on the use of volunteer inspectors to visit the poor in their homes, won a competition sponsored by the Academy of Lyons for the best proposal for identifying 'genuine indigence'. The second was a monumental study of the history, philosophy and methodology of public assistance.[49]

Gérando wrote from a Catholic perspective close to that of Villeneuve-Bargemont, whose writings he admired; secular philanthropy was not to his taste, although he held up the work of the Société Philanthropique as a practical model to emulate and rejected the common distinction between *bienfaisance* and charity. Inequality was part of a providential design, in which pity and charity would serve to restore lost harmony – provided that they were free, voluntary and individual: 'The voluntary, individual, direct guardianship [*tutelle*] of prosperity over poverty is the essence of good administration of public assistance.'[50]

Gérando saw *la bienfaisance* as the best response to what many feared would soon become a 'war of the poor against the rich'. Indigence, like great wealth, was the product of economic freedom in modern societies. The beneficiaries had a moral obligation to those who suffered, collectively rather than individually. Society could not simply wash its hands of the less fortunate, as radical Malthusians suggested. This did not mean 'legal charity', which was an oxymoron. A state guarantee of welfare would do more harm than good, and the government in any case could not replace private charity, *la prévoyance* (savings, insurance and other provisions against future contingencies) and self-help. Government could, however, supplement, guide and regulate. Responsibility began with the family. Higher collectivities would intervene only as needed – first, the occupational organisation, which Gérando called the 'tribe' (he missed the old guilds), then the municipality, the province or *département*, and, finally, the state. In the case of medical assistance, however, Gérando did not rely in the first instance on the charity of individual private practitioners but called for district physicians as found in Italy and elsewhere, and for ambulatory clinics on the German model. All these recommendations, Gérando argued, were based not on conjecture but on 'positive principles'. Despite, or rather because of, generations of debate over the poverty question, he saw *la bienfaisance* emerging as an objective science.[51]

Behind the partial consensus embodied in Gérando's writings lay the larger debate on the 'social question' in post-revolutionary France, where the dislocations associated with industrialism and rapid urban growth were a source of public alarm and the subject of much-discussed studies by Villermé, Buret and others. Villermé, writing from a liberal perspective, deplored the sufferings of the working class but hoped for salvation through prosperity; he distrusted state intervention, except for children, who could not help themselves. Liberal political economy drew fire both from the Catholic right and, increasingly, under the July Monarchy, from the Left.[52] Buret derided its complacent optimism.[53] The wide variety of socialists who irrupted into the public sphere after the Revolution of 1830 preached many alternatives to charity, including mutualism. Not all rejected Christianity – consider those among the Saint-Simonians who saw Jesus, the son of a carpenter, as a proletarian and socialist – and not all absolutely condemned private property, for that matter. In one way or another, though, they advocated new forms of social organisation to help alleviate poverty and its attendant ills, and scorned paternalism and liberal notions of self-help.

The charitable enterprise

Throughout all these debates, the development of French philanthropy continued apace. Although much influenced by foreign models, France produced several innovations, notably the *patronage* (youth club), which was Gérando's single greatest contribution. The French also pioneered day care for working mothers. The crèche movement began in Paris in the 1840s as a charitable programme for working-class women, with a medical component; doctors would monitor infant health and help instruct mothers in hygienic child care.[54]

A growing number of foundations addressed particular needs or groups of beneficiaries. Some specifically provided for the working class, rather than (or in addition to) the indigent; under the Second Empire, for example, the Société du Prince Impérial lent money to buy tools and materials.[55] The Société de Saint Jean-François Régis pour le Mariage des Pauvres de Paris sought to reduce 'concubinage by giving the indigent and workers and artisans of slender means the wherewithal to fulfil the duties that human and divine law require of them'.[56] Other organisations helped people with limited resources, especially the elderly, who were not poor enough to qualify for public assistance administered by the Hospital Council. Some catered for orphans, widows or elderly persons from comfortable backgrounds who had fallen on hard times. Highly specialised foundations of this kind included the Catholic and royalist Œuvres des Orphélines de la Révolution and the Association Paternelle des Chevaliers de Saint-Louis et du Mérite Militaire, for widows and orphans of the chevaliers.[57] The Swiss had their Société Helvétique de Bienfaisance; the Société Israëlite des Amis du Travail placed Jewish children in apprenticeships.[58]

One of the most generous bequests under the Restoration came from the industrialist Michel Brézin, mentioned earlier, who died in 1828; his foundation supported the Hospice de la Reconnaissance, established by royal ordinance the following year. Brézin, himself a poorly educated former worker, set up the foundation to express his gratitude to his employees. Candidates for admission had to be poor elderly workers who had 'practised an occupation like those of my employees, whose work helped increase my fortune' – smelters, miners, loggers, charcoal-burners, hammersmiths and others associated directly or indirectly with his ironworks. The foundation's resources grew substantially over the course of the century, thanks in part to subsequent donations; one gift came from the engineer Gustave Eiffel, five years after the completion in 1889 of the iron tower that bears his name.[59]

In order to perpetuate the principles of *la bienfaisance*, some philanthropists established associations to train the children of the propertied classes in the art of giving wisely. The most prominent was the Société des Enfants en Faveur des Vieillards, founded in 1803. The children saved money from their allowances to pay the weekly subscription which provided assistance in kind to the indigent elderly; some also contributed clothing they had made. Like all good members of an association, they elected a president, secretary and treasurer. As Gérando would have wished, they went out, accompanied by their mothers, to visit candidates for assistance and, after ascertaining whether they were of good character and genuinely needy, they duly reported back to the society. Older boys could join the Comité des Jeunes Gens, or Comité de Placement pour les Jeunes Orphelins (1822), designed to rescue young orphans from a life of vice and vagrancy. Young ladies could join the Association des Jeunes Économes (1823), where they would 'adopt' unfortunate girls, place them in an apprenticeship, and pay for their upkeep and instruction.[60]

Later establishments included the Hôpital de l'Institution des Diaconnesses (1843) for Protestant women, the Hôpital Rothschild, endowed in 1852 by Baron James de Rothschild for Jewish patients, and the Hôpital Hertford (1871), founded by Sir Richard Wallace for English patients of all religions. The Fondation Rossini (1889) was endowed by a bequest from the composer's French-born widow; Rossini had served as director of the Théâtre des Italiens in Paris. It was open to aged or infirm singers, French or Italian, of either sex. (In contrast, the Asile Léo-Delibes, located at Clichy-la-Garenne in Seine-et-Oise, was a public hospice subsidised by the Paris municipal council.) The Fondation Chemin-de-Latour (Ivry, 1891) took in elderly men, with a preference for those who had been dealers in scales and balances for at least five years.[61]

1848 and after

The debates over the social question intensified during the Revolution of 1848, much as Enlightenment discussions of poverty and mendicancy had taken on new urgency in 1789. The experience of 1848 and of the Second Republic, which lasted almost five years, is in some ways the experience of the great French Revolution writ small – high hopes quickly dashed. Socialism was soon contained. The national workshops for the unemployed, a pale reflection of the social workshops envisaged by the socialist Louis Blanc, who had been a member of the original provisional government, proved a disaster in the eyes of many; their dissolution provoked the bloody June Days, which seemed to demonstrate the folly of assembling vast masses of the unemployed in Paris. The preamble of the Constitution completed in November promised work or assistance, but legislative committees quickly undercut those commitments. The government did not reorganise welfare on national lines or reform health care. The Republic did produce a voluntary national pension fund, a new law on unhealthy dwellings, and a Conseil Consultatif d'Hygiène Publique (CCHP), which was to supervise the local health councils. In 1851 the CCHP began to coordinate the activities of the epidemic doctors. In Paris, 1849 marked a watershed year in the history of poor relief and health care provision: the functions of the old Hospital Council passed to a director-general of public assistance in Paris, aided by a council. The change, however, represented more a restructuring than a revolutionary reconceptualisation of welfare. The first director, H-J-B. Davenne, was an old-school liberal who invoked Thiers and feared that increasing assistance might engender new needs.[62]

The Second Empire

The role of the state expanded more significantly under the Second Empire (1852–1870). As Emperor Napoleon III, Louis-Napoleon Bonaparte enjoyed a freer reign than as president of the Second Republic to promote his Saint-Simonian vision of a partnership between the government and the private sector and his image as protector of the poor (as a young man he had published a work on ending poverty).[63] He encouraged, but continued to regulate, the mutualist movement, fully legalised by the Second Republic and, towards the end of his reign, in 1868, created voluntary state insurance funds for accidental injury and death. The Empire also saw some limited initiatives to encourage low-cost housing, but private enterprise was to shoulder the major burden.[64] Child welfare policy was adjusted to discourage abandonment; the by now infamous *tours* were eliminated – this happened in Paris in 1862 – or closely guarded. In the end, though, the regime did not substantially increase public assistance. In Paris, it was more closely identified with the extraordinary public works projects undertaken by the activist prefect of the Seine, Baron Haussmann, which provided employment and improved sanitation but also levelled much working-class housing to make way for the new boulevards, squares and monuments.

As for medical assistance, the government adopted measures in the mid-1850s that encouraged, but did not require, the departments to create systems of free medical care for the rural poor.[65] Many cities also moved to increase medical assistance, typically using the doctors attached to the *bureaux de bienfaisance*. Here, Paris led the way, building on the work of the medical aid stations during the cholera epidemic of 1849, when many hospitals had discharged patients for fear of infection. What was then the fifth *arrondissement* retained that service, as an experiment; in 1850 the government held it up as a model for other cities. Then, in 1853, Haussmann used it as the basis for a free medical service – including house calls – for all of Paris, independent of the hospitals and the existing programmes of public assistance; it was to cover a larger group of the needy than the *bureaux de bienfaisance*. The reform created a fully-fledged medical service with salaried physicians outside the hospitals and began the process of detaching medical assistance from the welfare system for the destitute.[66] In 1875 the prefecture of police added a night-time medical service funded by the municipal council.[67]

The Third Republic

It is not clear what further national reforms might have followed had the Empire not ignominiously collapsed, with its army, in the late summer of 1870. The Third Republic emerged inauspiciously from this defeat in the Franco-Prussian War. Paris, whose short-lived revolutionary *Commune* was crushed by the forces of the national government in the spring of 1871, found itself in an uncongenial environment, a country generally unsympathetic to Parisians, socialists, and the working class – whom some were inclined to lump together – governed by a national legislature whose majority wished at heart to return to some form of monarchy. In punishment for its misbehaviour, the capital lost its mayor, a position established by the Government of National Defence after the fall of the Empire in 1870, and closely linked to the revolutionary tradition. (The first mayors of Paris served from 1789 to 1794; thereafter, apart from a brief interlude following the Revolution of 1848, the capital was subject to special provisions that set it apart from other *communes* and deprived it of a chief executive officer.) The municipal council, which survived, became notorious for its truculent radicalism. The physician–politician Clemenceau, who became its president in 1875, is a not unrepresentative specimen. The council combined complaints about the growing population, whose needs overwhelmed the municipal budget, with earnest calls to increase free medical care for the sick poor and support for the aged and infirm. It pressed for ameliorating the living conditions of workers, although it stopped short of directly constructing new housing for them. It succeeded in opening the system of neighbourhood doctors for the poor to all physicians who wished to participate. It also vociferously demanded the secularisation of the hospitals, becoming a leader in the emerging Church–state conflict that was to dominate the politics of the Republic at the end of the century.

The Third Republic, which after 1879 was fully in the hands of convinced republicans, took up the French Revolution's commitment to welfare and medical assistance at the national level.[68] The debates began early, but the results were slow and piecemeal, starting with a law on wet nurses and foundlings in 1874. The key institutional development came in 1888 with the creation of a national welfare office, the Conseil Supérieur d'Assistance Publique within the ministry of the interior; its director, Henri Monod, became the head of the CCHP the following year, effectively linking welfare and medical assistance at the national level. It is not surprising, given this configuration and the extraordinarily disproportionate number of medical men who served both on the CSAP and in the Chamber of Deputies,[69] that the first major new welfare measure, in 1893, provided medical services under an arrangement very favourable to private practitioners, rather than food, shelter or money.[70]

By the 1880s, the network of medical services inherited from the Second Empire was in decline. The law of 1893 made medical assistance an obligation for the *commune*, the *département* and the state, though without prescribing a particular model or providing the requisite funding. The government envisaged the new programme essentially as a system of home medical care outside the urban areas covered by hospitals, and for patients officially identified as needy rather than the population at large – a few per cent of inhabitants at most. Local solutions varied widely, although under pressure from the medical profession, which insisted on a 'liberal' model, the *départements* tended to reject district physicians in favour of an arrangement in which the patient could consult the physician of his choice, who would then be reimbursed for services provided. Physicians' unions, or *syndicats*, which had been fully legalised only in 1892, proved a powerful lobby and used this issue to promote themselves to the profession. Although Paris was not directly affected – under a provision of the new law, *communes* with existing medical assistance programmes could opt out – the *syndicat* of the Seine played an important role in all the debates on medical assistance and on the related question of the growing role of mutual aid societies and insurance companies that signed contracts with physicians and used competitive pressures to drive down rates. The debates gained new intensity in 1898, which witnessed a workman's compensation law for industrial accidents[71] and another measure providing for home or hospital care for elderly invalids and completely incapacitated younger ones. The physicians complained about the new role of the government and 'collectivities', as they had complained earlier about dispensaries and hospitals with which they might have to compete for fee-paying patients. On the whole, however, they greatly benefited from third-party payments that underwrote an expanded demand for medical services.

If we were to pursue the story to the end of the century and beyond, we would see new national programmes and an increase in state funding for medical assistance and then welfare, particularly after the adoption of a new law on public assistance in 1905. How can we explain this pattern? Pronatalist pressures strongly influenced welfare legislation, especially the pro-family measures adopted in the early 20th century. At the national level, the period was marked by demographic stagnation and fears of falling even further behind the united Germany that had emerged from the Franco-Prussian war. (Paris, however, continued to grow; its region accounted for something like half the modest increase in the French population between 1870 and 1914.)

Equally important were class tensions and ideology – the development of socialism and labour militancy or, perhaps more accurately, the fear of those things and the desire for 'social peace'.[72] Classic liberalism evolved into a form more solicitous of the needs of the least advantaged and more accepting of government intervention. These developments have many parallels outside France. The paradigmatic French manifestation, known as solidarism, sought a middle way between classic liberalism and socialism that would balance the rights and duties of both the individual and society; it would respect both property and the needs of the disadvantaged. Its leading exponent, Léon Bourgeois, had served as chairman of the committee on social insurance in the Chamber of Deputies before becoming premier in 1895. Although open to a role for government, solidarists remained distrustful of state compulsion and the extension of what critics had come to call *l'Etat-providence*. They preferred voluntarist and local solutions and were fond of things like mutual aid societies, municipal baths and tram lines. They – and many others in France – were drawn to the model of social insurance developed in Belgium in 1899, which relied on state subventions to voluntary mutual aid societies and avoided the German model of compulsory insurance.[73]

The new social legislation in no way impeded the continued growth of the charitable enterprise within the larger framework of *l'assistance publique*, although voluntary associations now operated in a changed social and cultural landscape shaped by the conflict between the Church and the Republic. By the late 19th century, the Enlightenment terms *bienfaisance* and *philanthropie* enjoyed less currency than *charité*, which, as used by Catholic conservatives, had at the very least anti anti-clerical flavour. A book on private charity in Paris by Flaubert's friend Maxime du Camp, who had moved sharply to the right in reaction to the Commune of 1871, epitomises this counter-Enlightenment vision of public assistance. Much of what he had to say is familiar, but the thrust of his work was polemical in a new way. Charity is a social necessity, a form of self-defence, 'perhaps the best barrier against the invasion of evil and the tidal wave of perversity ... Whether it wishes or not, it is an instrument of social preservation. The suspension of charity in Paris contributed to the duration and violence of the Commune ... In this time of political equality and social inequality, charity is the safety valve of our civilisation.' Du Camp respected the work of the Société Philanthropique; he revered the mission of the institutions run by various religious orders. In the end it was a question of fundamental values. He championed faith, hope and charity, together with philosophical spiritualism, against coldhearted atheism, materialism, municipal secularization campaigns, Darwinism and the war of all against all. He insisted that he was defending religion, not the Church; it was the source of charity, and to attack it was to undermine the foundations of society itself. If religion did not exist, to paraphrase Voltaire's famous *mot*, it would be necessary to invent it.[74]

Conclusion

Overall, we have seen a pattern of localism, voluntarism and surprisingly limited direct involvement by the state in poor relief and the provision of medical care. The Revolution displaced the Church from its central role and imposed uniform regulation from above, but many of the old patterns persisted. State participation expanded toward the end of the 19th century, but hardly to the detriment of voluntary efforts; the explosive growth of charity and mutualism are as remarkable as the manifestations of *l'Etat-providence*.

Industrialisation and class tensions – in Paris or elsewhere – provide only a very partial explanation of this pattern and its transformations, however prominently they figured in public discourse on poverty and social welfare. Public assistance consistently targeted traditional groups such as children, the elderly, the sick or simply the indigent, rather than workers, who were largely left to the world of mutualism. There was never, in practice, a presumptive right to work. Susan Pedersen's recent analysis of the 20th century French welfare state, which stresses the family rather than class, would apply, *mutatis mutandis*, to its 19th century antecedents.[75]

Ideology and politics played a larger role, particularly at certain privileged moments, in the late 18th century, the late 19th century, and around 1848. But the transformations were less decisive than might be expected, and one is struck by the continuity of the tension between the competing claims of the individual and the community, forcefully articulated during the Revolution and never fully resolved. Similar dilemmas have emerged in every democratic polity, but in France the revolutionary legacy greatly complicated the task. Even more striking, though hardly surprising, is the continuity of practices, as opposed to discourses. Paris, rich in both institutions and ideologies, is simply a case in point.

Thanks to the prominence of local and voluntary assistance, certain groups benefited more than others. So did certain regions, notably Paris, led by its more prosperous *arrondissements*; charity tended to concentrate where it was least needed. In the absence of adequate funding, the state would have been hard pressed to intervene to even out the differences. A government which before the First World War lacked an income tax, and for which the excise on *pari mutuel* bets constituted one of the more important sources of revenue, could not embark on a major programme of social expenditures.

From the vantage-point of the beginning of the 21st century, 1945 seems a more crucial turning point than any we have encountered in our period. The social security system, though administratively decentralised, did eventually help reduce disparities among groups and regions. In more recent years French governments from different points on the ideological spectrum have begun a campaign of devolution and dispersal that has already moved significant institutions and some powers and resources from Paris to the provinces.

To the extent that they succeed they will have shown that it paradoxically took the stronger centralised state of the Fifth Republic to diminish Paris as a centre, and confirmed that the Paris of our period owed some part of its good fortune to imperfect political centralisation.

Notes

1. Benjamin titled an unfinished work 'Arcades', or 'Paris, Capital of the Nine-teenth Century'. See Johannes Willms, *Paris, Capital of Europe: From the Revolution to the Belle Epoque,* trans. Eveline L. Kanes, New York, 1997. Other great conurbations, of course, faced many of the same challenges; for a useful set of comparisons, see Peter Mandler (ed.), *The Uses of Charity: The Poor on Relief in the Nineteenth-Century Metropolis,* Philadelphia, 1990.

2. Catherine Duprat, *Usages et pratiques de la philanthropie: pauvreté, action sociale et lien social, à Paris, au cours du premier XIX*^e *siècle,* Paris, 1996, p. 8; Martha L. Hildreth, *Doctors, Bureaucrats, and Public Health in France, 1888–1902,* New York and London, 1987, p. 225.

3. C-J. Lecour, *Manuel d'assistance: La charité à Paris; des diverses formes de l'assistance dans le département de la Seine,* Paris, 1876, p. 8.

4. Ann F. La Berge, *Mission and Method: The Early Nineteenth-Century French Public Health Movement,* Cambridge and New York, 1992.

5. The archive and library (7, rue des Minimes), together with the Le Senne collection on the history of Paris at the Bibliothèque Nationale de France, are the fundamental resources for the history of poor relief and medical assistance in Paris. The Museum (47, quai de la Tournelle) regularly organises historical exhibitions, sometimes accompanied by publications; see, for example, the collection *Depuis 100 ans, la société, l'hôpital, et les pauvres,* Paris, 1996.

6. Evelyn Bernette Ackerman, *Health Care in the Parisian Countryside, 1800–1914,* New Brunswick, NJ, 1990.

7. For the 18th century, Shelby T. McCloy, *Government Assistance in Eighteenth-Century France,* Durham, NC, 1946, is still a useful conspectus. See also Camille Bloch, *L'Assistance et l'État en France à la veille de la Révolution: Généralités de Paris, Rouen, Alençon, Orléans, Châlons, Soissons, Amiens (1764–1790),* Paris, 1908.

8. Muriel Joerger, 'The Structure of the Hospital System in France in the Ancien Régime', in Robert Forster and Orest Ranum (eds), *Medicine and Society in France,* Selections from the *Annales,* **6,** Baltimore, 1980, pp. 104–36; Françoise Hildesheimer and Christian Gut, *L'Assistance hospitalière en France,* Paris, 1992; Laurence Brockliss and Colin Jones, *The Medical World of Early Modern France,* Oxford, 1997, ch. 11.

9. Michel Foucault, *Madness and Civilization: A History of Insanity in the Age of Reason,* trans. Richard Howard, New York, 1973. For a corrective, emphasising the hospitals' genuine contribution to the needs of the local poor, see Colin Jones, *The Charitable Imperative: Hospitals and Nursing in Ancien Régime and Revolutionary France,* London and New York, 1989, especially 'Introduction: the Charitable Imperative', pp. 1–28.

10. See Robert M. Schwartz, *Policing the Poor in Eighteenth-Century France,* Chapel Hill and London, 1988.

11. Jones, *The Charitable Imperative* (n.9), p. 8, calls the French hospital popula-

tion the largest of any European state under the ancien régime. On the fate of the provincial hospitals, see Daniel Hickey, *Local Hospitals in Ancien Régime France: Rationalization, Resistance, Renewal, 1530–1789*, Montreal and Buffalo, 1997.

12. On the many avatars of the latter, see Jean Delamare and Thérèse Delamare-Riche, *Le grand renfermement: Histoire de l'hospice de Bicêtre, 1657–1974*, Paris, 1990.

13. George D. Sussman, *Selling Mothers' Milk: The Wet-Nursing Business in France, 1715–1914*, Urbana, Ill., 1982.

14. McCloy, *Government Assistance* (n.7), p. 451.

15. Steven L. Kaplan, *Provisioning Paris: Merchants and Millers in the Grain and Flour Trade During the Eighteenth Century*, Ithaca, NY, 1984.

16. See Marcel Fosseyeux, *L'Hôtel-Dieu de Paris au XVIIe et au XVIIIe siècle*, Paris, 1912.

17. Jean-Pierre Goubert, 'Épidémies, médecine et État en France à la fin de l'Ancien Régime', in Neithard Bulst and Robert Delors (eds), *Maladie et société (XIIe–XVIIIe siècles), Actes du colloque de Bielefeld, novembre 1986*, Paris, 1989, pp. 393–401.

18. An excellent overview can be found in Catherine Duprat, *'Pour l'amour de l'humanité': Le temps des philanthropes: La philanthropie parisienne des Lumières à la Monarchie de Juillet*, Vol. 1, Ministère de l'Éducation Nationale et de la Culture, Mémoires et Documents, XLVII, Paris, 1993, Part I.

19. Louis-Sébastien Mercier, *Le Tableau de Paris*, ed. Jean-Claude Bonnet, 2 vols, Paris, 1994. See also Jeffry Kaplow, *The Names of Kings: The Parisian Laboring Poor in the Eighteenth Century*, New York, 1972.

20. Pierre-Samuel Dupont de Nemours, *Idées sur les secours à donner aux pauvres malades dans une grande ville*, Philadelphia and Paris, 1786.

21. Bernhard Groethuysen, *The Bourgeois: Catholicism vs. Capitalism in Eighteenth-Century France*, trans. Mary Ilford, New York, 1968. Colin Jones provides an excellent account of the broader debates in his local monograph, *Charity and bienfaisance: The Treatment of the Poor in the Montpellier Region, 1740–1815*, Cambridge, 1982. On the economic issues, see also Catherine Lis and Hugo Soly, *Poverty and Capitalism in Pre-industrial Europe*, Brighton, 1979.

22. See John Frangos, *From Housing the Poor to Healing the Sick: The Changing Institution of Paris Hospitals under the Old Regime and Revolution*, Madison and Teaneck, NJ, 1997, Part I; and the series of articles by Louis S. Greenbaum, for example, 'Measure of Civilization: The Hospital Thought of Jacques Tenon on the Eve of the French Revolution', *Bulletin of the History of Medicine*, **49** (1975), pp. 43–56.

23. Valérie Hannin, 'La fondation de l'hospice de charité: une expérience médicale au temps du rationalisme expérimental', *Revue d'histoire moderne et contemporaine*, **31** (1984), pp. 116–30.

24. On the medical aspects of the Society's work, see Dora Weiner, 'The Role of the Doctor in Welfare Work: The Example of the Philanthropic Society of Paris, 1780–1815,' *Historical Reflections/Réflexions historiques*, **9** (1982), pp. 279–304.

25. On the debates, see Duprat, *Temps des philanthropes* (n.18), part II. On the poor and poor relief, see Alan Forrest, *The French Revolution and the Poor*, New York, 1981. For a full treatment of the legislation and institutions, through the Napoleonic period, see Jean Imbert, *Le Droit hospitalier de la Révolution et de l'Empire*, Paris, 1954. A very useful account of hospitals, hospices, and their

clients in the Revolutionary and Napoleonic period is Dora B. Weiner, *The Citizen-Patient in Revolutionary and Imperial Paris*, Baltimore and London, 1993. For the Revolution, see also Robert Vial, *Mœurs, santé et maladies en 1789*, Paris, 1989, and Jean-Charles Sournia, *La médecine révolutionnaire (1789–1799)*, Paris, 1989, esp. ch. 2 on the hospital system.

26. Société Royale de Médecine, *Nouveau Plan de constitution pour la médecine en France*, Paris, 1790.

27. '"Le Droit de l'homme à la santé" – une belle idée devant l'Assemblée Constituante, 1790–1791', *Clio Medica*, **5** (1970), pp. 209–23.

28. Duprat, *Temps des philanthropes* (n.18), Part II, ch. 4. On the reconstruction of social welfare in the wake of the radical revolution, see also Colin Jones, 'Picking up the Pieces: The Politics and the Personnel of Social Welfare from the Convention to the Consulate', in Gwinne Lewis and Colin Lucas (eds), *Beyond the Terror: Essays in French Regional and Social History, 1794–1815*, Cambridge, 1983, pp. 53–91.

29. On assistance to mothers and infants, see Rachel G. Fuchs, *Poor and Pregnant in Paris: Strategies for Survival in the Nineteenth Century*, New Brunswick, NJ, 1992.

30. Ann Fowler La Berge, 'The Paris Health Council, 1802–1848', *Bulletin of the History of Medicine*, **49** (1975), pp. 339–52; Dora Weiner, 'Public Health under Napoleon: The Conseil de Salubrité de Paris, 1802–1815', *Clio Medica*, **9** (1974), pp. 271–84.

31. Nicolas Frochot, *Plan d'organisation de l'administration générale des hôpitaux et hospices de Paris*, Paris, nd.

32. Catherine J. Kudlick, 'Giving is Deceiving: Cholera, Charity, and the Quest for Authority in 1832', *French Historical Studies*, **18** (1993), pp. 457–81.

33. Augustin-François de Silvestre, *Annuaire de la Société philanthropique, contenant l'indication des meilleurs moyens qui existent à Paris de soulager l'humanité souffrante et d'exercer utilement la bienfaisance*, Paris, 1819, p. 23. On Paris hospitals, hospices, and outdoor relief in the first decades of the 19th century, see also C-E-J-P. de Pastoret, *Rapport fait au Conseil général des hospices, par un de ses membres, sur l'état des hôpitaux, des hospices et des secours à domicile à Paris, depuis le 1er janvier 1804 jusqu'au 1er janvier 1814*, Paris, 1816; idem, *Code administratif des hôpitaux civils, hospices et secours à domicile de la ville de Paris*, 2 vols, Paris, 1824; and idem, *Recueil de règlemens et instructions pour l'administration des secours à domicile de Paris*, Paris, 1829.

34. *Almanach royal et national*, 1840, ch. 8. It is an indication of Paris's singular position that the royal, imperial and national almanacs listed, in addition to royal, imperial and national institutions and officials, all the hospitals, hospices, and medical personnel of the capital.

35. *XIIIe Congrès International de Médecine, Paris, 1900: Paris médical, assistance et enseignement*, Paris, 1900, p. 268 and *passim*.

36. *Comptes généraux des hôpitaux, hospices civils, enfans abandonnés, secours à domicile, et directions des nourrices de la ville de Paris*, Paris, Year XI (1802–03), p. 27 and *passim*.

37. *Bal donné au profit des pauvres, le 22 janvier 1831 … *, Paris, nd.

38. Silvestre, *Annuaire* (n. 33), pp. 7–8; Guy Thuillier, *Aux origines des maisons de retraite: Sainte-Périne de Chaillot, 1800–1836*, Paris, 1997.

39. *Code administratif*, vol. 1, pp. 82, 331–2.

40. Pastoret, *Recueil de règlemens* (n.33), p. 1.

41. Lecour, *Manuel d'assistance* (n.3), p. 4.
42. David Johnston, *A General Medical, and Statistical History of the Present Condition of Public Charity in France ...* , Edinburgh and London, 1829, p. 60.
43. Frochot, *Plan d'organisation* (n.31), p. 1.
44. L. Althoy, *Promenades poétiques dans les hospices et hôpitaux de Paris, dédiées à M. le comte Chaptal*, Paris, 1826, p. xi.
45. On liberalism, see Lucien Jaume, *L'individu effacé, ou le paradoxe du libéralisme français*, Paris, 1997.
46. See, for example, Société des Raffineries et Sucreries Say, *Caisse de secours pour les malades et les blessés: statuts*, Paris, nd [1884].
47. See Ann F. La Berge, 'A Restoration Prefect and Public Health: Alban de Villeneuve-Bargemont at Nantes and Lille, 1824–1830', *Proceedings of the Western Society for French History*, 1977, pp. 128–37.
48. See Katherine A. Lynch, *Family, Class, and Ideology in Early Industrial France: Social Policy and the Working-Class Family, 1825–1848*, Madison, Wisc., 1988; and Carol E. Harrison, *The Bourgeois Citizen in Nineteenth-Century France: Gender, Sociability, and the Uses of Emulation*, Oxford, 1999, esp. ch. 6, 'Charitable Imperatives'.
49. Baron de Gérando, *Le visiteur du pauvre*, Paris, 1820; idem, *De la bienfaisance publique*, 4 vols, Paris, 1839.
50. Gérando, *Visiteur du pauvre* (n.49), pp. xiii, 5, 11–12, 32 (quotation at p. 12).
51. Gérando, *De la bienfaisance* (n.49), I, lxxvi, 205, 471, 486, 499, 503–11; IV, 247–53.
52. A very detailed account of the debates on assistance can be found in Duprat, *Usages et pratiques* (n.2). On public health, ideology, and Paris as a site of social investigation, see William Coleman, *Death is a Social Disease: Public Health and Political Economy in Early Industrial France*, Madison, Wisc., 1982. On the larger debate over the social question in the first half of the 19th century, see Giovanna Procacci, *Gouverner la misère: la question sociale en France (1789–1848)*, Paris, 1993. Frances Gouda develops an illuminating comparison in *Poverty and Political Culture: The Rhetoric of Social Welfare in the Netherlands and France, 1815–1854*, Lanham, MD, 1995. On the debates in the second half of the century, see Henri Hatzfeld, *Du paupérisme à la Sécurité sociale, 1850–1940, essai sur les origines de la Sécurité sociale en France*, Nancy, 1989.
53. Eugène Buret, *De la misère des classes laborieuses en Angleterre et en France ...* , 2 vols, Paris, 1840.
54. Ann F. La Berge, 'Medicalization and Moralization: The Crèches of Nineteenth-Century Paris', *Journal of Social History*, **25** (1991–92), pp. 65–87.
55. H-J-B. Davenne, *De l'organisation et du régime des secours publics en France*, 2 vols, Paris, 1865, II, 135.
56. Pastoret, *Recueil de règlemens* (n.33), p. 348.
57. Duprat, *Temps des philanthropes* (n.18), p. 431; Silvestre, *Annuaire* (n.33), p. 133.
58. Pastoret, *Recueil de règlemens* (n.33), pp. 350–51.
59. Marescot du Thilleul, *L'Assistance publique à Paris: ses bienfaiteurs et sa fortune mobilière*, 2 vols, Paris, 1904, I, pp. 573–74, 580 (quotation at p. 573).
60. Silvestre, *Annuaire* (n.33), pp. 135–36; Pastoret, *Recueil de règlemens* (n.33), pp. 344, 345–46.
61. *XIIIᵉ Congrès* (n.35).
62. Davenne, *De l'organisation* (n.55), pp. 5, 7.

63. *Extinction du paupérisme*, in *Œuvres de Napoléon III*, 5 vols, Paris, 1869, vol. 2.

64. Ann-Louise Shapiro, *Housing the Poor of Paris, 1850–1902*, Madison, Wisc., 1985.

65. On the development of medical assistance, see Olivier Faure, 'La médecine gratuite au XIXᵉ siècle: de la charité à l'assistance', *Histoire, économie et société*, **3** (1984), pp. 593–610.

66. Jeanne Gaillard, 'Une expérience de médecine gratuite au XIXᵉ siècle: l'arrêté d'Haussmann du 20 avril 1853', *Actes du 103ᵉ Congrès National des Sociétés Savantes, Nancy, 1978: Colloque sur l'histoire de la sécurité sociale, problèmes et méthodes, Paris*, Paris, 1978, pp. 61–73.

67. Lecour, *Manuel d'assistance* (n.3), pp. 142–43.

68. For a survey and a rather negative assessment of French accomplishments, see Allan Mitchell, *The Divided Path: The German Influence on Social Reform in France after 1870*, Chapel Hill and London, 1991. For a more positive interpretation, emphasising the Third Republic's pro-family and pronatalist legislation, see Philip Nord, 'The Welfare State in France, 1870–1914', *French Historical Studies*, **18** (1983), pp. 821–38.

69. Jack D. Ellis, *The Physician-Legislators of France: Medicine and Politics in the Early Third Republic, 1870–1914*, Cambridge and New York, 1990.

70. Martha L. Hildreth, 'Medical Rivalries and Medical Politics in France: The Physicians' Union Movement and the Medical Assistance Law of 1893', *Journal of the History of Medicine*, **42** (1987), pp. 5–29.

71. On workplace accidents and the general development of the French welfare state, see François Ewald, *Histoire de l'Etat providence: Les origines de la solidarité*, Paris, 1996.

72. Judith F. Stone, *The Search for Social Peace: Reform Legislation in France, 1890–1914*, Albany, NY, 1985.

73. Mitchell, *The Divided Path* (n.68), pp. 278–79.

74. Maxime Du Camp, *La Charité privée à Paris*, Paris, 1885, pp. 1–2, 9, 14, 533–34, 538–39.

75. Susan Pedersen, *Family, Dependence, and the Origins of the Welfare State: Britain and France, 1914–1945*, Cambridge and New York, 1993.

CHAPTER FIFTEEN

Health Care Provision and Poor Relief in 19th Century Provincial France

Olivier Faure

In such a brief chapter it is very difficult to describe provincial health care provision and poor relief in 19th century provincial France for many reasons. First, French centralisation and the many political changes which happened in France make it impossible to describe local situations without references to the national context, political debates and legislative framework. Second, despite centralisation (perhaps more an appearance than a reality) deep local differences existed among the French provinces and overall between cities and the countryside. Unfortunately, local situations have been unequally studied and it is difficult to give an overall survey. Third, private institutions seem to have played a big role that has been underestimated until recent years. Because of the lack of archival material (or difficulties in using it), scholars have tended to study public institutions and little is known about private societies.

In this short chapter I shall develop some main ideas. In France, more than anywhere else, the construction of poor relief services was closely bound up with the demographical situation and the fear of a popular revolution. France's particular demographical situation (the decline in the birth rate began a century before other European countries) was considered a national problem in connection with rivalry with Germany, especially after the 1870 war and the loss of the eastern provinces (Alsace-Lorraine). The numerous revolts and revolutions during the century (and not only in Paris) quickly made clear to the ruling élites that social measures should be implemented in order to avoid social revolution.

In this context, medical aid occupied an important and growing role in political reflections about social questions and in the implementation of poor relief. Medical aid was not only conceived as a means to improve health standards, but it was also considered as a means to reduce mortality rates and to 'civilise' the poor. In this view, physicians were treated like social go-betweens who had to foster the habits of cleanliness, temperance and prudence and to promote a rational and scientific conception of life among the poor.

Because of French centralisation, scholars often assume that the French state played a significant and growing role in the implementation of poor relief. I shall argue that, despite numerous acts and large powers given to the prefects, the French state manifested no will to act before the middle of the 19th century. The birth of a social policy at the end of the century was compelled more by the social and demographical situation than chosen for political and ideological reasons. Even at the end of the century, public action was always considered as a complement to that of charitable and voluntary organisations. Finally, one could argue that the late and restricted action of the state in this field was also the result of the strength of voluntary, charitable and friendly societies.

The revival of charity

The French Revolution was unhappy in its social and health policy even when its laws were generous.[1] The Constituent Assembly and the Convention invoked the principle of obligatory public assistance. The nation had to help its poorest members, but could require work in return. Unfortunately war and economic difficulties impelled the implementation of a real public relief system.[2] Revolutionary political men were also men of Enlightenment. They wanted to establish a rational and equal medical service for the poor. In order to apply these precepts, the *Comité de mendicité* of the Constituent Assembly proposed to nominate a medical officer in each *canton* (ten to 15 parishes). This doctor had to care freely for the poor and to survey the public health situation (such as vaccination against smallpox). Under the Convention three doctors were set up in each *arrondissement* (county) in order to care freely for the people registered on the lists of the poor (on the *Grand Livre de la bienfaisance nationale*). Under pressure of war and financial difficulties, the system quickly vanished.[3] At the same time medicine was deeply disorganised. To establish freedom of the professions, medical colleges, surgical communities, faculties and medical societies were suppressed and prohibited. In the years 1792–1793 revolutionary politicians, as well as doctors, were convinced that a free population would be able to choose the best healers. For example Vicq d'Azyr (former president of the Royal Society of Medicine) agreed with the principle of total freedom for people to choose whom they wanted to cure them. The result was, of course, quite different and many uneducated men became healers between 1792 and 1803.[4]

The revolutionary hospitals policy was even more unhappy. At the end of the ancien régime numerous hospitals (over 2000) were unevenly distributed all over the French territory. Forty per cent of the 1400 hospitals set up in the countryside or in very small towns had less than ten beds, which were occupied by sick people, by old poor people or by foundlings. The 400 Hôtels-Dieu, mainly devoted to the sick, had been set up in the big towns, especially in the north of the country.[5] General hospitals (177), created during the reign of Louis XIV as jails and workhouses for ablebodied beggars, were in fact full of old poor people and orphans. All the hospitals had been created by charitable people and they were unequally distributed and bore no connection with the number or degree of poverty of the local population. Some hospitals in small and decaying towns were very rich, while hospitals in growing cities with a working population had only restricted incomes. This irrational and unequal situation was strongly criticised by men of the Enlightenment. Hospitals were also criticised as expensive institutions, as houses of confinement managed by the clergy, and as unhealthy places. According to revolutionary politicians such as Bertrand Barère, free people didn't need hospitals any more. Outdoor relief was clearly preferable to indoor relief.

In order to promote equality and to restrict the number of hospitals, the National Convention decided that hospitals' properties would become national properties (Messidor, Year II – July 1794). The state then began to sell these properties and had to use the money to support hospitals and poor relief agencies with public funds according to local needs. Unfortunately, some of the money was diverted into war expenditures and to help soldiers' families, and the public funds actually given to hospitals and poor relief agencies partly vanished because of the strong depreciation in the value of the *assignats*, leaving hospitals in a difficult situation. However, the sale of properties was quickly interrupted in the period of the Directory, and unsold properties were returned.[6] In the event, most hospitals survived to the end of the Revolution and the unequal geographical spread inherited from the Middle Ages remained.[7] This single experience of effective centralisation had serious consequences throughout the whole century. After such an unhappy experience, further state intervention was hardly possible.

The unsuccessful revolution and the further political evolution towards the right led to the return of the earlier charitable organisation. The religious revival at the beginning of the 19th century gave the old system a new chance. Since 1796 hospitals had been public and municipal institutions. The mayor of the local *commune*[8] presided over the administrative commission, but the hospitals themselves were autonomous from the *commune*. From the Consulat (1799–1804) onwards, hospitals, like all French local institutions, were controlled by the prefects who represented the central state in the 83 *départements*. According to the importance of the hospitals, the members of the administrative committees were nominated by prefects or by the minister himself.

A part of the hospital's income could come from public institutions. The *communes* could give hospitals subsidies. Towns which operated a local custom tax (*droit d'octroi*) had to help hospitals facing financial difficulties. But all this was nothing other than appearance; very few *communes* gave subsidies to hospitals. Despite the law and decrees, *communes* forgot to return local taxes to hospitals. In 1833 a third of hospitals' income came from municipalities. In 1847 the proportion had fallen to 18 per cent (12 per cent for France outside Paris).[9] Because the government paid little attention to hospitals' problems and had no hospital policies, the prefects didn't use their right to nominate the members of the administrative commissons, who were in fact coopted. Members of the commmittees were thus recruited among the traditional local élite who considered themselves more as the representatives of the charitable benefactors than of society as a whole. They considered hospitals to be local charitable institutions rather than public institutions with a role of improving public health and of protecting social order and the welfare of the community. This political orientation was reinforced by the hospitals' continued financial independence. At least two-thirds of hospitals' incomes came from the exploitation of their own properties. Hospitals rented out farms and houses. They were independent and rich enterprises. They loaned money to people, to cities and to the state. As a rough summary it could be said that the state and the cities were more dependent on the hospitals than the hospitals were on the state. Hospitals continued with their various traditional tasks. According to their charitable purposes, hospitals could receive only poor people, but according to the legacies they had accepted, they assumed many tasks. Orphans, foundlings and old poor people outnumbered the sick within their walls. Some hospitals also had to manage elementary schools, infant schools, nurseries and even workhouses. Some of them had to organise outdoor relief.

On the other hand, some sick people could not be admitted to the majority of hospitals. People suffering from venereal or skin diseases were not admitted into the wards for moral reasons. Pregnant women were also not admitted, with exceptions at some larger hospitals. The different classes of patient were often lodged in the same wards. Even in big towns where there existed both a Hôtel-Dieu (devoted to sick people) and a Charité (devoted to old poor people and orphans), the separation was never an absolute one. In Lyons, in 1836, the new service devoted to sick infants was established in the old Charité (the former Hôpital-général) among the wards devoted to old poor people.[10] The only general separation was that which was established for the insane after the 1838 act that obliged départements to manage dedicated asylums. The distinction between hospitals (devoted to sick people) and hospices (devoted to disabled and old people) that the government tried to promote did not become a reality until the 1850s. Furthermore, local authorities considered hospitals as institutions à tout faire (general institutions), where they could send prostitutes, the insane, beggars, sick soldiers and, more generally, all people who might disturb social order. The official centralisation, the rigorous state regulations and the claims of physicians (describing hospitals as cure machines – 'machines à guérir' – in Tenon's words, as popularised by Foucault[11]) must not lead one to misunderstand hospital reality.

The bureaux de bienfaisance (benevolence agencies devoted to outdoor relief) were in exactly the same situation as hospitals. Officially founded by a

1796 (Year V) law as public and municipal institutions, they were partly suppported by entertainment taxes and by private gifts. Entertainment taxes did not exist everywhere. Where they existed, their product was often very low and divided betweeen different institutions, so that *bureaux de bienfaisance* were in fact financed by private charities. In 1871, 60 per cent of their income came from private gifts (20 per cent) and from their own properties (40 per cent). Consequently they were quite independent from the state and the cities and were never set up everywhere. At best, one-third of the French *communes* possessed such a *bureau* (13 367 out of 36 000 in 1871).[12] Managed by conservatives from the traditional bourgeoisie, they were little different from private charities.[13] They gave only a basic form of aid (bread, coal, clothes) to a small section of the poor population. On the national average, at best only 5 per cent of the population was helped by the *bureaux de bienfaisance*, where they existed.

The charity system was reinforced by the strong religious revival during the first half of the century. This revival was embodied in the creation and development of many orders of nuns and sisters of charity. The first ones, like the sisters of the Charité de Saint-Vincent-de-Paul, were originally founded during the 17th century,[14] but no less than 300 orders were created in France between 1810 and the end of the Second Empire. During the 1850s no fewer than 100 000 women worked in such orders.[15] Even when sisters were primarily devoted to elementary instruction, they took on roles in hospitals and *bureaux de bienfaisance*. Small communities were also set up in many villages. One or two sisters would be schoolmistresses, the third would visit the poor and the sick and the fourth would help the others. Visits to the sick poor quickly led to medical care. Sisters distributed remedies and some communities managed complete apothecary shops despite the legal prohibition.[16]

Charitable revival was also embodied in the creation of many philanthropic and charitable societies.[17] Some of them, such as the Société Philanthropique or the Société de Charité Maternelle, had been created during the years 1780–1789 and multiplied during the first half of the 19th century. Others joined them during the French Restoration (1815–1830). Some of them were politically liberal, like the Société de la Morale Chrétienne or the Société pour l'Enseignement Elémentaire. They encouraged the creation of infant schools, day nurseries,[18] saving banks, mutual societies and dispensaries. In order to fight them, conservative and Catholic societies were also created during the same period; examples were the Société des Bonnes Oeuvres or the famous Société de Saint-Vincent-de-Paul founded in 1833. As a result of this competition, the number of societies grew significantly, and not only in Paris. Some of the national societies had local agencies (Société de Charité Maternelle, Société de Saint-Vincent-de-Paul). Many local societies called Oeuvre des Messieurs, Dames de la Miséricorde, Oeuvres de la Marmite (soup kitchens) and others were created during the 1820s and 1830s, particularly in big cities such as Bordeaux or Lyons.[19] They distributed bread and meat, and managed some small homes for old poor people. A few of them were devoted to medical aid. The Dispensaire Général de Lyon, founded in 1818, imitated the Société Philanthropique of Paris. Its aim was to offer workers' families domiciliary medical aid (physicians' visits and distribution of free remedies). The dispensary aimed to limit the use of hospitals by honest workers' families. Hospitals were described as overcrowded with beggars, the 'professional poor' and members of the dangerous classes. This medical institution, by contrast, wanted to reinforce and improve relations between rich and poor. The subscriber had a card that he could give to 'his' poor people to allow them use of the dispensary. Because of a lack of income, the general dispensary did not have much success, but it is an example which shows very well the varying aims of a 'medical aid' institution.[20] The voluntary free medical aid by professionals did not lead to success. Health officers (*officiers de santé*) had been created by the 1803 act on medicine. They were second-class physicians with only a short and practical education. The legislators had hoped that these health officials would set up in the countryside and would treat the poor people at low cost. Unfortunately they preferred to set up in the towns where the wealthy society lived.[21]

The return of charity led to many inequalities – in particular, inequalities between town and countryside, between the poor who had the chance to live in towns with numerous institutions, and those who lived in poor towns. This traditional situation was not considered as a problem before the 1830s and the outbreak of social unrest.

The failure of charity and the search for new ways

The disadvantages of charity became clear only when social problems grew so great that it was no longer possible to ignore them. The growth of towns (the growth of Paris was particularly impressive, from 500 000 inhabitants at the beginning of the century to 1 million in 1850) depended on the arrival of newcomers. They were, of course, young, unmarried and relatively poor people. Immediately, the rates of criminality and prostitution grew. In regions where heavy industry took off, such as in the region of Saint-Etienne or in northern France, the number of injuries increased and hospitals were insufficient to treat them. Hospitals, *bureaux de bienfaisance* and private institutions were not devoted to newcomers and transient people but only to the well-known and domiciled poor. With the revolutions of 1830 and 1848, and with the revolts of the *canuts* (the silk weavers of Lyons) in 1831 and 1834, it was clear that charity could not cope with the new social issues.

The cholera epidemics in 1832–1835 and from 1849 to 1854, played a big role in the birth of a social and sanitary policy.[22] The lower social classes suffered much more than the wealthy, but affluent people were not completely protected. The death of the prime minister Casimir Périer in March 1832 showed that the common people were a biological menace for the wealthy and society as a whole. Public action against sickness and unhealthy conditions became necessary. Cholera struck France at a time when the social and political situation was very difficult. At the beginnning of the July Monarchy, republican rebellions against the new government were numerous and there was considerable social unrest. Cholera was considered as a source of the new disorders and rebellions. According to some rumours, public authorities were poisoning the wells in order to eliminate the revolutionaries. In turn, republicans and socialists were accused of spreading these rumours in order to provoke revolts. In this context, sanitary commissions were created, not only to fight unhealthy conditions and distribute alms and remedies, but also to establish a new social climate of confidence between the poor and the wealthy.

The experience of cholera epidemics (100 000 persons died in 1832 and 140 000 in 1854) also led to reflection about the implementation of a medical service for the poor. Many public assistance projects were discussed at the end of the July Monarchy and during the Second Republic, with particular reference to medical aid.[23] After 1848 the introduction of universal suffrage and the part played by countrymen during the June Days (1848), more attention was paid to the countryside population. Peasants and countrymen were described as the best part of the population; rural depopulation (even very relative) was described as a social tragedy. As lack of public assistance was, according to the politicians, one of the main causes of the migration to towns, the implementation of public assistance in the countryside was considered as a means of preventing further depopulation. However, other laws were called for in opposition to these projects. Liberal politicians, such as Thiers and Montalembert, vigorously opposed the principle of a compulsory welfare state system. They feared a growth of state bureaucracy, increasing public deficits and the demoralisation of the poor if they were able to be sure that they would be helped in all difficult situations. The medical profession, despite its financial difficulties, in its first national congress (Paris 1845) rejected state intervention and denied any dependence on state or local authorities.[24]

These debates led to some very restricted measures. The 1851 Hospital Act allowed the hospitals to admit poor people living outside the town where the hospital was established, when local councils agreed to reimburse hospitals for the cost of their stay. In any case, this system was compulsory. At the beginning of the Second Empire the government allowed the *conseils généraux* (elected councils for *départements*) and *conseils municipaux* (elected councils for *communes*) to organise medical aid services for the sick poor living in the countryside. At most, 48 *départements* organised such services. During

316   HEALTH CARE AND POOR RELIEF

1865 some 800 000 people were registered and 250 000 were cared for, but the services received only 1 million francs.

Local and national authorities and philanthropists were much more enthusiastic about the development of mutual societies (friendly societies). These were born under the ancien régime through associations of colleagues. Their primary aim was to guarantee a decent burial to their members. After the French Revolution these societies were illegal, but they were tolerated – even when they were a danger for the political order and for social relations when they encouraged the organisation of strikes or boycotts. But friendly societies taught their members to set aside one franc each month in order to care for themselves in old age and sickness. According to many philanthropists, such societies could foster habits of saving, prudence and temperance. They could contribute to 'moralisation' which was, according to philanthropists, the only solution to resolve social problems. During the first half of the 19th century these associations multiplied. In the middle of the century 2000 mutual societies were functioning, with 250 000 members. In 1850 the government created the *Caisse nationale des retraites pour la vieillesse* where honest workers could deposit money under the guarantee of the state in order to obtain pensions. But the state gave no subsidies to the new institution.

The decree of March 1852 was of greater importance in that it gave friendly societies legal recognition. Some of them could be recognised by the state and receive subsidies both from the state and local authorities. The mayors of each French *commune* were invited to create such a society. Of course, friendly societies were under the strict control of the police and prefects. Presidents of societies were nominated by the emperor, and police authorities could be present during their annual sessions. However, these societies were not led by the state and remained free. The real pressure came not from the state but from society. The proposed regulation of societies (*règlement modèle*) invited societies to give their members medical aid (and, above all, visits by doctors) and established two kinds of member. Active members were members who deposited regular contributions and received money and medical aid in case of sickness. The honorary members were recruited among the wealthy, paid high conributions without receiving benefit and were often members of the society's administrative commissions. The aim was clear. The main aim of friendly societies was not to promote public health or to improve standards of life but to protect social order. The honorary members were introduced in order to respect the law of philanthropy and to rule popular societies. Medical services were also conceived to oversee lower-class members and as a means to keep the quacks at bay. Briefly summarised, friendly societies were thought of as laboratories for a better social order.[25]

Mutual societies increased considerably in number after the decree of March 1852. Ten years later France had 4000 societies and half a million mutualist members. At the beginning of the 1880s France had more than 7000 societies and 1 million members. The outcome of the *caisse nationale des retraites* was not so good, with only 15 000 pensions awarded in 1882. If mutual societies grew, they still did not cover the greatest part of the poor population. Two-thirds of mutual societies were located in urban areas at a time when the majority of French people still lived in the countryside. However, it seems that rural societies grew more quickly than the others. With respect to the monthly fees, the mutual societies are said to have been limited to the workers' aristocracy although the one franc monthly fee does not seem to have been beyond the reach of a large majority of working people. In fact, although the sociological composition of mutual societies is not completely known, it seems to have been very mixed, and not restricted to skilled workers.

The principal limits of the development of mutualism lay elsewhere. In the 1850s and 1860s, wives and children were not covered by the society in case of illness. Societies were also so small that they could disappear when costs escalated during epidemics or when too many men lived to qualify for a retirement pension. Remedies were seldom paid for by societies and staying in a hospital led to the withdrawal of relief. Hospitals, however, did not consider mutualists as poor people because they were able to pay a one franc monthly fee to the society, and they refused to admit them, the rationale being that hospitals had been founded with money for the poor and money for the poor must be used only for the poor. On the other hand, mutualist administrators considered hospitals as dangerous places where a mutualist – that is, an honest and provident man – should not go.[26] At the same time, the public medical services did not function very well. In 1887 they existed in only 38 *départements*, registered 500 000 persons and cared for less than 200 000. Like charity, public voluntary services and friendly societies could not afford complete and equal care for the poor population.

Compromise at the end of the century

The general context and the laws are well-known, but the local applications are not. In this final section I shall try to describe some local practices. The main argument is that, despite the general laws, public assistance went on under local, municipal or voluntary management.

The defeat of Sedan (1870) in the Franco-Prussian War and the Parisian Commune in March 1871 led to a deep crisis and to much reflection among French élites. Rivalry with Germany and the possibility of, and concern about, a new war made the demographic problem a national one and it became an obsession. The depopulation problem led to the further idea that there had been a degeneration in the race. According to physicians, depopulation and degeneration were caused by social diseases (*fléaux sociaux*) such as tuberculosis, alcoholism and venereal diseases. This 'scientific' approach reinforced social fears, but it also offered solutions. When society could eradicate social diseases, then the social and demographic problems would be solved. This solution led to a bigger role for medical men and for medical aid. Medicine clearly became a social science during this time. The threat of socialist revolution grew with the Commune experience, the growth of socialist parties and the increase in strikes, particularly at the end of the century. The republican government was menaced both from the left and the right. The second menace became clear during the *affaire Boulanger* and with the Dreyfus crisis. If republican politicians were obliged to appease the population, they also sincerely wished to build a new society founded on a solidarity which would neither be capitalist nor socialist. But 'solidarism', despite the works of Léon Bourgeois, was more a collection of precepts than a real and complete doctrine.

The long discussion about the conditions of the poor population led to measures founded on the various principles of assistance, providence and social insurance. For the republican governments between 1879 and the end of the century, the growth of mutual societies and voluntary insurance remained the best solution to the social question. The rivalry between mutual aid societies and private insurance companies led to the passing of two contradictory laws in April 1898. The first encouraged the creation and development of mutual societies; the second decided that employers would always be responsible in case of accidents to employees,[27] but employers were free to take out accident insurance managed by private companies. A compromise had been found between mutual and private insurance.[28] The development of public assistance was the second adjustment of the republican social policy.[29] According to its promotors (such as Henri Monod, director of public assistance at the ministry of the interior between 1887 and 1905),[30] public assistance agencies were not created to replace private institutions but to complete them. At the end of the 19th century some organisations such as the Revue Philanthropique or the Alliance d'Hygiène Sociale tried to gather together philanthropists and bureaucrats interested in social reform.

After 1900 international and national congresses were organised by public administrations and private charities together. Just before the First World War it was generally admitted that private charities should remain free but had to work under the supervision of the state.[31] Nevertheless, certain laws set up public and compulsory assistance for poor sick people (*aide médicale gratuite*) in 1893, for old and disabled poor people (*Assistance obligatoire pour les vieillards, infirmes et incurables*) in 1905, and for poor pregnant women and poor families with more than three young children in 1913. At the beginning of the 20th century radical politicians like Léon Bourgeois, whose political role was growing, gradually came to prefer social insurance to public assistance. A law setting up a system of compulsory social insurance for mining workers had been passed in 1894. The law on retirement pensions for old workers and farm labourers (*loi sur les retraites ouvrières et paysannes*) was passed in 1910,[32] but radical politicians were unable either to promote a complete insurance system, or to apply the new law broadly.

These laws did not lead to a centralised system. Medical aid was managed by *départements* and *communes*. The state had only to make sure that the law was applied generally, and to give some complementary subsidies to poor *départements*. *Communes* had to register the destitute persons who were entitled to receive assistance. This list was established on the suggestion of *bureaux d'assistance* (some local members of the local élite, or members of both hospital and *bureaux de bienfaisance commissions*). *Communes* could also organise a quite independent service if they were able to afford sufficient aid (paragraph 35 of the 1893 law). Some large cities, such as Lyons, Reims and Saint-Etienne (often ruled by mayors who were medical men) had organised such systems after the 1884 municipal law which freed the *communes* from the oversight of the state. Thus the state was not the first to act – on the contrary, the 1893 law was inspired by municipal measures. *Communes* also had to provide for the main part of expenditures. They received subsidies from *départements* only when they made special efforts for financing (when they voted in new taxes called *centimes additionnels*) or when they were very poor. *Départements* had to organise medical services and deal with the medical trade unions and with local hospitals. Each hospital had to receive sick people from the surrounding *communes*. The price for a day's stay (*prix de journée*) was also negotiated between hospitals and *départements*. Hospitals and *bureaux de bienfaisance* were not suppressed by these laws and they kept their autonomy. They were allowed to contribute to the expenditures of the new system, but it was in any case obligatory. Private legacies or gifts could also support the new organisation. The same system was applied for the 1905 law and for the 1913 laws. It is clear that these laws took care to respect communal autonomy and the freedom of private charity. The construction of a state centralised system was not on the agenda of republican politicians.

The results of this very complicated system are not easy to describe or to explain. Research on this subject is not extensive and the situations differed widely between regions.[33] With the medical aid law, regional and local inequalities remained and assistance was very restricted. The law was not in force before 1897 and some *communes* and *départements* were not enthusiastic for it. Many *communes*, including small ones, demanded the benefit of paragraph 35 in order to escape the law or to gain some time before applying it. The others applied the law with timidity. No more than 5 per cent of the whole country's population was registered on the destitute people lists. In this way, the public assistance was no broader than the old system of the *bureaux de bienfaisance* with their traditional poor people. As far as one can tell, the destitute population had the traditional characteristics: old women, widows, old people. A clear majority of *départements* entered from 3 per cent to 7 per cent of the population on their list, but some of them (around ten) entered more than 8 per cent and one almost 20 per cent of its population. Others had very restrictive attitudes and entered only less than 2.5 per cent of their population. These departmental numbers were the results of highly variable results from different *communes*. Some *communes* entered a lot of their population but a clear majority were very cautious. It is very difficult to explain such differences without micro-historical studies. It seems that industrial *communes* and *départements* entered more people than the others, but this did not hold everywhere. The political, religious and ideological orientation of the local councils seemed to play as small a role as the richness of the *communes*. In the end, it is possible to think that the registration rate reflected the types of population. In the east of the Massif Central region, for example, whose population was composed of a majority of small independent landholders living in hamlets or in isolated houses with little contact with cities, the registration rate was very low. Regions with a strong religious practice and many communities of nuns did not apply the law very strongly. By contrast, regions with rural industry and with good connections with other regions applied the law with more enthusiasm. Many questions remain without answers because of a lack of intensive local studies. But roughly summarised, public assistance brought no large changes for the poor population.

Despite the organisation of a public assistance system, the number of benevolent associations and private charities increased significantly during the late decades of the century. In Bordeaux, for example, 70 charities existed in 1870 and in 1914 there were 115 benevolent associations functioning.[34] Many associations were still charitable and Catholic societies, stimulated by the political and ideological fight between the Church and the republic. The main innovation was a rather more rational approach toward benevolence. In some big cities central clearing houses (*offices centraux de bienfaisance*) were created in order to investigate all supplicants and to prevent abuse of assistance.

The creation of lay associations is nevertheless more interesting. Using the new liberal attitudes of the state for creating associations, many specialised societies were created during the 1870s and during the 1880s in order to fight social diseases such as tuberculosis or venereal diseases, or to cope with social problems like depopulation. These societies often brought together physicians, politicians, lawyers and manufacturers. Assistance and social hygiene was at this time the single sector where Catholics, Protestants, Jews, republicans (some of them freemasons) worked together.

The relations between associations and the public agencies were compli-cated but not unfriendly. Theoretically, according to the 1901 law on associations, such societies were subject to the supervision of the state.

They had to send to the prefects their statutes and the list of their administrators. This supervision was in fact only a formal and a jurisdictional one. Lay associations more often completed than competed with public assistance agencies. This was particularly clear in the field of assistance towards endangered infancy or against juvenile deliquency. In Bordeaux or Lyons such societies as the *Oeuvre du refuge des enfants abandonnés ou délaissés*[35] or the *Société lyonnaise pour l'enfance abandonnée* took charge of young people condemned by the courts or children under the guardianship of public assistance. They established extensive placement networks in the countryside and managed specific institutions for these abandoned or endangered children.[36]

The fight against tuberculosis offered another kind of relationship between private and public institutions. Provincial associations created in Lyons, Bordeaux and other cities like Lille, organised new kinds of dispensaries (the first of them opened in Lille in 1901 under the leadership of Calmette). Dispensaries had several functions. They were established in order to survey working-class quarters of towns, identify the people suffering from tuberculosis and convince them to go to the sanatorium or to the hospital. Visiting nurses had to promote hygienic habits in order to fight tuberculosis. Dispensaries distributed food (meat) in order to improve the resistance of men to the spread of disease.[37] Provincial associations also managed sanatoriums for poor sick men and women. For example, in the region of Lyons, the Mangini (an important manufacturer) sanatorium opened in 1903.[38] At the beginning, such institutions were supported by private legacies and funds, but these private funds very quickly proved insufficient and the associations demanded public subsidies from municipal and departmental councils; because they were tightly linked to politicians, they received them. Just before the First World War, public subsidies were more important than private funds. But this growing role of public financing did not lead to a greater oversight by the public authorities. Moreover, further laws (*loi Bourgeois* in 1916; *loi Honnorat* in 1919) against tuberculosis took the private organisations as their model. The first one established departmental commmitees managed by local authorities in association with private institutions, to fight tuberculosis. The second one required departments to create public sanatoriums for the poor sick. Here, private initiative did not complete but preceded the intervention of the state.

Conclusion

The French social system established during the 19th century was, and remains today, a very complicated one. It is based on private charity, public assistance, compulsory social insurance, mutual and voluntary aid. Each component of the system was created by one of the numerous social and political forces acting during the 19th century. Private charity was supported by traditional and conservative Catholics. Mutual aid societies and philanthropic societies were managed by liberal philanthropists (sometimes Catholics). Public assistance was supported by republicans; social insurance by radical political men like Bourgeois. At the end of the century, a general compromise was reached between these political orientations in the general framework of the 'republican synthesis'. Republicans did not want to fight Catholics on both the fields of education and assistance. The social issue was the only one on which all political groups could work together and find a compromise.

The compromise was easier because all partners shared the same major aim. The different political groups all considered the particular French demographic situation (strong decrease of birth rates and relatively high mortality rates) as a dangerous threat to the nation in view of a possible war against Germany. The will to increase the population, to reduce infant mortality and to fight social diseases (tuberculosis, venereal diseases and alcoholism) was stronger than political rivalries. Private associations, the state and mutual aid societies constituted a real united front, a first *union sacrée*, to fight these main social dangers. The situation explains the major role played by medical aid, family and child benefits in French social policy.[39]

Notes

1. Jean Imbert (ed.), *La protection sociale sous la Révolution Française*, Paris, 1990.
2. Alan Forest, *The French Revolution and the Poor*, Oxford, 1981. French edition: *La Révolution française et les pauvres*, Paris, 1986.
3. Olivier Faure, *La médicalisation de la société dans la région Lyonnaise au XIXe siècle*, thèse d'Etat, Lyons, 1989, pp. 585–86.
4. Jacques Léonard, *Les médecins de l'ouest au XIXe siècle*, 3 vols, Lille, 1978, Vol 1, pp. 196–253.
5. Muriel Jeorger, 'La structure hospitalière de la France à la fin de l'Ancien Régime', *Annales, Economies, Sociétés, Civilisations* (5), (1977), pp. 1025–51.
6. Jean Imbert (ed.), *Histoire des hôpitaux en France*, Toulouse, 1982.
7. Forest, *The French Revolution* (n. 2).
8. The smallest administrative district in France. Villages, like towns, are *communes*. France possessed 36 000 *communes* during the 19th century and has 33 000 today.
9. Olivier Faure, 'Municipalités et hôpitaux dans les villes françaises au XIXe siècle', in Yannik Marec and Jacques Petit (eds), *Le Social dans la ville en Europe (XVIIe–XXe)*, Paris, 1996, pp. 63–74.
10. Olivier Faure, *Genèse de l'hôpital moderne*, Lyons and Paris, 1982.
11. Michel Foucault (ed.), *Les machines à guérir*, Paris, 1976.

12. André Gueslin, 'L'évolution du bureau de bienfaisance jusqu'en 1914', in Marec and Petit, *Le Social dans la Ville* (n. 9), pp. 239–49.

13. Pascale Lefebvre-Quincy, 'Le bureau de bienfaisance de Nancy (1850–1914)', in André Gueslin and Pierre Guillaume (eds), *De la charité médiévale à la Sécurité Sociale*, Paris, 1992, pp. 91–96.

14. Colin Jones, *The Charitable Imperative: Hospitals and Nursing in Ancien Régime and Revolutionary France*, London, 1989.

15. Claude Langlois, *Le Catholicisme au féminin: les congrégations françaises au XIXe siècle*, Paris, 1984.

16. Olivier Faure, *Les français et leur médecine au XIXe siècle*, Paris, 1993, pp. 30–33.

17. Catherine Duprat, *Le temps des philanthropes: Pour l'amour de l'humanité. Le philanthropie parisienne des lumières à la Monarchie de Juillet*, Paris, 1993.

18. Jean-Noël Luc, *L'invention du jeune enfant au XIXe siècle : de la Salle d'Asile à l'École Maternelle*, Paris, 1997.

19. Faure, *Les français et leur médecine* (n. 16), pp. 112–20.

20. Ibid., pp. 119–20.

21. Jacques Léonard, *La médecine entre les savoirs et les pouvoirs*, Paris, 1981.

22. Patrice Bourdelais and Yves Raulot, *Une peur bleue : Histoire du choléra en France (1832–1854)*, Paris, 1987; Catherine J. Kudlick, *Cholera in Post-Revolutionary Paris: A Cultural History*, Berkeley, Cal., 1996.

23. Olivier Faure, 'La médecine gratuite en France au XIXe siècle : de la charité à l'assistance', *Histoire, economie et société*, 3 (1984), pp. 593–610.

24. Léonard, *Les Médecins de l'Ouest* (n. 6), Vol. 2, pp. 787–822.

25. On the history of mutual aid societies see Bernard Gibaud, *De la mutualité à la Sécurité Sociale*, Paris, 1986. André Gueslin, *L'invention de l'economie sociale. Le XIXe siècle français*, Paris, 1998 (1st edn 1987); Allan Mitchell, *The Divided Path: the German Influence on Social Reform in France after 1870*, Chapel Hill and London, 1991. Idem, 'The functions and misfunctions of mutual aid societies in 19th century France', in Jonathan Barry and Colin Jones (eds), *Medicine and Charity before the Welfare State*, London and New York, 1991, pp. 172–89.

26. Faure, *Les français et leur médecine* (n. 16), pp. 121–44.

27. François Ewald, *Histoire de l'Etat providence:Les origines de la solidarité*, Paris, 1986.

28. Bernard Gibaud, *Mutualité et assurances (1850–1914): les Enjeux*, Paris, 1998.

29. Colette Bec, *Assistance et République*, Paris, 1994.

30. Didier Renard, 'La direction de l'Assistance publique', in Colette Bec et al., *Philanthropies et politiques sociales en Europe (XVIII– XIXe siècles)*, Paris, 1994.

31. Bec, *Assistance et République* (n. 29).

32. Bruno Dumons and Gilles Pollet, *L'état et les retraites*, Paris, 1994.

33. Studies of this kind are only devoted to the medical aid law. See Faure, *Les français et leur médicine* (n. 16), pp. 194–205; idem, 'La médecine gratuite' (n. 23).

34. Steven M. Beaudoin, 'Without Belonging to Public Service: Charities, the State and Civil Society in Third Republic Bordeaux, 1870–1914', *Journal of Social History*, (2) (1998), pp. 671–99.

35. Pierre Guillaume, *Un siècle d'histoire de l'enfance inadaptée: l'oeuvre du refuge des enfants abandonnés de Gironde*, Paris,1989.

36. Dominique Dessertine, *La Société Lyonnaise pour le Sauvetage de l'Enfance (1890–1960)*, Toulouse, 1990.
37. Pierre Guillaume, *Du désespoir au salut: histoire des tuberculeux*, Paris, 1986.
38. Olivier Faure and Dominique Dessertine, *Combattre la Tuberculose, (1900–1940)*, Lyons, 1988.
39. Catherine Rollet-Echallier, *La politique à l'egard de la petite enfance sous la IIIe République*, Paris, 1990.

Index

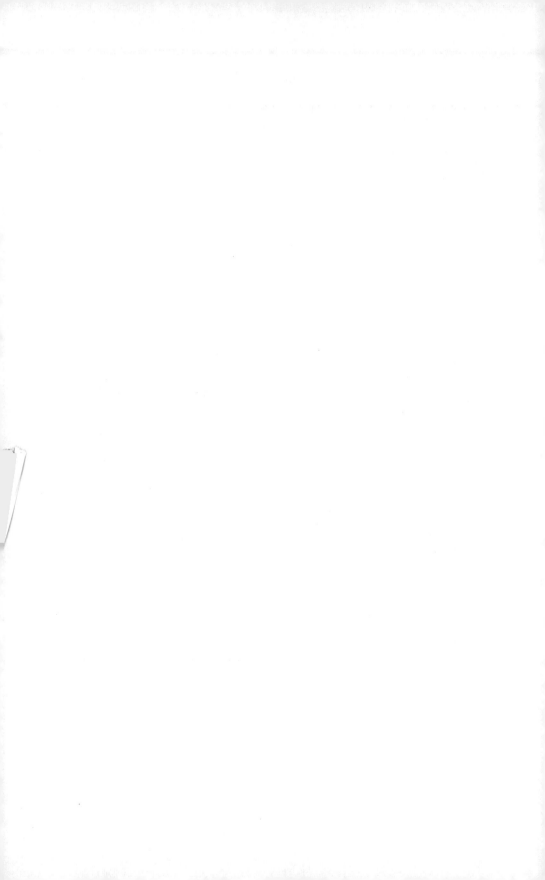